ESSENTIAL PAPERS IN PSYCHOANAL

Essential Papers on Borderline Disorders
   Michael D. Stone, M.D., Editor

Essential Papers on Object Relations
   Peter Buckley, M.D., Editor

Essential Papers on Narcissism
   Andrew P. Morrison, M.D., Editor

Essential Papers on Depression
   James C. Coyne, Editor

Essential Papers on Psychosis
   Peter Buckley, M.D., Editor

Essential Papers on Countertransference
   Benjamin Wolstein, Editor

Essential Papers on Character Neurosis and Treatment
   Ruth F. Lax, Editor

ESSENTIAL PAPERS ON CHARACTER NEUROSIS AND TREATMENT

Ruth F. Lax
Editor

NEW YORK UNIVERSITY PRESS
NEW YORK AND LONDON
1989

Library of Congress Cataloging-in-Publication Data

Essential papers on character neurosis and treatment / Ruth F. Lax,
    editor.
      p.   cm. — (Essential papers in psychoanalysis)
    Includes bibliographies and indexes.
    ISBN 0-8147-5041-9   ISBN 0-8147-5042-7 (pbk.)
    1. Personality disorders.   2. Character.   I. Lax, Ruth F.
II. Series.
    [DNLM: 1. Character.   2. Neurotic Disorders—therapy.
3. Personality Disorders—therapy.   4. Psychoanalytic
Interpretation.   5. Psychoanalytic Therapy.   WM 460.5.P3 E78]
RC554.E88   1988
616.85′2—dc19
DNLM/DLC
for Library of Congress   88-38247
                                                              CIP

New York University Press books are printed on acid-free paper,
and their binding materials are chosen for strength and durability.

Book design by Ken Venezio

To Ari

Contents

Introduction

The term *character,* derived from the Greek *charassein* and *charakter,* refers to the engraving instrument and its product, the *sign.* Applied to personality, the term denotes those features considered indelibly engraved upon it. Depicted in world literature from ancient times on, character was considered the most important aspect of a person and was judged in accordance with prevailing ethical and moral codes. Religion, philosophy, medicine, psychology, and sociology proposed a variety of theories—genetic and/or environmental—to account for character structure. In each of these theories, the interaction between endowment and nurture varies. Depending on the specific theoretical bias, views differ regarding the origin, development, and specific factors that influence and shape character.

In the historical development of psychoanalytic theory and technique, interest in character followed the investigation of neurotic symptoms and their treatment. The recognition of the role of character as a source of resistance led to an intensified study of both pathological and normal character structures, as well as to experimentation with various treatment techniques.

This volume is intended as a contribution to the continuing search for increased understanding and precision in defining the constituents of character and its disorders. It also elucidates some of the persistent controversies regarding the treatment of character neurosis. These essays likewise explore the difficulties in the achievement of therapeutic goals.

Chapters of this volume follow the progress of analytic thought regarding these issues.

OVERVIEW

Character represents the typical regularities in a person's behavior, including a wide range of stable patterns of thought, attitude, and affect that are singular and unique for a given person. This accounts both for the evaluation by others of the "kind of person" an individual is and for the expectation of predictability. Character has an adaptive function. It comprises the totality of a person's stable ego-syntonic functioning. It "is an individual, unique, and idiosyncratic synthesis, manifested in behavior, of the ego's ways of retaining, restructuring, and satisfying its impulses and their objects, to achieve gratifications and sublimations and insure self-esteem" (Panel, 1983, p. 216).

Fenichel (1945) views a person's character as socially determined. The mores of a given society are transmitted from generation to generation via parents and other familial objects. In this way the environment enforces specific frustrations, blocks certain modes of reaction to these frustrations, and facilitates others. Certain specific ways of dealing with conflicts between instinctual demands and the fear of further frustrations are encouraged. Additionally, because of the formation and promulgation of particular ideals by a given society, it could even be maintained that society creates the desires expressed by its members. "Different societies, stressing different values and applying different educational measures, create different anomalies. Our present unstable society seems to be characterized by conflicts between ideals of individual independence . . . and regressive longings for passive dependence" (p. 464).

For Fenichel, character is a function of the ego, the constant organized and integrating part of the personality. The particularity of character thus relates to the question of "when and how the ego acquires the qualities by which it habitually adjusts itself to the demands of instinctual drives and of the external world, and later also of the superego" (Fenichel, 1945, p. 467).

Baudry takes issue with Fenichel's view of character as almost identical with the ego. He suggests that "even though character is best understood as the result of many ego functions, *once it becomes established as an entity,* it is an organization on a different order, *one way of describing the unchangeable basic core of the individual and expressing all aspects of his ego-syntonic functioning* (editor's italics; Panel, 1983, p. 214). Character achieves completion only after major ego and superego identifications are stabilized. Baudry emphasized that character must be differentiated from behavior.

There is an ongoing controversy as to whether character should be considered as a superordinate concept (Panel, 1983). Schafer (1983) points out that we as yet do not have a satisfactory conceptualization or a definite place for character in psychoanalytic theory.

Historically, there are two main trends in psychoanalysis leading toward the development of a theory of character. The first stems from Freud's discoveries of psychosexual development and focused on the significance of erotogenous zones in the determination of specific character traits. The second trend incorporated the findings following the formulation of the structural hypothesis. Freud states in the *New Introductory Lectures* (1933):

> what is known as "character," a thing so hard to define, is to be ascribed entirely to the ego. We have already made out a little of what it is that creates character. First and foremost there is the incorporation of the former parental agency as a superego, which is no doubt its most important and decisive portion, and, further, identifications with the two parents of the later period and with other influential figures, and similar identifications formed as precipitates of abandoned object-relations. And we may now add as contributions to the construction of character which are never absent the reaction-formations which the ego acquires—to begin with in making its repressions and later, by a more normal method, when it rejects unwished-for instinctual impulses. (p. 91)

During the twenties, the exploration of character and its development as well as the impact of character on the analytic situation occupied analysts.[1] It was Wilhelm Reich's (1949 [1933]) contribution, however, which led to a greater precision and delineation of this concept.

According to Reich, the development of a child's character depended on the character of his parents. Deep-reaching analysis revealed that many of the traits considered "hereditary" actually were the results of early identifications. Reich acknowledged hereditary predispositions but pointed to character changes due to analysis as proof that the vicissitudes of predispositions were shaped by environmental forces. Reich maintained that character is the sum total of modes of reaction specific to a given personality. Thus, fundamentally, character is functionally determined, expressing itself in specific ways of walking, manner of speaking, posture, etc. Reich referred to the formal aspects of character as "character armor." While the content of "character armor" was of social origin and the principal reason for its formation was protection against the external world, it subsequently also served to protect the individual from inner, i.e., instinctual dangers. Thus "the task of character [was] to master stasis anxiety [actual anxiety] caused by the energies of the impulses which [were] barred from expression" (Reich, 1949 [1933], p. xxiv). Reich affirmed that the formation of character was motivated by the unconscious fear of instinctual gratification. He recognized, however, that character is not only a defensive formation but, like symptoms, it also provides avenues for disguised instinctual gratification.

Influenced by Reich's findings, A. Freud (1936) refers in her discussion of "permanent defence-phenomena" to "bodily attitudes such as stiffness and rigidity, personal peculiarities such as a fixed smile, contemptuous, ironical, and arrogant behavior . . . all these are residues of very vigorous defensive processes in the past, which have become dissociated from their original situations (conflicts with instincts or affects) and have developed into permanent character-traits, the 'armour-plating of character' [*Charakter-panzerung*, as Reich calls it]'' (p. 35).

Fenichel (1945) formulated a psychoanalytic characterology into which he incorporated Freud's views and subsequent analytic findings. Fenichel distinguished between sublimatory character traits, in which, after some alteration of aim and object, the original instinctual energy is discharged freely, and reactive character traits. The latter are defensive and employ countercathexis to check the original instinctual attitude, which is contrary to the manifest attitude.

Relative mental health prevails in those people who have an optimal amount of sublimatory-type character traits, since adequate discharge of instinctual drives is then possible and there is a minimal amount of defensive countercathexis. Under such circumstances, gratification is forthcoming, and the development of stasis precluded. In addition, as Hartmann (1939, 1950, 1952, 1955) points out, during the process of psychosexual maturation a given defensive activity may acquire pleasure in its own right and thereafter function independently of the original source of conflict. Such an activity has the characteristics of secondary autonomy. As such, it becomes resistant to regression and may become a trait and/or ego interest. Traits characterized by secondary autonomy contribute to the stability of mental functioning and to mental health.

Laplanche and Pontalis (1973) state that a character disorder is a "type" of neurosis in which defensive conflict, instead of being manifested by the formation of identifiable symptoms, appears in the shape of character traits, modes of behavior, and the pathological organization and structure of the "whole personality." Thus the patient's behavioral modes lead to permanent difficulties in his relationship with the environment. These maladaptations preclude good love relationships, happiness, and frequently creative productivity. The patients complain about a sense of isolation and loneliness, a sense of insufficiency, of mistrust that interferes with intimacy, of an inability to love. These and other similar feelings account for the psychic pain and difficulties such patients experience when coping with the exigencies of living.

In character neurosis defensive traits predominate, manifesting themselves as attitudes of avoidance (phobic) and/or of opposition (reaction formation). These responses become rigid, stereotyped, and are no longer selectively responsive to the specificity of external stimuli. Thus, flexible adaptability is lost. In such cases the optimal limits of a character trait have been transgressed, and pathological exaggeration occurs. Examples are haughtiness, self-righteousness, overpoliteness, exaggerated shyness, obsequiousness, overgenerosity, impudence, habitual mistrustfulness, and so forth.

Analytic observation indicates that in the genital character the attainment of genital primacy provides the best basis for successful sublimations. On the other hand, in pregential characters with intense ambivalence conflicts, reactive traits usually prevail. Fenichel classified such character pathology by analogy to the psychoneuroses (phobic, hysteroid, obsessional, etc.), since mechanisms similar to those present in the various forms of symptom formations likewise operate in the development of character traits. In character neurotics, especially of the obsessive type, it can be seen that a reaction formation directed against a specific instinctual threat has a tendency to generalize into a behavior pattern. When reaction formation is used for the resolution of psychic conflict, the return of the repressed is precluded and therefore the need for subsequent secondary repression is avoided. Reaction formation is a "once and for all solution" that leads to definite personality changes. The character in such cases appears as an essentially defensive formation designed to protect the individual against instinctual threat and outer danger (Fenichel, 1945).

Character traits and constellations can also be classified in accordance with different stages of libidinal development, such as oral, anal, urethral, phallic, and genital. In addition, character can be categorized according to the predominating psychic structure.

The reaction to symptoms differs greatly from a person's response to character traits and constellations. Symptoms are circumscribed, regarded as "foreign," even shameful. The patient wishes to rid himself of them as soon as possible and "by all means." In contradistinction, pathological character traits, since they become integrated into the ego and vested with narcissistic cathexis, are not recognized by the individual as pathological. They are experienced as ego-syntonic, and rationalizations are used to account for them.

Broadly defined, character neurosis (Waelder, 1930) represents in large measure a malformation of the ego, resulting from compromise formations attempted to accommodate conflicting demands impinging upon the individual from reality, the superego, the drives, and the repetition compulsion. Specific characteristics of particular compromise formations depend on the relative strength of these conflicting demands, the level of psychic maturity at the given time, the type of former identifications with significant objects, or the need to disidentify.

TREATMENT CONSIDERATIONS

In the analytic situation, neurotic character traits manifest themselves as resistances. Reich (1949 [1933]) was the first to attempt ''a consistent application of the newer method of resistance analysis to the analysis of the character, corresponding to the progress of analytic therapy from symptom-analysis to the analysis of the total personality'' (p. 10). As leader of the seminars on psychoanalytic technique held in Vienna (1924 through 1930) and subsequently in Berlin (1930 through 1933), Reich wanted to create a psychoanalytic technique that was exact and replicable. He mistrusted intuition. Reich maintained that chaos and prolonged stalemates stemming from unsystematic interpretations were avoided when his technique was used.

According to Reich (1949 [1933]), character resistance manifested itself in the formal aspects of behavior, not in the content of the material. Thus the specifics of character are in *how* the patient talks, acts, and censors, not in *what* the patient says or does. The patient's character resistance always remains the same irrespective of the material against which it is directed. The roots of character resistances are in infantile experiences and instinctual drives. Character armor serves as a psychic protective mechanism. Reich claimed that the consistent analysis of character resistance ''provides an infallible and immediate avenue of approach to the central infantile conflict'' (this volume, p. 93).

Reich introduced the useful distinction between transference resistance and character resistance. In contrast to the former, character resistance reflects general and diffuse responses that are characteristic of the patient's reactions to people in general and not to the analyst specifically. These reactions are the patient's response to unconscious danger stemming from his intrapsychic conflicts. According to Reich, the negative transference is present in character neurotics from the beginning of treatment and has to be analyzed relentlessly. An initially positive transference must be regarded as a ''cover-up'' and analyzed to reveal the hostile aggressive feelings transferred upon the analyst. As will be seen, Nunberg (1928 [this volume, chap. 5]) differed strongly with Reich on this point.

Reich stressed that in the process of analysis the patient has to discover:

1. that he unconsciously defends himself against something he considers dangerous;
2. what means he uses for the purpose of defense;
3. against what this defense is directed.

In character analysis, as Reich saw it, "we isolate the character trait and confront the patient with it repeatedly until he begins to look at it objectively and to experience it like a painful symptom; thus, the character trait begins to be experienced as a foreign body which the patient wants to get rid of" (this volume, p. 95).

Reich maintained that character analysis must be consistent, systematic, and historic to attain the desired dynamic and economic goals. He acknowledged[2] that the consistent character analytic approach caused the patient great suffering and could even result in a temporary breakdown. However, Reich insisted, such an approach was necessary since a "healthy" personality could only develop after the character resistances were "dissolved."

Reich's extreme position evoked strong opposition in the analytic community. The main controversy was between advocates of content interpretation and proponents of resistance interpretation. Fenichel (1953 [1935, this volume, chap. 6]) argued against the extremes of both positions and formulated principles of technique anchored in ego psychology. He emphasized the need for an optimal balance between interpretations of defense and interpretations of content. Fenichel was opposed to Melanie Klein and Theodor Reik, who gave id interpretations without regard for the appropriate readiness of the ego; he was likewise opposed to Reich and more so to Hellmuth Keiser (1934), who wished to limit all interpretations to those of character resistance only.

Fenichel's view of Reich's theory and technique was critical and selective. Fenichel agreed with Reich's insistence that the interpretation of defense always precedes the interpretation of content. Likewise, Fenichel's familiar principles of analytic technique—namely, that the patient be helped to recognize that he is defensively resistive, how he does it, why he does it, and against what the defense is directed—are the legacy of Reich.[3] Fenichel, as will be seen from his papers in this volume (chaps. 6 and 7), was opposed to Reich's extreme one-sidedness and to his aggressive approach to the patient.

Fenichel (1941) pointed out that Reich did not take into account the consequences of his approach on the patient's psyche and some patients' trauma-
tophilia. Reich thus did not recognize the extent of the deleterious effects of
his therapeutic stance.

The currently prevalent point of view expressed by Arnold Cooper (Panel,
1982) considers the distinction between psychoanalysis and character analysis as no longer useful. From the dynamic, structural, genetic, and developmental vantage points, analysis of character is basic to psychoanalytic technique. The psychoanalytic task requires an understanding of the formation of
psychic structure and fantasies and the knowledge and understanding of their
sources and vicissitudes during the process of development. Cooper states:
"The adaptive maneuvers created under the stimuli of frustration and desire
and their compromise in the particular matrix of objects for that individual
are the sources of behavior which appear as character in the analysis and
provide the evidences of transference. We know today that all important
communications are nonverbal as well as verbal, and that free association is
always impaired by chronic characterologic modes as well as by acute conflictual issues" (p. 110).

According to Fenichel (1945), in the treatment of character neurosis a
"mobilization of conflicts" must take place that, when successful, changes
the "character neurosis into a symptom neurosis, and character resistances
into . . . transference resistances" (p. 538). This recommendation is generally accepted. The achievement of such a transformation, however, is a very
complicated process. Even with our current understanding that an empathic
stance is necessary when dealing with the patient's characterological defenses, the beginning phase in the treatment of these neurotics nonetheless is
most difficult. As Schafer (1979) clearly points out, the ego-syntonicity one
encounters in character neurosis implies a closed, perpetually self-confirming
system that poses a formidable obstacle to treatment. This system, based on
unconsciously held convictions dating from childhood, defines the nature of
self, others, and of the world and is used also to make sense of one's
existence and interactions. Complete consistency of this system would preclude the possibility of analysis. Fortunately, however, such homogeneity
does not prevail at all times and in all areas. Some inconsistency is usually
present, at least in some areas, as well as some experiential diversity and the
ability to perceive contradictions.

In cases where ego-syntonicity is particularly persistent, the initial analytic
task is to strengthen dystonic elements and to encourage curiosity. Of utmost

importance in this process is the highlighting and exploration of contradictions (Kernberg, 1980, 1984; Schafer, 1982, 1983), since this enables patients to become aware of ego-dystonic elements.

The analytic aim of treatment, at this time, is the disturbance of the neurotic equilibrium. This is necessary to increase the patient's accessibility to treatment.

Even when the patient is motivated by a sense of unhappiness and seeks analysis, the tactful yet consistent analytic attention to incongruities and inconsistencies arouses his anger. This is understandable since such an analytic stance evokes in the patient a feeling that his narcissistically invested character patterns are being criticized. Eventually, however, such a method leads to and does facilitate the exploration of unconscious conflicts (Lax, 1988).

Regardless of whether the analytic approach is basically nonadversarial and affirmative (Schafer, 1982) or "confrontational" (Kernberg, 1984), the patient feels criticized and/or assaulted when his narcissistically invested character patterns appear to be scrutinized. Thus, any analytic intervention that threatens the neurotic equilibrium is perceived by these patients as an attack. This is one of the factors contributing to the negative transference, which plays such a prominent role in the analysis of character neurotics. Scrutiny by the analyst of his countertransference and awareness of his own characterologic tendencies is necessary to avoid provocation of the patient's justified anger. This is an important prerequisite for an eventually successful analysis of the necessary negative transference.

Even though optimism is guarded, successful character analysis that eventuates in meaningful structural change is possible. Such a process, however, is long, arduous, and painful.

Reich (1949 [1933]) did not think that qualitative changes—namely, changes in character style—are possible. He recognized, however, that quantitative changes could "equal qualitative change" (p. 118) when these were substantial. In such cases patients experienced increased gratification from work and sex.

Fenichel's goal in character analysis was the transformation of reactive character patterns into sublimatory type traits. This, he believed, would enable the person to discharge instinctual drives via acceptable channels, diminish stasis, and attain gratification.

In addition to the analysis of unconscious conflict, the current emphasis is on the analysis of the superego and its introjects, the analysis and reconcilia-

tion (synthesis) of conflicting identifications based on the archaically con-
strued characters of each parent, and the analysis of pregenital fixations and/
or arrests. With the advent of ego psychology, an increase in ego and
superego autonomy and the development of ego interests became the additional goals of psychoanalysis.

Most analysts acknowledge that the core-character pattern will not change
due to treatment, and thus an obsessive or compulsive personality will not
become hysteroid and vice versa. An analysis, however, which includes the
exploration of the psychic structures will lead to changes in each one of them
and to the resolution of psychic conflicts. As a consequence of such a
process, the nature of the unconscious psychic dangers will change, as will
the unconscious means of coping with them. This will result in the evolve-
ment of new compromise solutions leading to more adaptive ego and superego autonomy.

In summary, though the gains of character analysis may lead only to
relative attainments, they increase the possibility of greater flexibility, adaptability, and availability of energy. Consequently, the joy in love and work is
enhanced.

THE SELECTION AND ORGANIZATION OF ESSAYS

The editor's aim was to present a volume of essays that would reflect specific
contributions to the development of psychoanalytic concepts of character and
would also contain discussions of clinical and theoretical issues.[4]

The first two chapters in part 1 are overviews. In chapter 1, Francis Baudry
(1983) discusses the historic evolution of the concept of character in Freud's
thinking. Robert Liebert (1988), in chapter 2, somewhat critically presents
Freud's views and thereafter briefly examines the views of leading analysts
who expanded and/or diverged from Freud's position. His article presents a
review of nearly a century of analytic thought about character. From this
study the scope of divergence will become apparent. In part 2, the reader
learns about the extent to which the increased knowledge of psychic development enriched the dynamic and structural understanding of character. In
chapter 3, Maxwell Gitelson (1963) differentiates clearly between symptom
neurosis and character neurosis, indicating the relevant dynamic elements
leading to the development of each kind of pathology. Different character
types are sketched. Peter Blos (1968) discusses maturational and genetic

aspects, the impact of the environment, and the consequences of the interaction of all these factors on character formation.

The growth in Freud's clinical acumen led to his recognition of the negative therapeutic reaction. On the basis of this observation, Freud postulated the existence of unconscious guilt and developed the concept of the superego. These clinical findings served as a basis for Freud's conceptualizations which resulted in the formulation of the structural theory. This fundamental theoretical revision was also reflected in changed therapeutic approaches and goals. The emphasis shifted from the "making of the unconscious conscious" to an increased appreciation of the role played by the ego in psychic conflict and in the defensive process. The new methods and goals are conveyed by the phrase "where id was there ego shall be" (Freud, 1933, p. 80).

Part 3A presents in chapter 4 Wilhelm Reich's (1949 [1933]) theory of psychoanalytic technique. Reich in this essay attempts to incorporate into psychoanalytic practice the new discoveries regarding resistance and defense and to convey the essence of his theoretical and technical recommendations. This chapter is also replete with excellent clinical illustrations. Unlike Freud, Reich maintains that most patients cannot free associate. This makes it useless to demand of them that they follow the "basic rule." Reich also stressed that all patients have a tendency to remain ill. Consequently, telling a patient "you don't *want* to get well" is meaningless. According to Reich, unresolved interruptions of analysis are caused by the analyst's inability to analyze the character resistances correctly. Reich viewed character as a layering of resistances—id impulses being opposed by ego impulses (character resistances). Reich asserted that all neuroses were caused by the damming up (stasis) of sexual energy and followed Freud's model of the "actual neurosis."[5] According to Reich, only those patients who attained orgastic potency in the course of their analysis would remain free from neurosis. For Reich, the neurotic character was the opposite of the genital character.

Criticisms of Reich's position are presented in part 3B. Herman Nunberg (1928) was one of the first analysts to take issue with Reich. He especially disagreed with Reich regarding the role of positive transference in the initial phase of treatment. In chapter 5, Nunberg maintains that with establishment of positive transference a true collaboration with the analyst begins. In his analytic work, Nunberg stresses the unconscious and not the relationship of the ego to the unconscious. He considers the modification of the superego, which results, according to Nunberg, from the internalization of the benign image of the analyst, as most important for psychoanalytic technique.

Otto Fenichel (1953 [1935]) had been a member of Reich's technical seminars and was his friend. Fenichel's discussion of Reich's position in chapter 6 is mostly positive and sympathetic: he criticizes Reich's style rather than the substance of his views. In chapter 7, Fenichel (1954 [1941]) elaborates on his own theoretical views and technical recommendations and gives a detailed discussion of character analysis.[6] Fenichel illustrates his recommendations by two vignettes indicating how resistance analysis and content analysis should be interwoven.

Part 3C begins with Otto Kernberg's (1976 [1970]) classification of character pathology, which incorporates the propositions of the structural theory, ego psychology, and object relations theory. Kernberg proposes "(1) to establish psychoanalytic criteria for differential diagnoses among different types and degrees of severity of character pathology; (2) to clarify the relationship between a descriptive characterological diagnosis and a meta-psychological, especially structural, analysis; and (3) to arrange subgroups of character pathology according to their degree of severity" (this volume, p. 191). Such classification, according to Kernberg, "incorporates three major pathological developments: (1) pathology in the ego and superego structures; (2) pathology in the internalized object relations; and (3) pathology in the development of libidinal and aggressive drive derivatives" (p. 193).

D. W. Winnicott (1965) views early parental deprivation as the root of character disorders. The antisocial tendency is a reaction to parental deprivation marked by inconsistency. Antisocial behavior, however, still contains an element of unconscious hope; it is an SOS, a *cri de coeur,* a signal of distress.

To be successful, therapy with this type of patient must reach the original traumas. During the analytic process, the therapist must acknowledge his mistakes to enable the patient to become angry rather than retraumatized.

Whereas Winnicott's therapeutic approach has an analytic-reparative quality, Otto Kernberg's is strictly analytic. In chapter 9, Kernberg (1983) integrates his ideas on ego psychology and object relations theory with Fenichel's theory of technique. According to Kernberg, conflict always occurs between two opposing units of internalized object relations in which both impulse and defense find expression. "All character defenses consist of a defensive constellation of self and object representations directed against an opposite dreaded, repressed self and object constellation" (p. 211). The therapeutic aim is the reactivation of conflicting, internalized object relations, preferably in the transference, and their analyses. Kernberg presents a clinical vignette to illustrate his propositions and deftly discusses strategies of character analysis.

Peter Giovacchini's (1972) topic in chapter 10 is therapy with patients designated as character disorders and described as suffering from problems related to existential questions of identity. Giovacchini considers specific therapeutic approaches that are variations of the psychoanalytic method but are not seen by him as deviations or parameters.

Types of character pathology and treatment techniques are discussed in part 4. Karl Abraham (1920), in "Manifestations of the Female Castration Complex," describes the genesis and developmental vicissitudes of penis envy, as well as the concomitant narcissistic injuries. In this connection, contrary to Freud, Abraham stresses that "the undisturbed enjoyment of early genital sensations[7] will . . . aid in facilitating the renunciation of masculinity, *for by this means the female genitals will regain a narcissistic value"* (editor's italics; p. 342). Since menstruation, defloration, and fantasies about childbirth remind the girl of her "defect," it is not surprising, according to Abraham, that traces of the castration complex can be found even in normal women.

B. Ruth Easser and Stanley Lesser (1965) reevaluate the hysterical personality. Present-day analysts do not see the florid symptom picture described by the early psychoanalysts. Careful diagnostic criteria are presented by the authors to differentiate the "hysterical personality," which is more mature, better integrated, and whose core conflict revolves around oedipal issues, from the "hysteroid" group, in which pregenital issues predominate. On the basis of careful clinical observations, Easser and Lesser (1966; this volume, chap. 11), make specific recommendations for the treatment of the hysterical personality. Easser and Lesser caution analysts that the hysterical personality has the capacity to evoke in others emotional interest, responsiveness, and pleasure. Such a countertransferential response, according to the authors, occurs frequently. When this happens, the patient has a repetitive rather than a corrective experience. To attain therapeutic goals, the analyst must guard against this type of countertransference and fully analyze the child-role assumed by this type of patient.

Within the normal range, the obsessional character is considered by Humberto Nagera (1976) as a desirable form of personality organization which he contrasts with the obsessional character disorder. In chapter 12, the obsessional neurosis is described and differentiated from other pathological entities. Nagera points to factors which account for a transition from character to symptom neurosis and suggests that a reversal of this process is also possible. In chapter 13, Nagera (1976) compares the obsessional and the hysterical personalities with regard to the level of ego development attained by each.

In its normal form, masochism may be considered a ubiquitous aspect of human nature. In its pathological form, masochism has confronted psychoanalysis with many challenges regarding theories of pleasure, pain, and motivation. The preponderance of masochistic-character pathology in present-day practice prompted the inclusion of the next four chapters. In these, a variety of points of view concerning the formation of the masochistic character as well as different theoretical and technical approaches to issues arising in the treatment of this type of patient are discussed.

Charles Brenner (1959) summarizes Freud's ideas and presents the views of subsequent authors who add to or diverge from Freud's position. Oedipal as well as pregenital issues are considered. According to Brenner, the analysis of masochistic patients does not differ in principle from any other character analysis. However, special problems arise from the sadomasochistic transference and the negative therapeutic reaction. Countertransference factors are of crucial importance.

In chapter 14, Theo Dorpat (1982) emphasizes the object relations model, the role of behavioral disturbances, and faulty relationships with external objects. Using a clinical example, Dorpat indicates how primitive aspects of the ego express themselves in part-object relations. These adaptations are the outcome of defective integrations and can be seen in the transference. The patient attempts to re-create the traumatic infantile ambience in the analytic situation. Dorpat presents a case of masochistic perversion treated psychoanalytically.

In chapter 15, Arnold Cooper (1988) explores issues in separation-individuation, self-esteem regulation, and the nature of early object relations to reexamine, clarify, and thereby increase our understanding of masochistic phenomena. Narcissism and masochism are ubiquitous in psychic growth and achieve their specific individual character from the viscissitudes of pregenital development. According to Cooper, narcissism and masochism reveal a structural unity and should therefore be considered as a single nosological entity. Clinically, Cooper points out, the interpretation of masochistic behavior results in narcissistic mortification, and the interpretation of narcissistic defenses results in a sense of masochistic victimization. Cooper presents two vignettes to illustrate difficulties inherent in the treatment of such cases.

The pathological consequencs of internalized, disharmonious and uninte-
grated identifications with maternal and paternal imagos are discussed by
Ruth Lax (1977) in chapter 16. In these cases two conflicting identification
systems develop simultaneously, each with its own wishful self-image. Consequently, these patients' self-representation has a faulty structure since it
contains two diverse, split-off imagos. Such a constellation has a disruptive
effect since it interferes with the development of a harmonious ego ideal
necessary for integrated and cohesive character formation.

Though all aspects of the masochistic constellation must be analyzed, it is
important to recognize the current and predominant function masochism
serves for a given patient. In chapter 17, Helen Meyers (1988) discusses
appropriate variations in technique necessary to achieve this aim. Meyers
examines the function of masochism in relation to guilt, the maintenance of
object relations, self-esteem, and self-definition.

In her discussion of the relationship of gender and masochism, Meyers
states that masochism is equally distributed among men and women. However, there may be differences in the content of masochistic fantasies for
each sex due to cultural factors. The therapist's gender, according to Meyers,
affects only the sequence and intensity of certain transference reactions.

The negative therapeutic reaction, a major obstacle in the treatment of all
character neurosis, plays a predominant role in the analysis of the masochistic
character. This is not only due to unconscious guilt but also to unconscious
sadism and narcissism. A combination of these factors seems to mandate the
patient's unconscious wish to defeat the analyst. Envy of the analyst's superior power, the wish for omnipotence, the wish for autonomy and mastery,
the fear of passivity and submission have, among other reasons, been proposed as explanatory factors for this paradoxical, self-defeating, antithera-
peutic reaction.

Stuart Asch (1976) expands the concept of oedipally related unconscious
guilt by which Freud sought to explain the negative therapeutic reaction.
Asch includes: (1) masochistic ego distortions in response to a special pathology of the ego ideal; (2) defense against the regressive pull toward symbiotic
fusion with a depressed mother; (3) the defensive role or oral and/or anal
negativism; and (4) pregenital "crimes."

According to Asch the analysis of the negative therapeutic reaction is
essentially an analysis of introjects that the patient in part projects onto the
analyst. Attempts to provoke the analyst into a punitive response occur often.
Intense countertransference reactions are frequent.

In chapter 18, Ruth Lax (1980) describes the formation of a specific type of self-pathology, the rotten core, which originates as a reaction to a depressed mother's lack of libidinal availability to the child during the rapprochement subphase. The child experiences such a mother as rejecting. The internalization of the interaction with this type of mother results in a specific kind of identification with the aggressor. Such an identification leads to the formation of a rotten core, which represents on the most primitive level the fusion of the "bad" (angry-rejecting) maternal introject with the "bad" (rejected) aspects of the self. A consolidated and integrated self representation does not develop in patients with this pathology. The specific split in the self representation that contains the good self and the rotten core evokes in these patients the subjective awareness of a duality of their selves.

In the next two chapters, the analysts discuss their specific reactions to certain types of patients and the subsequent effect on their technique. Joyce McDougall, in chapter 19 (1972), describes the analyst's experience ranging from frustration to helplessness and guilt when faced with a "model patient" who goes through the motions of an analysis without feeling. McDougall is tempted to name such a patient a "robot analysand" but realizes this would be inaccurate since such patients are unconsciously "active" in their "uninvolvement." These are patients who follow all the analytic rules, seemingly develop no transference, and show no change as a result of treatment. McDougall calls the process a "nonanalysis" and examines what led her to take such patients into analysis, the course of such treatment, and what she experienced in the process.

Annie Reich (1973 [1958]) discusses active intervention in the treatment of impulse-ridden characters[8] in chapter 20. In these cases the ego appears weak, caught between powerful drives and a relentless superego. The patients seem driven by uncontrollable outbursts of libidinal and aggressive impulses, and are unable to pursue ego-syntonic, gratifying activities. To become therapeutically effective, the analyst in such cases must "take sides with the patient . . . against the object: demasking and dethroning it" (p. 386). Annie Reich presents a patient in whom both instinctual and ego development was repressed by obedience to a mother who forbade expression of either. Mother, internalized, became the "ideal" (superego and ego ideal), thus making autonomous development impossible. Reich describes her therapeutic procedure as a "frontal attack on the original superego model; i.e., as a systematic devaluation of the idealized mother" (p. 391). This method, in the editor's view, is comparable to the analyses of introjects discussed by Asch (1976).

Reich, however, found that it was insufficient to demask and analyze mother to enable the patient to understand and tolerate her own libidinal and aggressive impulses. Reich expressed value judgments in regard to the mother, thus offering herself as a "new object of identification to the patient" (p. 393). Though Reich considers her approach an unanalytic way of attacking the malignant object, she does believe that this "variation of classical technique . . . is often necessary in cases of this kind" (p. 386). Such a procedure, Reich cautions, is only permissible when "combined with a careful analysis of the conflict" (p. 393) to prevent it from becoming an educational experience.

The essays in part 5 examine the effect of the analyst's character on the analytic situation and the analytic process. This topic, until quite recently, has received little attention in analytic literature, possibly because of the strength of the idealization of the analyst's character and the corresponding illusion that the analytic process is value-free (Hartmann, 1960, pp. 20–21). A differentiation must be made between the analyst's character and countertransference, which is "the whole of the analyst's unconscious reaction to the individual analysand—especially the analysand's transference" (Laplanche and Pontalis, 1973, p. 93). Thus, countertransference is specific as to source of arousal and the unconscious motives for the reactions. Contrasted with the specific and circumscribed nature of countertransference, the analyst's character refers to ego-syntonic, always present attributes and attitudes. The analyst's character is evident in his way of being, which is pervasive in all interactions with patients and is not fine-tuned or responsive to a given individual or situation. The ramifications, consequences, and problems related to the role and the significance of the analyst's character for the treatment process are discussed in the next four chapters.

In chapter 21 Francis Baudry (1982) asks: "How does the analyst's character permeate his technique?" To obtain the answer, Baudry explores the role of the analyst's self-syntonic general ways of being, the effect of his analytic style, and his reaction to the patient's affects.

The relevance of Maxwell Gitelson's (1973 [1954]) essay, chapter 22, which deals with problems inherent in the analysis of the "normal candidate," increases with our sharpened understanding of the role of the analyst's character in assuring and safeguarding the integrity of the analytic process. Gitelson considers the vicissitudes of the analysis of a candidate who lives in terms of a *facade* structured and patterned by the environment. Such a candidate has an *"adopted"* personality appropriate to his culture; and he, therefore, passes for normal.

According to Gitelson, such a personality is not appropriate for psychoanalysis. Since psychoanalysis is "incompatible with opportunism and compromise," it must be free from the biases of a particular culture (p. 424). Thus, in the course of an analysis, the culturally determined "normal behavior" of the candidate must be regarded as a resistance. The integrity of the analytic situation, according to Gitelson, provides an opportunity to "test out a new reality," (p. 424) in which the conflicts made latent by the culture can be mobilized and the vicissitudes of the libido[9] analyzed.

Winnicott (1960), discussing ego distortions in terms of the true and false self, warns that analyses dealing with the false self are unending—a point also made indirectly by Gitelson. Winicott stresses that careful diagnostic assessment of such pathology must be made, especially of candidates in the mental health field.

In chapter 23, Heinrich Racker (1958) demonstrates the extent and different ways in which the analyst's characterological masochism influences his conduct of an analysis. In such instances, psychoanalytic technique expresses the analyst's unconscious pathology, which may collude with that of the patient.

In chapter 24, Arnold Cooper (1986) suggests that in addition to the analyst's character "therapeutic burnout" may seriously diminish the quality of an analyst's work with patients and limit its therapeutic effectiveness. Cooper points out the great emotional demands and isolation of analytic work, which contribute to the development of the burnout syndrome. He describes two variations: the masochistic defense schema and the narcissistic one. In each case, characterological factors are of great significance. Further analysis is the only remedy that can alleviate the burnout syndrome and characterological impediments in the analyst. Cooper's essay brings to our attention the need for continuous monitoring via self-analysis to forestall mistakes caused by characterological factors or burnout.

NOTES

1. Abraham, 1921, 1924, 1925; Glover, 1924, 1925; Nunberg, 1928.
2. See Reich, 1949 [1933], 67–76 and 114–18 in which Reich discusses the ethical problems related to his technique of character analysis.
3. See Reich, 1933, p. 28; Fenichel, 1941. See also chap. 7, this volume.
4. For a more detailed historical survey, see also chapter 2 in Bergmann's (1976) *The Evolution of Psychoanalytic Technique.*

5. For a discussion of actual neurosis, see Fenichel, 1945, *The Psychoanalytic Theory of Neurosis.*
6. See also chapter 30 in Fenichel's (1945) *The Psychoanalytic Theory of Neurosis,* especially 538–40.
7. That is, masturbation.
8. Also referred to as acting-out hysterics.
9. As well as aggression, which Gitelson does not mention in this connection.

REFERENCES AND SUGGESTED READINGS

Abraham, K. 1920. Manifestations of the female castration complex. In *Selected Papers on Psychoanalysis,* 338–69. New York: Basic Books, 1953.
———. 1921. Contributions to the theory of anal character. In *Selected Papers on Psychoanalysis,* 370–92. See Abraham, 1920.
———. 1924. The influence of oral erotism on character formation. In *Selected Papers on Psychoanalysis,* 393–406. See Abraham, 1920.
———. 1925. Character-formation on the genital level of the libido. In *Selected Papers on Psychoanalysis,* 407–17. See Abraham, 1920.
Asch, S. 1976. Varieties of negative therapeutic reaction and problems of technique. *J. Amer. Psychoanal. Assn.* 24:383–407.
Barnett, J. 1981. Character, cognition, and therapeutic process. In *Changing Concepts in Psychoanalysis,* ed. S. Klebanow, 47–58. New York: Gardner Press.
Baudry, F. 1984. Character: A concept in search of an identity. *J. Amer. Psychonal. Assn.* 32(1): 455–477.
Bergmann, M. S., and Hartman, F. R. 1976. *The Evolution of Psychoanalytic Technique.* New York: Basic Books.
Blos, P. 1968. Character formation in adolescence. *Psychoal. Study Child* 23:245–63.
Brenner, C. 1959. The masochistic character: Genesis and treatment. *J. Amer. Psychoanal. Assn.* 7:197–226.
Easser, B. R., and Lesser, S. R. 1965. Hysterical personality: A re-evaluation. *Psychoanal. Q.* 34:390–405.
Eissler, K. R. 1953. The effect of the structure of the ego on psychoanalytic technique. *J. Amer. Psychoanal. Assn.* 1: 104–43.
———. 1958. Remarks on some variations in psychoanalytic technique. *Int. J. Psychoanal.* 39: 222–29.
Fenichel, O. 1941. *Problems of Psychoanalytic Technique.* New York: *Psychoanal. Q.*
———. 1945. Character disorders. In *The Psychoanalytic Theory of Neurosis,* 463–540. New York: W. W. Norton.
Freud, A. 1936. *The Ego and the Mechanisms of Defense.* New York: International Universities Press, 1946.
Freud, S. 1908. Character and anal eroticism. *Standard Edition,* 9.
———. 1923. The ego and the id. *Standard Edition,* 19.
———. 1926. Inhibitions, symptoms and anxiety. *Standard Edition,* 20.
———. 1931. Libidinal types. *Standard Edition,* 21.
———. 1933. New introductory lectures. *Standard Edition,* 22.
Glover, E. 1924. Notes on oral character formation. In *On the Early Development of Mind,* Vol. 1, 25–46. New York: International Universities Press, 1956.
———. 1925. The neurotic character. In *On the Early Development of Mind,* vol. 1, 47–66.

Hartmann, H. 1939. *Ego Psychology and the Problem of Adaptation.* New York: International Universities Press, 1958.

————. 1950. Comments on the psychoanalytic theory of the ego. *Psychoanal. Study Child* 5:74–96.

————. 1952. The mutual influence in the development of ego and id. *Psychoanal. Study Child* 7:9–30.

————. 1955. Notes on the theory of sublimation. *Psychoanal. Study Child* 10:9–29.

————. 1960. *Psychoanalysis and Moral Values.* New York: International Universities Press.

Keiser, H. 1934. Probleme der technik, *Internat. Zeitschr. f. Psychoan.* 20:490–522.

Kernberg, O. F. 1980. *Internal World and External Reality.* New York: Jason Aronson.

————. 1984. *Severe Personality Disorders and Psychotherapeutic Strategies.* New Haven, Conn.: Yale University Press.

Khan, M. M. R. 1972. The finding and becoming of self. In *The Privacy of the Self: Papers on Psychoanalytic Theory and Technique,* 294–305. New York: International Universities Press. Reprint. *Int. J. Psychoanal. Psychotherapy* 1(1), 1972.

Laplanche, J., and Pontalis, J. B. 1973. *The Language of Psycho-Analysis.* New York: W. W. Norton.

Lax, R. F. 1975. Some comments on the narcissistic aspects of self-righteousness: Defensive and structural considerations. *Int. J. Psychoanal.* 56:283–92.

————. 1988. Comments on the narcissistic investment in pathological character traits and the narcissistic depression: Some implications for treatment. *Int. J. Psychonal.* Forthcoming.

Moore, B. E., and Fine, B. D. 1968. *A Glossary of Psychoanalytic Terms and Concepts.* New York: American Psychoanalytic Association.

Panel. 1982. Problems of technique in character analysis. Discussion by A. M. Cooper. *Bulletin Assn. Psychoanal. Medicine* 21(3): 110–18.

————. 1983. Theory of character. Reported by S. M. Abend. *J. Amer. Psychoanal. Assn.* 31(1): 211–24.

Reich, W. 1927. On the technique of interpretation and of resistance analysis. Chap. 3 in Reich, *Character Analysis,* 3d enl. ed, 20–38. Translated by P. Wolfe. New York: Orgone Institute Press, 1949. Reprint *Internat. Zeitschr. f. Psychoan.*

————. 1949 [1933]. *Character Analysis.* 3d enl. ed. Translated by P. Wolfe. New York: Orgone Institute Press.

Schafer, R. 1979. Character, ego-syntonicity, and character change. *J. Amer. Psychoanal. Assn.* 27:867–90.

————. 1982. Problems of technique in character analysis. *Bulletin Assn. Psychoanal. Medicine* 29:91–99.

————. 1983. *The Analytic Attitude.* New York: Basic Books.

Sterba, R. F. 1953. Clinical and therapeutic aspects of character resistance. *Psychoanal. Q.,* 22:1–20.

Waelder, R. 1930. The principle of multiple function. In *Psychoanalysis: Observation, Theory, Application,* ed. S. A. Guttman. New York: International Universities Press, 1976.

Winnicott, D. W. 1960. Ego distortions in terms of true and false self. In *The Maturational Processes and the Facilitating Environment: Studies in the Theory of Emotional Development.* New York: International Universities Press, 1965.

————. 1965. Psychotherapy of character disorders. In *The Maturational Processes and the Facilitating Environment,* 203–16. New York: International Universities Press.

PART I

HISTORICAL OVERVIEW

1. The Evolution of the Concept of Character in Freud's Writings

Francis D. Baudry

Among the few papers written by Freud (1908a, 1916, 1931) specifically devoted to the topic of character, there exists a rather rich weaving and slow development of the concept. In this section, I shall spell out the unfolding of Freud's thinking and show how the major strides in his clinical and metapsychological works made possible the evolution of character theory, or at least of some of its components since an overall conceptual framework is lacking. In a subsequent section, I shall attempt to summarize the evolution of the concept and its shifting emphasis and definition in the course of Freud's work. I shall purposely delay an overall formulation, as I believe it might detract from my description of the unfolding of Freud's thinking.

A problem in proceeding through isolation of the term "character" in the index and following up on the text references is that some short passages including the term may be difficult to evaluate unless placed in context. In addition, certain papers dealing indirectly with issues related to character but not under that label could be left out entirely—a consequence of the rather mechanical aspect of retrieval. This will be remedied by occasional reference to other papers that seem relevant to the topic. I shall, somewhat arbitrarily, divide the material of Freud's work into three sections: (1) works preceding the paper on anal character (Freud, 1908a); (2) papers leading up to the paper on the three character types (Freud, 1916); and (3) later writings, including the libidinal types classification (Freud, 1931). In what follows, I shall omit obvious repetitions and dwell only on those references indicating a change— either progress or regression in the use of the term.

EARLY DEVELOPMENT AND USAGE (1895–1907)

Early in the development of the theory and technique of analysis, character plays essentially no role. The reasons for this are several. (1) The main

Reprinted from the *Journal of the American Psychoanalytic Association* 31:3–31 by permission of International Universities Press, Inc. Copyright 1983 by American Psychoanalytic Association.

interest was focused on symptoms—what stood out—rather than on character—the matrix. (2) The concept of resistance and transference central to the
manifestation of character in the analytic situation had not yet burgeoned. (3)
Freud was more concerned initially with the sexual drives *per se* and their
multiple manifestations than with adaptation and reality. (4) Psychoanalysis
was first concerned with the unconscious rather than with exploration of the
conscious.

Until the *Three Essays* (Freud, 1905b), all references to character are
incidental and may be omitted from this survey, except for a brief allusion
(Freud, 1904) which makes a connection between character and resistance.
This is not the only instance of a major discovery that is buried and unearthed
some years later as in Freud's (1916) paper on character types. Here is the
1904 passage: "if the physician has to deal with a worthless character, he
soon loses the interest which makes it possible for him to enter profoundly
into the patient's mental life. Deep-rooted malformations of character, traits
of an actually degenerate constitution, show themselves during treatment as
sources of a resistance that can scarcely be overcome" (p. 254). This formulation recalls the then prevalent theory of personality disorders of 19th-
century German psychiatry which included theories of hereditary determinism of human behavior. It may be recalled that in the early formulations, the
socially deviant aberrations received the greatest attention; hence, the distinctive judgmental quality which emerges at this time. The contamination of the
lay usage of the term and its moral connotations are apparent. This passage
also suggests the operation within the analyst of countertransference resistance—that is, the reaction of dislike to the patient, rather than being seen as
a source of data, is conceptualized as a source of resistance "that can scarcely
be overcome"—the theory at this point then serves a protective function for
the analyst.

The first major development is to be found in the *Three Essays* (Freud,
1905b) in the section on sublimation, in the summary. It anticipates the paper
on anal character by showing how instincts and impulses that have been
transformed by processes of reaction formation and sublimation fuel and
contribute to the person's character traits. Freud also hints that in an artist
one may find a mixture of perversion, efficiency, and neurosis—presumably
according to the formula in usage at the time, equating perversion with the
direct expression of impulse, the neurosis with its negative, and the efficiency
with reaction formation or sublimation.

What we describe as a person's 'character' is built up to a considerable extent from the material of sexual excitations and is composed of instincts that have been fixed since childhood, of constructions achieved by means of sublimation, and of other constructions, employed for effectively holding in check perverse impulses which have been recognized as unutilizable. The multifariously perverse sexual disposition of childhood can accordingly be regarded as the source of a number of our virtues, in so far as through reaction-formation it stimulates their development [pp. 238–239].

One gains the impression that by "constructions," Freud had in mind some stable structure, anticipating the ego. This passage also foreshadows the future division of character traits into reactive and sublimatory. Freud assumed at this time that efficiency (presumably referring to socially acceptable instinctual derivatives such as character traits), perversion, and neurosis were equivalent potential outcomes of the transformation of instincts.

A note of caution is necessary in placing Freud's emphasis on drive manifestations in the context of the overall development of his theory. Freud's portrayal of character as originating in the transformation of drives should not be taken to mean that character is nothing but transformed instinctual derivatives; rather, Freud approached all of mental functioning from this viewpoint at that particular time. The implication of the historical approach, particularly for a term as inclusive as character, is that the evolution of the concept recapitulates the history of the development of psychoanalysis itself.

In another passage, Freud briefly introduces the role of masturbation during the oedipal phase; referring to this second phase of infantile sexual activity, Freud (1905b) writes: "But all its details leave behind the deepest (unconscious) impressions in the subject's memory, determine the development of his character, if he is to remain healthy, and the symptomatology of his neurosis, if he is to fall ill after puberty" (p. 189). Freud seems to imply that the person's character is a healthy development in contrast to the symptoms of a neurosis. This idea will be rapidly modified in the next few years.

The last theoretical formulation before Freud's (1908a) paper on anal character is to be found in 1907. Freud stated, at a meeting of the Vienna Psychoanalytic Society, "In general, the human being cannot tolerate contrasting ideas and feelings in juxtaposition. It is this striving for unification that we call character" (Nunberg and Federn, 1962, p. 236). Thus Freud introduced the synthetic function of character formation, the problem-solving aspect, later developed by Nunberg (1931).

As Stein (1969) reminds us, by 1908 Freud had the elements of a fairly complete theory of symptom formation as elaborated in the remarkable paper "Hysterical Phantasies and Their Relation to Bisexuality" (1908c). The paper on anal character (1908a) does not present the same concision and depth of understanding of the processes of character formation. I shall summarize, through a few formulas, Freud's theory in 1908 as it applied to patients with anal character.

1. On a descriptive level, this category includes orderliness, parsimony, and obstinacy (the three character traits).

2. These patients had unusual difficulty in controlling direct expression of instinct in childhood (i.e., they were born with unusually strong constitutional anal propensities).

3. During the period of latency, strong reaction formations formed "at the expense of the excitations proceeding from the erotogenic zones," opposing "like dams" direct expression of instincts (p. 171).

4. The traits mentioned above are direct results of the sublimation of the instincts—defined as a deflection of excitation from sexual aims to other aims.

5. Character is formed out of the constituent instincts—either as unchanged prolongation or as sublimations or reaction formations against them.

6. Other component instincts such as the urethral instinct can undergo a similar fate. The theory described so far comprises (a) clinical description and isolation of recurring groupings; (b) constitutional predisposition and factors in early history; (c) some hints of a developmental process occurring during latency; (d) an attempt to describe the process by which the transformation occurs and to generalize from this clinical instance.

It is tempting to speculate why the obsessional character was the first to be described. On the clinical level, obsessional patients have a great propensity to verbalize. It may be that a clear organizational structure is the formal counterpart of the clinical manifestations, and thus was easier to isolate.

We may wonder about the reasons for the more simplistic theory of character development as contrasted to the theory of symptom formation. It is due in part to the relative neglect of character in clinical work at this stage of development of psychoanalyis. Although it is possible to describe some of the disagreeable character traits that colored Dora's treatment (Freud, 1905a) —her wish for revenge, her manipulativeness—these are not related by Freud to other manifestations of her pathology and, of course, not yet to the course of the transference which has a close relationship to character. Character traits being experienced as self-syntonic are not brought by the patient as something to be analyzed. It is left to the analyst to bring them up for consideration. Freud did not do this in the case of Dora because he did not realize that her character attitudes would serve the purpose of resistance and would bring a premature end to his efforts.

SECOND PERIOD OF DEVELOPMENT (1908–1916)

Excessive masturbation was given a role in weakening character. Initially masturbation was understood to represent a close derivative of the sexual drives. However, Freud (1908b) was beginning to depart from his previous mechanistic emphasis, as this passage suggests:

> The sexual behavior of a human being often *lays down the pattern* for all his other modes of reacting to life. If a man is energetic in winning the object of his love, we are confident that he will pursue his other aims with an equally unswerving energy; but if, for all sorts of reasons, he refrains from satisfying his strong sexual instincts, his behavior will be conciliatory and resigned rather than vigorous in other spheres of life as well [p. 198].

There follows a passage relating the inhibition of women in intellectual matters to the taboo against their interest in sexual issues. This finding expressed in clinical terms the primacy of the sexual instincts in determining patterns of behavior—this at a time when the theory of the ego had not yet been developed.

A brief sentence in the Leonardo paper (1910a) alludes to the constitutional aspect of character—its roots in the organic matrix. "We are obliged to look for the source of the tendency to repression and the capacity for sublimation in the organic foundations of character on which the mental structure is only afterwards erected'' (p. 136). This is one of the very few references Freud makes to the inborn biological roots of character.

Freud's paper on object choice (1910b) is a good example of the papers that deal indirectly with the concept of character and yet do not mention the word *per se*. He isolates a clinical picture, describing certain men with consistent characteristics in their conditions for loving: the presence of an injured third party, the selection of a woman of ill repute, the high value the man sets on her, and finally the urge to rescue the woman who is loved. Freud is able to unite these apparently diverse and puzzling attributes as derivatives of the psychic constellations connected with the mother. Freud's explanation remains at a clinical level. He refers to the Oedipus complex and the position of the boy looking for revenge. At the end of the paper, he alludes to his method of classification:

I have in the first place aimed at singling out from the observational material extreme and sharply defined types. In both cases we find a far greater number of individuals in whom only a few features of the type can be recognized, or only features which are not distinctly marked, and it is obvious that a proper appreciation of these types will not be possible until the whole context to which they belong has been explored [pp. 174–175].

This paper is the first to introduce the term "types" as a classification concept referring to some aspect of object relations. The term will recur again in his (1931) paper "Libidinal Types." This paper enriches the concept of character by broaching the important topic of object relations—novel at the time. It deals in clinical fashion with the outcome of the Oedipus complex and with character in other than instinctual vicissitudes. It also illustrates the shaping influence of unconscious fantasies on the character and behavior of the mature individual.

In this relatively brief review, I can mention only in passing two metapsychological papers whose concepts lay the groundwork for much of the theory of character formation: the paper on "Two Principles of Mental Functioning" (1911) and the paper on "Instincts and Their Vicissitudes" (1915a). The former paper, by clearly identifying the reality principle, foreshadows the adaptive point of view and spells out the development of critical ego functions—memory, judgment, attention, and thought. The latter paper, concerning the processes of change in the aims of instincts—reversal into the opposite, turning around on the subject, repression, and sublimation—lays down broad principles which will play a role in determining the shape of character traits.

From 1914 on, we find rather precipitous and momentous developments following each other. Probably the key concepts determining such an explosion of discoveries include the elaboration of narcissism and the formulations of the concept of transference in the paper "Remembering, Repeating and Working Through." The key passage introducing the concept of repetition compulsion (in the clinical sense) is as follows:

We have learnt that the patient repeats instead of remembering, and repeats under the conditions of resistance. We may now ask what it is that he in fact repeats or acts out. The answer is that he repeats everything that has already made its way from the sources of the repressed into his manifest personality—his inhibitions and unserviceable attitudes and his pathological character-traits. He also repeats all his symptoms in the course of the treatment [Freud, 1914, p. 151].

The central issue of repetition was already hinted at in his previous paper, "The Dynamics of the Transference," in which Freud refers to the individual's acquisition of "a specific method . . . in his conduct of his erotic life— that is, in the preconditions to falling in love which he lays down, in the instincts he satisfies and the aims he sets himself in the course of it. This produces what might be described as a a stereotype plate (or several such), which is constantly repeated—constantly reprinted afresh—in the course of the person's life, so far as external circumstances and the nature of the love-objects accessible to him permit, and which is certainly not entirely insusceptible to change in the face of recent experiences" (Freud, 1912, pp. 99–100).

Although the process of repetition is first related to the strength and tendency of the unsatisfied instincts which are repressed and dominate the object-seeking behavior, the next step involves the discovery of resistance to the analytic process, as it manifests itself in the transference.

The second major discovery concerns the substitution of action for memory; behavior (or character trait) is a communication—in another language —about the individual's past which needs to be analyzed and becomes, via the transference, the most useful tool and the source of the strongest resistance; the struggle at this point is dynamically active and, therefore, subject to interpretation.

The concept of the "stereotype plate reprinted afresh" seems to apply a metaphor drawn from the original literal meaning of the term character. This term does not appear anywhere else. Since character is ego-syntonic, the patient will not bring it up. The analyst however, cannot afford to do the same, he is forced to pay attention to resistances anchored in the patient's character. He is also confronted with the clinical fact of repetition of "unserviceable attitudes and pathological character traits."

A subsequent paper, "The Disposition to Obsessional Neurosis" (1913), allows Freud to stand back and contrast the process in character formation and symptom formation.

In the field of development of *character* we are bound to meet with the same instinctual forces which we have found at work in the neuroses. But a sharp theoretical distinction between the two is necessitated by the single fact that the failure of repression and the return of the repressed—which are peculiar to the mechanism of neurosis—are absent in the formation of character. In the latter, repression either does not come into action or smoothly achieves its aim of replacing the repressed by reaction formations and sublimations. Hence, the processes of the formation of character are more obscure and less accessible to analysis than neurotic ones [p. 323].

Thus, reasons for the difficulty in understanding character formation emerge—some practical, some theoretical. The process is silent, ego-syntonic and not obviously involved in conflict with various signposts indicative of the struggle. In his theory building, Freud had attempted until then to apply the same model for the formation of character trait and symptom. This could lead only to confusion, as each obviously arose from different exigencies; i.e., a neurotic symptom is always a pathological process, whereas character formation is a normal developmental process which, though involved in conflict, is not necessarily pathological.

Yet another reason complicating the comparison between symptom and character (pointed out by Rosen [Panel] 1957) lies in the dichotomy apparent in early analytic writings: symptom formation is understood in terms of regression from oedipal conflicts, whereas character, at least in its instinctual components, is seen in terms of pregenital fixations. This oversimplification was not to be rectified until the 1930's, with the interest in female sexuality. By then analysts became sensitized to the distorting effects of the pregenital phases on the oedipal one.

There is no question that a character trait is not as clearcut an entity as a symptom. Hence, it is more difficult to delineate and to study. There remained to develop the concept of the ego before new advances could be made in the field. In the paper on repression, Freud (1915b) describes the evolution of a character trait from the transformation of a repressed hostile impulse.

It is this hostile impulsion against someone who is loved which is subjected to repression. The effect at an early stage of the work of repression is quite different from what it is at a later one. At first the repression is completely successful, the ideational content is rejected and the affect made to disappear. As a substitutive formation there arises an alteration in the ego in the shape of an increased conscientiousness, and this can hardly be called a symptom. Here . . . repression has brought about a withdrawal of libido; but here it has made use of *reaction-formation* for this purpose, by intensifying an opposite. . . . Here substitute and symptom do not coincide [pp. 156–157].

In this passage dealing with obsessional neurosis, Freud is probably referring to the formation of a character trait, should the alteration in the ego persist. The same impulse whose transformation gives rise to symptoms according to the classical formulations can also give rise to another type of substitute formation, namely, an alteration in the ego. As the role of aggression in human development becomes better understood, its key role in character formation will emerge.

"Mourning and Melancholia" (1917), though not directly referring to character formation, alludes to those processes through which an object cathexis under the influence of loss is replaced by an identification. The role of identification will, of course, be elaborated in 1923 in *The Ego and Id,* as will be described later. The setting up of the superego as a critical agency spit off from the ego is also hinted at.

In "Thoughts for the Times on War and Death," Freud (1915c) tackles the issues of the prerequisite leading up to a completed character formation. In a section describing reaction formation and the presence in the unconscious of opposite impulses which are eventually synthesized in the personality, Freud writes:

Psycho-analysis adds that the two opposed feelings not infrequently have the same person for their object.
  It is not until . . . these 'instinctual vicissitudes' have been surmounted that what we call a person's character is formed, and this, as we know, can only very inadequately be classified as 'good' or 'bad'; . . . most of our sentimentalists, friends of humanity and protectors of animals have been evolved from little sadists and animal tormentors [281–282].

Freud's concern with good and bad has to be placed in context of the timing of this paper and its subject matter—disillusionment and war. He again takes up an idea first quoted in 1907—the synthetic aspect of character formation. As the most common mode of transformation was reaction formation (in theory) Freud deals mostly with obsessional neurosis. The allusion to surmounting instinctual vicissitudes as a prelude to character formation is an important early step in indicating the way-stations to completion of character formation.

The last paper in this period is the second major paper of Freud's (1916) devoted entirely to our topic, "Some Character-Types Met with in Psycho-Analytic Work." The classification of character is unsatisfactory to this day. Often a literary allusion (Don Juan character) or a brief description (the exceptions) may capture the flavor of certain individuals and encapsulate the essence of their make-up better than a more scientific term. Of the three categories described by Freud, only the "exceptions" could describe a general type of character; the other two, "those wrecked by success" and "criminals from a sense of guilt" do not easily lend themselves to translation into character traits. The former deals more with onset of illness, the latter with antecedents of a particular behavior. Both describe patterns of a very general order. All three are in one way or another related to issues of guilt. Freud makes the following specific points: (1) Analysts are forced to pay attention to character because some major resistance to analytic work is a manifestation of character—a reemergence of a point first made in passing in 1904. (2) The character traits that show up in the analytic situation as resistance are not necessarily the ones that are outstanding outside the analysis. This latter point highlights the difficulty confronting analysts in evaluating the observations they may make about their patient's character in the office. This paper illustrates the problems of a classification scheme. Freud suggested one approach for the practitioner—the evaluation of character from the point of view of resistance.

THIRD PERIOD OF DEVELOPMENT (1916–1939)

We now come to the last period in Freud's work on character. With the shift in clinical work toward more detailed analysis of resistance and its subtle manifestations, interest in character was bound to increase. This third period saw the evolution of the structural theory, the understanding of masochism and increased interest in the general role of aggression, and finally the delineating of the functions of the superego and ego ideal. Increased clinical experience led to the delineation of certain clinical syndromes and the influence of key fantasies (e.g., beating fantasies) on character and behavior, and also the beginnings of the theoretical relation between character and neurosis. Many of the clinical examples given by Freud will be drawn from the obsessional neuroses (really character manifestations of these patients).

In his lecture dealing with transference resistance, we find the following passage.

It may . . . be said that what is being mobilized for fighting against the alterations we are striving for [in the analysis] are character-traits, attitudes of the ego. In this connection we discover that these character-traits were formed in the relation to the determinants of the neurosis and in reaction against its demands, and we come upon traits which cannot normally emerge . . . which may be described as latent [Freud, 1916–1917, p. 291]

A later section implies that an essential function of analysis lies in bringing these resistances to light and overcoming them.

Emphasis is laid on the latent aspect of some of these traits. A point made previously is that the traits which contribute most heavily to the resistances are not necessarily the most obvious or manifest in the person's functioning outside the analysis.

The relation between character and transference neurosis deserves a longer discussion than can be given here. There are complicated connections between the view of the analyst in the transference (e.g., punitive father, seductive mother), the character traits that arose as solutions to conflicts with the original objects, and compromise formations arising out of the current transference neurosis with an analyst who represents all these images in conflict with the adult personality and its character rigidities.

In another section, speaking of the form the castration complex takes in the little boy, Freud states that it "plays a great part in the construction of his character if he remains normal, in his neurosis if he falls ill, and in his resistance if he comes into analytic treatment" (1916–1917, p. 318).

From a developmental point of view, the solution to the Oedipus complex is the last infantile watershed. From it emerges a new structure, the superego, which will give character its own stamp.

The paper "A Child Is Being Beaten" afforded one illustration of the effect of an unconscious fantasy on character formation, specifically the second, unconscious masochistic phase.

. . . we can also detect effects upon the character, which are directly derived from its unconscious form. People who harbor phantasies of this kind develop a specific sensitiveness and irritability towards anyone whom they can include in the class of fathers. They are easily offended by a person of this kind, and in that way (to their own sorrow and cost) bring about the realization of the imagined situation of being beaten by their father [Freud, 1919, p. 195].

The structural theory allowed Freud to formulate more stringently the mechanisms of character formation, specifically the role of identification in both ego and superego formation. It also allowed for a more thorough understanding and description of the dynamic relations in the mind. This was developed in *The Ego and the Id* (1923). An entire chapter, "The Ego and the Superego (Ego Ideal)," deals with this topic—the view of the ego as the precipitate of object cathexis replaced by identifications.

The main points relevant to our topic are: (1) The replacement of object cathexis by identifications "has a great share in determining the form taken by the ego and that it makes an essential contribution towards building up what is called its 'character' " (p. 28). (2) The character of the ego is a precipitate of abandoned object cathexis and contains the history of those object choices. (3) There are various degrees of capacity for resistance which decide the extent to which a person's character fends off or accepts the influence of the history of his erotic object choices. (4) In some cases the alteration in character may precede the loss of the object. (5) "the transformation of object-libido into narcissistic libido which . . . takes place obviously implies an abandonment of sexual aims, a desexualization—a kind of sublimation" (p. 30). (6) If the various identifications are incompatible with each other, a pathological outcome may occur. (7) The effect of the first identification made in childhood will be general and lasting. (8) The ego ideal (in the boy) is derived from identification with the father. (9) Identifications are influenced by two major organizers—the Oedipus complex and the constitutional bisexuality. (10) The dissolution of the Oedipus complex consolidates the masculinity of the boy's character. (11) The superego is not simply a residue of the earliest object choices of the id; it also represents an energetic reaction formation against those choices.

Freud stresses the motives for the formation of psychic structure as an attempt to deal with object loss (negative) and also loving, admiring feelings (positive). Both may lead to identification. In this process, energy is desexualized—an issue pursued by Hartmann, among others. The crucial role of identifications (or struggles against identifications), both ego and superego, the greater influence of the earliest identification, and the timetable of character formation, including the necessary resolution of the Oedipus complex before the identifications are sufficiently stabilized, explain the clinical facts.

The introduction of the structural theory presages much of the contemporary view of character and the development of ego psychology. It lays much of the groundwork for the clarification of the key role of identification and inter- and intra-systemic conflicts. It also presents some hints of a developmental line that can be contrasted with the early version (Freud, 1908a) and its primary emphasis on vicissitudes of the libido as a prime organizer. In contrast, the structural theory presents largely an object-relations model.

Although dealing with other topics, *Beyond the Pleasure Principle* (Freud, 1920) elaborates in greater detail than the paper on "Remembering, Repeating and Working Through" (Freud, 1914) the concept of repetition compulsion as it applies to character.

What psycho-analysis reveals in the transference phenomena of neurotics can also be observed in the lives of some normal people. . . . The compulsion which is here in evidence differs in no way from the compulsion to repeat which we have found in neurotics, even though the people we are now considering have never known any signs of dealing with a neurotic conflict by producing symptoms. Thus we have come across people all of whose human relationships have the same outcome: such as the benefactor who is abandoned in anger after a time by each of his *protégés,* however much they may otherwise differ from one another, and who thus seems doomed to taste all the bitterness of ingratitude . . . or, again, the lover each of whose love affairs with a woman passes through the same phases and reaches the same conclusion [Freud, 1920, pp. 21–22].

This description was to be elaborated later in Alexander's concept of the fate neurosis. Although it purports to demonstrate the strength of the repetition compulsion as it applies to pathological character traits—particularly those involving some unpleasure—there is no fundamental reason to assume that other phenomena in mental life are not directed by repetitive strivings, character being such a phenomenon.

In *Group Psychology,* Freud (1921) stresses the unifying or synthetic aspect of character formation—an idea that had first arisen in 1900 and then been lost sight of, though the later version is more complicated than the former. Freud compares those processes in the formation of the ego with the coordination of all the sexual instincts into a definitive genital organization. He states further that the unification of the ego is liable to the same interferences as that of the libido. Freud takes pains to show that unless there is a special situation, such as the increase in cathexis of an unconscious fantasy, the unconscious will tolerate conflicting tendencies without production of a pathological outcome—an important point in considering the relation between character and normality.

An important passage in *Inhibitions, Symptoms and Anxiety* clarifies the relation between character and neurosis. Freud contrasts the end results of reaction formations in obsessional neurosis with those in hysteria. In the former, one may speak of widespread effect, having the universality of a character trait, whereas in the latter, the reaction formations are confined to particular relationships. "A hysterical woman, for instance, may be specially affectionate with her own children whom at bottom she hates; but she will not on that account be more loving in general than other women or even more affectionate with other children" (Freud, 1926, p. 158). Freud then deals with the obvious question—what then are the characteristics of the hysterical personality? He refers to their tendency to scotomize as the particular way the anticathexis operates. Though this mechanism is described in general terms, it is possible to derive a number of character traits from it.

At this time, the model for character formation was still derived from analogies made with the processes in obsessional neurosis. This has obvious important consequences. "These reaction-formations of the obsessional neurosis are essentially exaggerations of normal traits of character formation . . ." (p. 157). They should be regarded, according to Freud, as yet another mechanism of defense and placed alongside regression and repression. The reasons for this choice lie in the greater clarity with which it is possible to observe the fate of some of the ideational representatives of the forbidden instincts: "the ego is . . . much more . . . the scene of action of symptom-formation in obsessional neurosis than it is in hysteria . . ." (p. 119).

As Freud examines in greater detail some of the common defense mechanisms in obsessional neurosis, he anticipates the principle of multiple function as he realizes that the behaviors of undoing and isolation also express the very instincts they are attempting to avoid. As the mechanisms of defense are thus described and broadened, their distinction from character traits blurs; one may say that they are a slightly more abstract way of describing a person's behavior and that, on a more directly observational level, it would be possible to infer the operation of a number of character traits derived from them. A careful reading of Freud's use of the term obsessional neurosis suggests that what he has in mind is more the total personality organization of such individuals than just the symptoms.

At this time in his life, Freud's illness made it almost impossible for him to participate in scientific discussions. Nevertheless, he held irregular meetings in the waiting room of his office. Waelder quotes the following anecdote from one of these sessions held some time in 1926 or 1927. Schilder had just presented a multidimensional system of characterology:

As was customary on these occasions, Freud opened the discussion, and in the course of his comments said that he felt like the skipper of a barge who had always hugged the coast and who now learned that others, more adventurous, had set out for the open sea. He wished them well but could no longer participate in their endeavor: "But I am an old hand in the coastal run and I will remain faithful to my blue inlets" [Waelder, 1958, pp. 245–246].

In the last phase of his thinking on character, Freud became concerned with broader issues involving adaptation to one's fate and happiness. A very beautiful passage in *Civilization and Its Discontents* aptly describes this aspect of his work.

Happiness, in the reduced sense in which we recognize it as possible, is a problem of the economics of the individual's libido. There is no golden rule which applies to everyone. . . . All kinds of different factors will operate to direct his choice. It is a question of how much real satisfaction he can expect to get from the external world, how far he is led to make himself independent of it, and, finally, how much strength he feels he has for altering the world to suit his wishes. In this his psychical constitution will play a decisive part, irrespectively of the external circumstances. The man who is predominately erotic will give first preference to his emotional relationships to other people; the narcissistic man, who inclines to be self-sufficient, will seek his main satisfactions in his internal mental processes; the man of action will never give up the external world on which he can try out his strength . . . Any choice that is pushed to an extreme will be penalized by exposing the individual to the dangers which arise if a technique of living that has been chosen as an exclusive one should prove inadequate [Freud, 1930, pp. 83–84].

The word constitution as used by Freud is a bit misleading. I originally believed it referred to the biological inborn element, but the passage, then, would make no sense—the man of action is not inborn. In this paragraph, Freud uses the word constitution as synonymous with make-up. It includes both biological inborn factors and experiential ones. This is taken up later in his paper on libidinal types (1931), wherein Freud makes a significant contribution in spelling out the requirements for a classification: (1) It "should not merely be deduced from our knowledge or our hypotheses about the libido . . ."; (2) "it should be easily confirmed in actual experience . . ."; (3) "it should contribute to the classification of the mass of our observations and help us to grasp them"; (4) the types should "not coincide with clinical pictures [but] must comprehend all the variations which . . . fall within the limits of the normal" (p. 217).

The rest of the paper dealing with the attempted working out of a classification based primarily on libidinal types has largely fallen into oblivion. The concept of libidinal types refers mostly to a combination of object relations and innate predisposition. Freud was trying to arrive at a character make-up independent of pathology. The paper's main drawback is its lack of dynamic framework and its distance from more clearly observable character traits. We are fortunate in that Freud saw fit to attempt to summarize some of his more important views in a passage in the *New Introductory Lectures:*

You yourselves have no doubt assumed that what is known as 'character,' a thing so hard to define, is to be ascribed entirely to the ego. We have already made out a little of what it is that creates character. First and foremost, there is the incorporation of the former parental agency as a super-ego, which is no doubt its most important and decisive portion, and, further, identifications with the two parents of the later period and with other influential figures, and similar identifications formed as precipitates of abandoned object-relations. And we may now add as contributions to the construction of character which are never absent, the reaction-formations which the ego acquires —to begin with in making its repressions and later, by a more normal method, when it rejects unwished-for instinctual impulses [Freud, 1933, p. 91].

The important aspects of this section are the relegation of character as an aspect of the ego, the primary importance attributed to the role of the superego, and the role of identification as shaping external influences. The internal aspects relate to the defense of reaction formation as the most important mechanism—both in terms of form and content (the incorporation of unwished-for instinctual impulses). This last defense, derived from the early days of analysis and its study of obsessional neurosis, thus remained a cardinal point in Freudian theory. Fenichel, much later (1941, p. 91), classifies character traits into reactive and sublimatory, still attesting to this point of view. I could not be entirely sure of what Freud had in mind when he wrote about the ego's "normal" methods of rejecting unwished-for instinctual impulses. Was Freud alluding to conscious repudiation on the basis of established reaction formation or had he some other mechanism in mind— suppression? secondary repression? Beyond this passage there are only scant references in Freud that add anything to the above.

In the last few papers, Freud was preoccupied with two themes. (1) The role of trauma in character—in the sense of the overcoming of trauma as playing a role in shaping character and the fixation to trauma which "may be taken up into what passes as a normal ego and, as permanent trends in it, may lend it unalterable character-traits, although, or rather precisely because, their true basis and historical origin are forgotten" (Freud, 1937b, p. 75). This passage describes the working of the repetition compulsion but in a new way, i.e., character as remnants of forgotten events. (2) The last major paper, "Analysis Terminable and Interminable," deals with therapeutic impasses and indirectly with some of the dynamics of unalterable ego states which can take the form of character resistances. Freud hovers between consideration of traumatic versus constitutional factors as limiting factors to the therapeutic effect of analysis. He considers the fixations of defense mechanisms "regular modes of reaction of [a person's] character, which are repeated throughout his life whenever a situation occurs that is similar to the original one" (Freud, 1937a, p. 237).

The constitutional factors described such as adhesiveness of libido, psychical inertia or, in case of women, insoluble penis envy, are open to question as explanatory statements. As Grossman and Stewart (1976) have shown, the so-called resistance of penis envy is capable of further analysis in its pregenital roots of narcissistic hurts. It is not necessarily the bedrock of analytic resistance Freud considered it to be in 1937, when analysis was devoted largely to the understanding of neurotic disorders viewed as regressions from an oedipal situation. In terms of the process of theory building, it may be that when a gap exists in our clinical understanding of a condition, it becomes useful to fall back on "explanations" of a higher degree of generalization. Freud, when faced with certain intractable resistances in analysis introduced into his theory the concept of psychic inertia, adhesiveness of libido, excessive mobility of libido, and the need to hold on to illness or suffering. Freud hypothesized that these are attributes of the ego, either innate distinguishing characteristics, dispositions, or trends early in life which will, in part, determine the choice of defense mechanisms. This brings us back to the question of temperament—in contrast to that of character.

By this time, Freud had applied many aspects of the theory of neurosis to the form and content of character traits (early trauma, defense, latency, outbreak of neurotic illness, partial return of repressed via character traits either expressing or avoiding trauma, and identification with parents). The major difference would seem to lie in whether pathological outcome, alterations, take place in the ego itself or whether they confront it as alien to it.

In the *Outline of Psychoanalysis,* Freud (1940) added to the above list of traumas "Derivatives and modified products of . . . early masturbatory phantasies [which] make their way into his later ego and play a part in the formation of his character" (p. 190).

We are fortunate in possessing a brief case history of Freud's, cited as an example of a neurosis including character traits resulting from the combination of several traumas. It is presented in a brief section in *Moses and Monotheism* (Freud, 1937b, pp. 79–80). Briefly, the illustration (which I assume to be the Wolf Man), deals with a little boy witness to the primal scene at an age when he had scarcely learned to speak. Following his first spontaneous emission, neurotic symptoms consisting of insomnia and sensitivity to noises developed; in addition, the little boy's identification with his father aroused his aggressive masculinity; he masturbated frequently and attempted to attack his mother sexually. Following a castration threat, the boy "gave up his sexual activity and altered his character." He became passive and provocative toward the father; he also clung to his mother and became an exemplary boy in school. In puberty, the manifest neurosis emerged with sexual impotence, avoidance of women, sadomasochistic fantasies and, secondary to the pubertal intensification of masculinity, there emerged "furious hatred of his father and insubordination to him . . . reckless to the pitch of self-destruction. He must be a failure in his profession because his father had forced him into it. [He made no] friends and he was never on good terms with his superiors." After his father's death, he married and "developed a completely egoistic, despotic, and brutal personality, which clearly felt a need to suppress and insult other people. It was a faithful copy of his father as he had formed a picture of him in his memory: that is to say, a revival of the identification with his father which in the past he had taken on as a little boy from sexual motives." Freud considered this last fact an example of the return of the repressed.

Can we refer to the traditional view of neurosis: early trauma—defense, latency, outbreak of neurotic illness, partial return of the repressed—and see where the concept of character fit in Freud's view? The first reference to character modification—the substitution of passivity for activity and the development of a masochistic provocative attitude during the latency period—is a consequence of the castration threat, experienced as a narcissistic mortification. In this context, Freud described a behavioral change as a result of the activation of certain unconscious fantasies. These fantasies could also be described as secondary to new identifications with the boy's view of the mother and abandonment of the identification with the father followed by its replacement by an object tie. The alteration in behavior could also be understood as a negative reaction to the threat, an avoidance. Freud (1937b) states, "These negative reactions too make the most powerful contribution to the stamping of character" (p. 76). He also refers to the compulsive quality of the symptoms, the inhibitions, and the stable character changes (implying, of course, that some changes, as in the case cited, are not stable) to be replaced by others when new conditions (e.g., puberty) prevail.

This compulsive quality refers to the great psychical intensity of the trait and its far-reaching independence of the organization of the other mental processes adjusted to the demands of the real world. When Freud refers to the "inhibition upon the life of those who are dominated by a neurosis" (p. 78), it is clear that he has in mind a global concept combining symptoms, inhibitions, and ego alterations or character traits. As Freud conceptualizes it, the emergence of the character traits of egoism, despotism, and brutality is clearly a consequence of the reappearance of an aspect of identification with the father under the sway of increasing masculine strivings at puberty.

One could say that the sadistic coloring reflected an identification with the punitive father and the child's misunderstanding of the primal scene.

Freud also implied that the character traits were a solution to the previous neurotic adjustment (failure in life and in a profession forced on him by the father). The character trait, then, has a more complicated origin than the symptom, representing the result of certain identifications and the attempt of the ego to adjust to previous neurotic illness. The opposite may also be true, that is, "defensive mechanisms, by bringing about an ever more extensive alienation from the external world and a permanent weakening of the ego, pave the way for, and encourage, the outbreak of neurosis" (Freud, 1937a, p. 238). It is important to dwell on this last point because, until then, Freud thought that neurotic character was a consequence and not a causative factor in neurosis. This argument formed the basis of his disagreement with Adler. Freud considered that unconscious sexual conflicts forcing themselves on a relatively weak ego were more fundamental than the ego's attempt to compensate for inferiority as a causative factor. The last passage quoted suggests that a chronic fixity in defense mechanisms, something close to character traits, could, by weakening the ego, encourage the outbreak of neurosis. This, toward the end of his career, represents a considerable enrichment in Freud's views.

DISCUSSION AND SUMMARY

There now remains the task of recapitulating the route that has been followed. As many of the references to character in Freud's work are minor statements interspersed among other current preoccupations, it is unavoidable that the preceding survey leaves one with the impression of a patchwork quilt. Any attempt to synthesize may thus stem more from the writer's need for closure than from any valid description of the evolution of Freud's theory. However, I believe there is some purpose to be served in recalling some of the main way stations previously covered.

The early usage of the term character was nearly synonymous with its lay origin, not being clearly distinguished from behavior. Aside from a few minor references, we find the first serious effort to delineate a truly psychoanalytic concept of character in the section on sublimation in the *Three Essays* (Freud, 1905b). It introduces the concept of transformation of instincts and their relation to individual character traits. As the concept of ego was not developed fully, it was pretty much used interchangeably with that of character. Beyond minor references to the role of masturbation and synthetic aspects of a person's character, we find little until the key paper on anal character (Freud, 1908a). It is hard to appreciate the breakthrough of this short paper—the concept of character as an organization of character traits, belonging together because of certain common origins. A process of development and its timetable were introduced. That much has been added since to our understanding of anal character should not detract from the audacity of the concepts and Freud's idea of establishing a relation between a superficial attribute (a trait) and an underlying organization (the drives). I consider "A Special Type of Object Choice" (Freud, 1910b) an important landmark; it was the first time that a clinical constellation of repetitive behavior was explained on the basis of unconscious fantasies derived from the Oedipus complex. While not clearly characterological, the paper introduces the concept of object relations and types. The next decade witnessed one major advance after another. The cornerstone of this edifice is the paper on "Remembering, Repeating and Working Through" (Freud, 1914). The clinical delineation of, and interest in, resistance, transference, and repetition opened the door to an understanding of character as resistance and as a communication about the repressed past. In addition to the clinical interest which led to additional formulation of character types, Freud began to address himself to a question which is still of interest today—the relation between character formation and repression. He differentiates the formation of character from that of neurosis in his paper on "The Disposition to Obsessional Neurosis" (Freud, 1913). Until that time, Freud had not found it necessary to make this differentiation as long as character traits were thought to be largely determined by instinctual vicissitudes. Additional data on the role of aggression and its fate and the key paper, "Mourning and Melancholia," offered a formulation linking identification, object loss and thereby hints of a developmental process of the ego (Freud, 1917). This was finally clarified with the emergence of the structural theory. Freud (1923) indicated that the character of the ego was a precipitate of abandoned object cathexis and contained the history of those object choices. This view was later to be altered in that it was not deemed necessary to have an abandoned object cathexis as a precondition for identification. The development of the concept of ego ideal and superego allowed more precise formulations, showing the combination of identifications with parental objects and reaction formations to the child's own aggressive strivings. The increasing focus on aggressive drive manifestation led Freud (1920) to a sobering outlook concerning the limits of analysis: *Beyond the Pleasure Principle* introduces the repetition-compulsion. This same caution is again highlighted in the final paper, "Analysis Terminable and Interminable" (Freud, 1937a), with such concepts as psychical inertia and adhesiveness of the libido. Another limiting factor is the impact and effect of trauma. We see offshoots of this in the current controversy between conflict and developmental defect.

As a way of summarizing, I shall list the major determinants of character as they were developed by Freud, more or less historically. These comprise character as (1) a derivative of libidinal drives; (2) reflecting the influence on behavior of certain unconscious fantasies, often masturbatory in nature; (3) an outgrowth of identifications with significant parents; (4) the outgrowth of certain solutions to critical complexes (castration and Oedipus); (5) influenced by constitution; (6) an expression of certain mechanisms of mental functioning—denial, projection, reaction formation, introjection, displacement; (7) a reaction to trauma (positive and negative); (8) a derivative of a conflict involving the superego; (9) a result of an attempt to deal with neurosis or an ego distortion, or representing the equivalent of well-recognized neurotic symptom formation.

Although we are lacking an overall theory of character, it is possible to organize the above list into a primitive schema. If we conceive of character as an amalgam—an attempted compromise between inner and outer—then a natural ordering presents itself. Constitution and the libidinal drives would be the bedrock. On the most primitive level, these would be influenced by interaction with significant adults, largely through mechanisms of identification. This interaction could be described along several different axes—one would be the organization of unconscious fantasies; another, more complex and implying a developmental thrust, would be the major complexes (Oedipus, castration); still another would be the selection of certain preferred mental mechanisms as methods of solution (denial, reaction formation, projection, and the like). The latest factor, from a developmental point of view, would be the superego. Trauma combines the accidental factor and an economic point of view. Finally, as preferred solutions lead to neurosis or ego distortions, character formation has to deal with these disturbances as further raw material.

Many of the above elements are found in combination; they do not operate in isolation. Nevertheless, some character traits are more easily related to one factor. Thus, obstinacy is certainly clearly an outgrowth of drive transformation and the character type. The exceptions reflect the pressure of the superego.

I believe it is a tribute to Freud that, without meaning to, he outlined the basic elements contributing to character formation. Although the forty years since his death have seen many refinements in his formulations, the core remains as valid today as when it was first described.

REFERENCES

Fenichel, O. (1941). Psychoanalysis of character. *Collected Papers,* Second Series. New York: Norton, 1954.

Freud, S. (1904). Freud's psychoanalytic procedure, *S. E.,* 7.

———. (1905a). Fragment of an analysis of a case of hysteria. *S. E.,* 7.

———. (1905b). Three essays on the theory of sexuality. *S. E.,* 7.

———. (1908a). Character and anal erotism. *S. E.,* 9.

———. (1908b). 'Civilized' sexual morality and modern nervous illness. *S. E.,* 9.

———. (1908c). Hysterical phantasies and their relation to bisexuality. *S. E.,* 9.

———. (1910a). Leonardo da Vinci and a memory of his childhood. *S. E.,* 11.

———. (1910b). A special type of object choice made by man. *S. E.,* 11.

———. (1911). Two principles of mental functioning. *S. E.,* 12.

———. (1912). The dynamics of the transference. *S. E.,* 12.

———. (1913). The disposition to obsessional neurosis. *S. E.,* 12.

———. (1914). Remembering, repeating and working through. *S. E.,* 12.

———. (1915a). Instincts and their vicissitudes. *S. E.,* 14.

———. (1915b). Repression. *S. E.,* 14.

———. (1915c). Thoughts for the times on war and death. *S. E.,* 14.

———. (1916). Some character types met with in psychoanalytic work. *S. E.,* 14.

———. (1916–1917). Introductory lectures on psychoanalysis. Lecture 19, resistance and repression. *S. E.,* 16.

———. (1917). Mourning and melancholia. *S. E.,* 14.

———. (1919). A child is being beaten. *S. E.,* 17.

———. (1920). Beyond the Pleasure Principle. *S. E.,* 18.

———. (1921). Group psychology and the analysis of the ego. *S. E.,* 18.

———. (1923). The ego and the id. *S. E.,* 19.

———. (1926). Inhibitions, symptoms and anxiety, *S. E.,* 20.

———. (1930). Civilization and its discontents. *S. E.,* 21.

———. (1931). Libidinal types. *S. E.,* 21.

———. (1933). New introductory lectures, *S. E.,* 22.

———. (1937a). Analysis terminable and interminable. *S. E.,* 23.

———. (1937b). Moses and monotheism. *S. E.,* 23.

———. (1940). An outline of psychoanalysis. *S. E.,* 23.

Grossman, W. & Stewart, W. (1976). Penis envy: from childhood wish to developmental metaphor. *J. Amer. Psychoanal. Assn.,* 24 (suppl.):193–213.

Nunberg, H. (1931). The synthetic function of the ego. In *Practice and Theory of Psychoanalysis.* New York: Int. Univ. Press, 1948, pp. 120–136.

——— & Federn, E., Eds. (1962). *Minutes of the Vienna Psychoanalytic Society,* Vol. I. New York: Int. Univ. Press.
Panel (1957). Preoedipal factors in neurosogenesis. V. H. Rosen, reporter. *J. Amer. Psychoanal. Assn.,* 5:146–157.
Stein, M. H. (1969). Problems of character theory. *J. Amer. Psychoanal. Assn.,* 17:675–701.
Waelder, R. (1958). Neurotic ego distortion: opening remarks to the panel discussion. In *Psychoanalysis: Observation, Theory, Application,* ed. S. A. Guttman. New York: Int. Univ. Press, pp. 244–247.

2. The Concept of Character: A Historical Review

Robert S. Liebert

It is my purpose to examine the concept of character, principally by means of presenting its history in psychoanalytic thought.

It has become customary that any paper on character begin by emphasizing the confused conceptual status of the term—a term that comes down to us from ancient Greece. Its etymological roots, significantly, refer to that which is carved or engraved. Character has been a subject of concern for Aristotle, the Stoics, and every theologian, dramatist, gossip, Boy Scout leader, and psychoanalyst ever since. Our exploration of character is further complicated by the fact that the term has technical meaning in our discipline and also has varied connotations that are established in common parlance.

Within psychoanalytic usage certain distinctions have usually been maintained with respect to *character traits, character types,* and *character.* Traditionally, in specking of "character traits" our referent is clearly delineated, typical, and stable behavior that is readily observable and, importantly, is selected for attention because of its implications for the broader fabric of psychic organization and social adaptation. But even here with the seemingly simple notion of "traits" the problem is complicated by issues involving: (1) the context in which the behavior appears; (2) the values of the observer; (3) the adaptive function for the individual; and (4) distinctions that must be made from *symptoms* with respect to a continuum into which the trait fits— one end of the continuum being that the particular behavior is conflicted, a source of subjective distress, and has little adaptive value, namely, a symptom; the other end being that it is a trait and is ego syntonic. But even with ego syntonicity, which has commonly been regarded as a hallmark of character and character traits, we must be aware, as Schafer (1983) has argued, "What is consciously self-syntonic may, unconsciously, be exceedingly dystonic" (p. 144). Despite these problems, when we speak of character traits, we are usually in the realm of common sense observations about which there would be general agreement and which then lend themselves to interpretive inference.

Character types simply refers to the grouping of individuals who have enough shared and overlapping specific behavioral patterns, such as the "masochistic character" or the "narcissistic character," to enable us to generalize about their comon developmental situation, psychic structure, object relationships, self-imagery, and controlling fantasies.

In contrast with character traits, the term *character* is generally regarded as an ill-defined structure, an organization that must be communicated through the language of metapsychological abstractions. Thus, character is frequently spoken of as a supraordinate entity that integrates dark impulses with external reality, id with superego, conflicted pregenital fantasies, largely unconscious, with a smoothly regulating set of defenses. Moreover, its origins are in the flux of a particular stage of development, and it expresses identification with certain internalized imagos. This tendency, exemplified by the definition given for "character" in the American Psychoanalytic Association's *Glossary of Psychoanalytic Terms and Concepts* (Moore and Fine, 1968), has led us to confuse character as observable behavior with character as a set of abstractions. These abstractions are then tied to and vary with the theoretical orientation to which one is partial in explaining behavior. It is as if character determines behavior rather than that it is the codification of a constellation of related behaviors.

HISTORY OF THE CONCEPT

I will begin my survey with Freud's treatment of the topic. He explicitly addressed the subject of character in only three, widely spaced papers (1908b, 1916, 1931) and of these, the first alone commands our attention—*Character and Anal Erotism* (1908b).[1] In addition, the foundation stones for the theory of character were set in place in crucial papers at each stage of his thinking in papers that did not, however, deal directly with character.

Freud's formulation of anal character is the crystallization of a remarkable mixture of clinical observation and theoretical abstraction. It grew directly out of his analysis of the Rat Man, begun the year before. It is significant to note that in reporting the first month of treatment of the Rat Man to his small

1. Baudry (1983) has offered a comprehensive review of the evolution of the concept of character in Freud's writings.

following in the Psychological Wednesday Society, Freud had said: "In general a human being cannot bear opposite extremes in juxtaposition, be they in his personality or in his reactions. It is this endeavor for unification that we call character" (quoted in Jones, 1955, p. 263).

Freud never offered a definition of "character," but at the outset, he clearly asserted his view of the conflictual basis of character, or, to be more accurate, the *function* of character as a means of resolving conflict. This primacy given to resolution of conflict remained an unchallenged proposition for decades, until modified by Hartmann (1939) and now largely contested by Kohut's followers. At the early period, Freud conceived of the instinctual drives as the energic basis and moving force of the otherwise inert psychological organism. The person evolved through a series of invariable psychobiological stages in which successful adaptation and progress to the next was governed by the reality principle, with repression serving as the major means of transforming the person from primary process beast to civilized being. At this point, aggression had not yet been accorded a companion role to libido as the instinctual driving force.

In his seminal work on character, Freud chose the anal zone and the transformation of the intense erogenicity of this tissue at a specific phase of development into a constellation of related character traits. These traits—orderliness, parsimony, and obstinacy—formed a pattern of observable behavior that was functionally adaptive and endured over time as the person moved through progressive stages of psychosexual development. The characterological outcome of this particular stage was variable, depending on the interaction of constitutional factors and the predominance of the defensive process employed—sublimation or reaction formation (an issue which he treated in "Three Essays," 1905). At the conclusion of the paper, Freud summarized his conceptual model, stating that he had provided:

A formula for the way in which character in its final shape is formed out of the constituent instincts: the permanent character-traits are either unchanged promulgations of the original instincts, or sublimations of those instincts, or reaction formations against them [p. 175].

I will not belabor the extent to which Freud's biological orientation informed this early conception of character, but we note that totally absent is the role of the mother or caretaker, and the imprint of the distinctive behavioral interaction between child and mother over the bodily zone and its taming into the use of the toilet. Absent, too, is a consideration of the process of identification with the parents—all hallmarks of later thinking about character.

The revolutionary model presented in "Character and Anal Erotism" (1908a) became the paradigm for the other stages of the natural sequence of psychosexuality—oral, phallic, and genital—with each stage holding the potential for generating a specific set of related character traits. Adult character emerged as a fabric woven with threads consisting of traits derived from each epoch of development. It was a progression marked by fixations and regressions, as well as advances. Once firmly based at the level of genitality, the person became relatively insulated from a regressive reintegration.

Freud's model of a progression in stages of psychosexual development to the final ideal of the genital character has been criticized (most notably by Reiff, 1959) as being a conflation of moral attitude and scientific observation. The criticism is that inherent in this model is that the genital heterosexual character is the only normal adaptation. Thus, other pathways and endpoints of psychosexual development, such as homosexuality, are failures in development, regardless of whether the particular individual meets the other criteria usually applied to measure subjective satisfaction, external functioning, and fulfilling object relations.

As has often been noted, at this 1908 mark, Freud's view of character was hardly comparable in its depth, detail, and complexity to the theory of symptom formation he spelled out in "Hysterical Phantasies and Their Relation to Bisexuality" (1908a), which is as close to the fulcrum of our thought on symptoms today as it was then.

In the years between the introduction of the concept of anal character and the great leap forward in establishing the tripartite structural theory in 1923 in "The Ego and the Id," Freud enunciated several more integral elements in theory of character. In "Remembering, Repeating, and Working Through" (1914), the concept of the *repetition compulsion* emerged in relation to both the choice of love objects and the form in which love is expressed, which are shaped by the nature of repressed and unfulfilled libidinal instincts. The repetition compulsion was to receive its full due later in "Beyond the Pleasure Principle" (1920). The other factor relevant to character theory was Freud's formulation of *acting out,* which referred to a pattern of substituting actions of particular symbolic meaning for repressed conflicted memories.

Thus, with the introduction of the repetition compulsion and acting out, Freud clarified two attributes of character—its consistency and regularity and its modality of expression.

The third element I wish to underscore is the role of unconscious and conscious *fantasy* in dictating the behavior that becomes each individual's uniquely characteristic adaptive mode. These issues were raised in the paper "A Child Is Being Beaten" (1919), although limited to the dynamic explanation of a specific fantasy. Yet this small model held large import for the subsequent thinking about moral masochism and represented a significant stepping stone from the formula, "Anatomy is destiny" to "Fantasy is destiny."

"The Ego and the Id," which appeared in 1923, ushered in the modern era of psychoanalytic thinking with the introduction of structural theory. Its implications for character formation were profound. In brief, the view of the ego as the heir to abandoned object cathexis, but now assuming the form of structured *identifications* with these lost objects, anticipated the central concern of contemporary object relations theory and heralded our present interest in the complex processes of internalization. Thus, Freud executed a sweeping shift in emphasis—from character as derivative of libidinal drives to character as derivative of identifications with the parents in the form of structured ego representations. The final major step in Freud's thinking was his introduction of superego and ego ideal (1923). With these concepts, the process of identification became more refined with respect to what aspects of the parents were internalized in the ego and what later aspects of them in the superego and ego ideal, and then how distinctive patterns of adaptation grow out of the tension between these two agencies.

Thus, there was a consistent direction to Freud's construction of a theory of character. He began by postulating the force of constitution and libidinal drive. Then he emphasized the function of character in resolving conflict. These concepts were followed by the introduction of the nature of the mechanisms of defense, the role of fantasy, the structures of ego and superego, and the process of identification.

The next analytic thinker to command our attention is Wilhelm Reich. Inasmuch as his contributions to technique were so new and radical with respect to the confrontation of resistance in order to reveal in workable form the negative transference, we might examine some of the theoretical underpinnings to his *Character Analysis* (1933). For Reich, character was the adversary. His very use of the term "armor" underscores its defensive nature. His conception was rooted in Freud's recently elaborated structural theory. He regarded the purpose of character as "primarily and essentially a narcissistic protection mechanism" (1929, p. 125), which developed in response to the dual threats of dangers in the external world and the claims of the id. Psychic energy played a major role in Reich's formulations. He spoke of character as a means of avoiding pain through its capacity to absorb that quantity of instinctual energy which has undergone or escaped repression. From the economic point of view, the main functions of character were "the binding of free-floating anxiety, or . . . the release of dammed-up psychical energy" (1930, p. 147).

Like symptoms, character was the conservator of the infantile past, alive in the present. Through its analytic dissection the central infantile conflicts became accessible and subject to resolution. In this pursuit, the adaptive, creative, and non-conflictual aspects of character are relatively disregarded.

Anna Freud's *The Ego and the Mechanisms of Defense* (1936) may be viewed in part as a reaction to Reich, with whom she taught side-by-side in Vienna until his expulsion from the movement shortly before her book went to press. The contrast between the two was captured by Jenny Waelder-Hall who, reflecting on the climate in Vienna at the time, informally stated at a meeting, "For Wilhelm, resistance [that is, character] was the enemy who was to be smashed in battle; for Anna it was the enemy who was to be treated with respect and won over as an ally."

The contribution of Anna Freud to the theory of character was not simply in the more differentiated description of the defenses and their coordination with specific sources of psychic danger. She also greatly refined the ordering of the mechanisms of defense in a developmental sequence. For example, in addressing *sublimation,* she wrote (1936):

Sublimation, i.e., the displacement of the instinctual aim in conformity with higher social values, presupposes the acceptance or at least the knowledge of such values, that is to say, presupposes the existence of the super-ego. Accordingly . . . repression and sublimation could not be employed until relatively late in the process of development [p. 56].

Refinement of the concept of defense in relation to development was taking place concurrently in the mid-1930s in the work of Melanie Klein. Beginning in 1934 she deviated from Freud's tripartite model with her own structural concept of *positions* (Klein, 1935). In so doing, she took the revolutionary step of changing the emphasis in psychoanalytic from father-dominated oedipal theory to the role of mother in preoedipal development. She also asserted that from the very beginnings of infancy an inner world of fantasy existed that was object relational. For Klein the concept of "position" defined the structure of the ego and superego and the dynamics of their relationship in terms of the *paranoid-schizoid* and *depressive* positions (cf. Klein, 1946; Segal, 1974). That is to say that the form of the resolution of these two fundamental psychic positions in relation to mother characterize all of one's personal relationships thereafter. Position, therefore, connoted much more than a stage in development. It implied a specific configuration of object relations, anxieties, and defenses that persist throughout life and substantially define the character of the individual.

Klein, in contrast with all of the later Object Relations theorists, conceived of the infant as perceiving in the mother and outer world what he has projected onto them, and then internalizing it anew. What is projected and reinternalized is a raging instinctual drama of sex and aggression. Thus, character for Klein is ultimately more a psychobiological entity than an interpersonal or culturally determined one.

Before the post–World War II modifications of Freud's thought had significantly progressed, Otto Fenichel, in 1945, integrated the structural and dynamic aspects of analytic theory into a conceptual model of character. He defined character as "the habitual mode of bringing into harmony the tasks presented by internal demands and by the external world, which is necessarily a function of the constant, organized, and integrating part of the personality which is the ego" (1945, p. 467). In the final outcome of character, Fenichel attributed crucial significance to the strength and nature of the superego while also acknowledging the importance of cultural variations. The form of the resolution of the structural intrapsychic conflict became the basis for a general classification of character. Fenichel's two broad categories were the *sublimation type* and the *reactive type*. In the former, the ego succeeds in replacing an original instinctual impulse with one that is compatible with the ego, one that is organized and inhibited as to aim. In the reactive type, countercathectic forces block the instinctual discharge and the result is character formation in one of two main directions: *avoidance* and *inhibition* on the one hand, or *opposition,* on the other, distinguished by processes of reaction formation. Within this schema, Fenichel was able to develop a relatively elaborate classification of pathological character types, depending on the dominance of instinctual forces, *superego* (as in the masochistic character), or *external objects* (as observed in extremes of social anxieties and pseudointimate sexuality).

The refinements of classical theory and contributions to the understanding of character of Heinz Hartmann (1939), and then Hartmann, Kris, and Loewenstein (1964), do not lend themselves readily to summary. In contrast to the path taken at the same time by Object Relations theorists, who emphasized the personal identificatory processes and content of the ego, Hartmann wrote impersonally of the *ego* as an integrating organization of apparatuses and automatisms that served the function of internal control and external adaptation. Hartmann introduced the concept of *ego apparatuses*— products of endowment and maturation that were part of our basic adaptive equipment and formed the nucleus of adaptive psychological functioning, which operated relatively free of intrapsychic conflict. Perception and memory are examples. The relative strengths and balance of these apparatuses are manifest in the patterns of conflict resolution, which is identifiable as character.[2]

Another concept of importance to character is Hartmann's discussion of the change in function of a behavioral form, leading to its *secondary autonomy*. Thereby, characterologic patterns that originated in one period of development, primarily serving a defensive function, later become relatively independent structures that operate in a highly adaptive way and also become an integrating feature of personality. An example of this principle is the manner in which intellectualization functions defensively during adolescence and then continues as a newly flexible and creative autonomous character pattern after the instinctual forces that resurged during adolescence have become successfully integrated.

A natural laboratory for testing psychoanalytic postulates regarding character was the study of non-Western cultures. Early studies by Roheim (1919) and others confirmed that there did indeed appear to be certain universal patterns, such as incest taboos and oedipal dynamics. Before long, however, psychoanalytic anthropology was pursuing a closed circle. This state of affairs changed dramatically with the investigations of Abram Kardiner in the late 1930s (e.g., 1939). He simply turned the question around from what is the *same* to what is *different* and *why?* Kardiner was faithful to the structural model of the mind, but he also demonstrated, in a way that no one had before, that cultural changes are registered by describable alterations that take place unconsciously in the agencies of the mind (cf. Marcus, 1982). Thus, Kardiner and his associates (1945) introduced the concept of a *basic*

2. Greenacre (1957) has persuasively applied Hartmann's line of thought to the study of individuals with extraordinary creativity.

personality type, which had characterologic specificity and was shared by the members of any given culture. It reflected the cultural needs and institutional patterns of that society and, in turn, served to sustain the culture. Kardiner emphasized the form and content of the superego as the variable psychic agency that served this individual and collective function. Kardiner and Ovesey (1951) applied this approach in their pioneering study of the characterologic consequences of the racial oppression of blacks in America.

After World War II, as Hartmann and his co-workers embarked on systematically refining and developing psychoanalytic theory largely according to the model of a biological science, it seemed almost inevitable that an additional conception of mind would have to emerge—one that devoted long due attention to the consequences of the dynamic interplay between particular flesh-and-blood mothers and children on the one hand, and the force of social and historical factors, on the other, in the shaping of character. Thus, with the publication of *Childhood and Society* in 1950, and for the following two decades, Erik Erikson was destined to fulfill this role complementary to Hartmann, Kris and Loewenstein.

Whereas Harry Stack Sullivan (1953) as far back as 1925 had with considerable perceptiveness addressed individual mother–child interactions through sequential stages of development and spelled out some of the consequences for character formation, his lack of an overall theory of mind limited any broader impact. Sullivan's relatively isolated position stood in marked contrast to the appeal of Erikson, both within psychoanalysis and in the social sciences.

Erikson offered a psychosocial theory of ego development, in which the individual's social development was traced through the unfolding of his *social character* in the course of his encounters with the environment at each phase of his epigenesis (cf. Rapaport, 1958). Erikson explored the social context of each phase with respect to the radius of significant relations, first with mother, then the basic family, followed by a progression of extrafamilial social institutions. Erikson focused on the process by which society influences the manner in which each individual solves phase-specific developmental tasks in a sequence of phases. These parallel stages of libidinal development continue throughout the whole life cycle. This ego epigenesis culminates at the end of adolescence in an individual *identity.* Erikson prefers the term "identity" or "ego identity" to character and defines identity as expressing "both a persistent sameness within oneself and a persistent sharing of some kind of essential character with others" (1959, p. 102). He elaborates:

At one time . . . it will appear to refer to a conscious sense of *individual identity*, at another to an unconscious striving for a *continuity of personal character;* at a third, as a criterion for the silent doings of *ego synthesis;* and, finally, as a maintenance of an inner *solidarity* with a group's ideals and identity [p. 102].

Erikson's graphic schemata of psychosocial crises, with their polarities in resolution, have become firmly integrated as part of our collective view of character. The grand scale of his work is captured in his own words:

From a genetic point of view . . . the process of identity formation emerges as an *evolving configuration*—a configuration which is gradually established by successive ego syntheses and resyntheses throughout childhood; it is a configuration gradually integrating *constitutional givens, idiosyncratic libidinal needs, favored capacities, significant identifications, effective defenses, successful sublimations* and *consistent roles* [p. 116].

In the end, however, it must be said, as Schafer has said (1968, pp. 39–41), that Erikson's use of the term "identity" communicates more the spirit of his overall approach than a clearly definable concept.

The importance of the period of adolescence in character formation was elaborated by Peter Blos (1968), who, along with Erikson, emphasized that the extent to which the developmental challenges of adolescence have been met and successfully negotiated will determine how autonomously character will function thereafter, stabilizing the experience of the self and protecting psychic structure from internal and external stresses.

It is surprising to realize that the current attention to the interaction between infants and young children and their mothers as the crucial matrix for the later development of character and psychic structure is entirely a post-Freudian phenomenon. The emphasis on this as the appropriate field of observation has been the unifying bond among the somewhat varied thinkers grouped together as the Object Relations School. The more prominent names associated with this school are Balint, Fairbairn, Guntrip,[3] Kernberg, and Winnicott. Kernberg, among this group, has endeavored also to maintain a strong link with ego psychology.

Sutherland (1980) has delineated what is common to the group in pointing to their belief that there exists an innate developmental potential, which, if activated by the input of loving, empathic care, will become the psychological matrix for the later capacity to love and enjoy. These theorists view later character formation and patterns of motivation primarily as a function of the

---

3. Guntrip (1971) has written a survey of central ideas of a number of major psychoanalytic theorists, which is valuable for the comparative study of the concept of character.

adequacy or inadequacy of the fit between the needs of the infant and young child and the responses of the mother. Traditional notions of drive are suspended, though not categorically rejected, thereby distinguishing them from the mainstream of Ego Psychology.

While mindful that clear differences exist between each of the major figures, to illustrate the general approach of this group I will briefly summarize an aspect of a model of character formation offered by Balint. In 1968, Balint wrote a book entitled *The Basic Fault*. This ''fault'' refers to a subjective sense of something lacking or missing within oneself and is the result of the impaired harmony in the early dyad. Out of this basic fault the individual will develop in one of two typical directions in subsequent object relations. In one, objects are clung to with a primitive intensity, lacking in mutuality and characterized by a pathological hostile dependency. The other line of development involves a reliance on an inner world of fantasy for sustenance, counterposed against precarious and tenuous relations with ''real'' people. Thus, in this schema, character is largely defined by the nature of the person's later relations with objects and, in the examples given, are directly based on the failure of adequate early mothering. Winnicott's (1960) schema of the *True Self* and the *False Self* has much in common with Balint's concept of the Basic Fault.

The richness of the experiential aspects of the British School has left its imprint on all of us in our thinking about character. At the same time, the relative looseness of their metapsychological formulations has catalyzed the work of such theorists as Kernberg (1976), Meissner (1979), and Schafer (1968, 1976, 1983) in the direction of creating a fuller psychology, particularly with respect to exploring the concept of structure—that is, what is structured, by what process is it structured, and, finally, what are the forms and fates of these structures.

In the 1970s in America, a new approach to character—self psychology —found enthusiastic receptivity. Self psychology is the virtually singular creation of Heinz Kohut (1971, 1977). Its clinical base is almost entirely derived from the treatment of patients that we now classify as narcissistic character disorders. For Kohut, the ''self'' was conceived of as a separate and organized entity in development and mature behavior and as the locus of disturbance in most forms of character pathology. As his work has evolved, self has increasingly become the superordinate concept in the structure of mind. The traditional elements of psychoanalytic metapsychology—drives and the complexities of ego and superego—are subsumed and treated as constituents of the self. Thus, Kohut and Wolf (1978) spoke of the self as an "independent center of initiative." As an amalgam of inherited and environmental factors, the self "aims toward the realization of its own specific program of action—the program that is determined by the specific, intrinsic pattern of its constituent ambitions, goals, skills and talents, and by the tensions that arise between these constituents" (p. 414).

Whereas classical theory has conceptualized all neurotic behavior as the outgrowth of *intrapsychic conflict*—that is, the resolution of the dialectic between drives and defenses—Kohut shifted the emphasis to *deficit*, by which he meant the arrest in the healthy maturation of the self due to failures of the nurturing environment to provide sufficient empathic care. The narcissistic pathology we observe clinically is the consequence of this early failure in *empathy*. In his focus on the crucial importance of the role of the mother's empathic attunement to the infant and young child for the healthy formation of character, Kohut bore close kinship with the Object Relations School.

Before Kohut, narcissism had been viewed as a way station along a single axis of development, beginning with autoerotism and ending in object love. According to this model, primary narcissism yielded to the formation of the ego ideal, which then became the object of the libidinal cathexis originally directed toward the self. In contrast, Kohut proposed a dual axis model in which narcissism itself followed an epigenetic sequence and evolved into mature narcissism, along with a parallel development of object love. This healthy progression along both axes takes place unless arrested by inadequate early care.

A crucial issue in the study of the narcissistic pathologies is the fate of what Kohut termed the "bipolar self." Through the observation of two predominant forms of transference in his clinical work—the "mirror" transference and the "idealizing" transference—Kohut reconstructed the normal development of narcissism. At an intermediate stage, objects who are needed to supply the functions that the immature self cannot autonomously execute are viewed as parts of, or extensions of the self and are referred to as "selfobjects." These selfobjects are experienced in two fundamental ways: (1) as "mirroring," that is, as affirming the fragile self; and (2) as "idealized," that is, as omnipotent and protective. In healthy development of narcissism, the mirroring aspect of selfobjects yields to a characterologic self-assertiveness and realistic ambition; and the idealizing aspect of selfobjects yields to a flexible set of internalized ideals and values. In contrast, in pathology, as a result of the arrest in development, the child's early objects are maintained as internalized selfobjects to provide psychic cohesion.

A final point to be stressed in discussing Kohut's contributions to the subject of character is his abolition of the pejorative connotation of narcissism. In its final transformation, narcissism achieves a secondary autonomy and becomes an intrinsic component in such higher human functions as creativity, wisdom, and empathy.

One more approach to character should be noted—that of Jacques Lacan (1966, 1977). It was Lacan who offered the boldest rethinking of Freud of any of the schools represented. Although he has had virtually no impact on American and British clinicians, Lacan has influenced non-English speaking analysts, particularly in France, where his following is widespread. His psychoanalytic concepts are deeply rooted in the complex ideas of the movement in structural linguistics, particularly in the works of Ferdinand de Saussure, Claude Levi-Strauss, and Roman Jakobson.

A fundamental postulate of Lacan's (1977) is that "the unconscious is structured . . . like a language, that a material operates in it according to certain laws, which are the same laws as those discovered in the study of actual languages . . ." (p. 234).

Thus, in his almost singular reliance on language and speech as the means for understanding human behavior, Lacan moved far from traditional neurobiological concepts of instinctual drive and need, and psychic energy. His orientation, as Leavy (1978) has pointed out, brought Lacan close to Sullivan and Erikson insofar as a person's identity or character is completely enmeshed in the symbolic structures that hold currency in the particular culture as laid down in his or her unconscious. Finally, American psychoanalysts tend to be bewildered by Lacan's taking issue with Ego Psychology in his view that ego is merely a system of defenses that serves as a barrier to the individual's access to his unconscious, the understanding of which is ultimately essential if one is to achieve true selfhood.

CONCLUSIONS

It is apparent as I conclude my summary of close to a century of analytic thought about character that there is not an agreed upon definition, not even agreement about the locus of description. As one path toward some resolution, I will suggest not more definitions, but rather that we look at the paradigm of dreams. We recognize that the dreamer is playing many, perhaps all the roles in a dream. Regardless how large the cast of characters, it is basically a one-person show—the dreamer's. In a similar way, we are none of us simply one character type; we are all, rather, a number of coordinated subcharacters. Or, to put it slightly differently, we have many characters, each the manifest behavioral representation of a unified constellation of our conscious and unconscious life of fantasy. Character is observable, and fantasy is obtainable, particularly in the clinical situation. And I cannot overstress the crucial role in my own thought to which I assign fantasy as the meaningful and workable substratum of character. Now, will this personal repertoire of characters be reasonably healthy or tainted with pathology in a particular individual? The answer to that question depends on outcomes along a number of abstract continua that we find very useful in organizing our thought on the matter. For example, the outcome depends on the predominant balance of *defenses*—say the higher developmental ones such as repression and sublimation, rather than more primitive ones such as projection and splitting. It depends on the nature of such ego capacities as frustration tolerance, thinking, and remembering, rather than impulsively acting. It depends on the stability or instability, the constancy or inconstancy of self and inner object representations. Thus our personal repertoire of characters either will be a harmonious ensemble of players or will be in conflict with one another, making contradictory claims, and suffering in palpable ways.

If we shift our metaphor to the theatre, each character is observable to the audience, known and defined by a coherent set of actions. Thus, Hamlet is known to us as a definable character who is reproducible by actors over centuries, because of the way he acts toward the king, his mother, Ophelia, his deceased father, and others; and also by the way he talks *of himself* in soliloquies, and by the emotion he displays when alone. Hamlet makes sense, and we experience something of ourselves in him and through him. This, then, is the character of Hamlet. His character is not his tripartite psychic structure, his balance of drives and defenses, his ego appartuses, nor the stage of psychosexual development he has achieved. These latter concepts are metapsychological narratives that explain the character or, more accurately, the many different dimensions of character that comprise Hamlet. Our ability to make sense of his character by employing these explanatory devices is what distinguishes us as psychoanalysts from others in the audience, who employ their respective explanatory devices. What is so exciting about psychoanalysis is that, as rich as our theoretical concepts are for understanding, they are, as we have seen, ever-changing, ever-growing to enable us to better grasps what has been indomitable in man since our prehistory—character.

REFERENCES

Balint, M. (1968). *The Basic Fault*. London: Tavistock.
Baudry, F. (1983), The evolution of the concept of character in Freud's writings. *J. Amer. Psychoanal. Assn., 31*:3–32.
Blos, P. (1968), Character formation in adolescence. *The Psychoanalytic Study of the Child*, 23:245–63. New Haven: Yale University Press.
Erikson, E. H. (1950). *Childhood and Society*. New York: W. W. Norton.
———. (1959), Identity and the life cycle. *Psychological Issues*, Monogr. 1. New York: International Universities Press.
Fenichel, O. (1945), *The Psychoanalytic Theory of Neurosis*. New York: W. W. Norton.
Freud, A. (1936), *The Ego and the Mechanisms of Defense*. New York: International Universities Press, 1946.
Freud, S. (1905), Three essays on the theory of sexuality. *Standard Edition*, 7:123–243. London: Hogarth Press, 1953.
———. (1908a), Hysterical phantasies and their relation to bisexuality. *Standard Edition*, 9:155–66. London: Hogarth Press, 1959.
———. (1908b), Character and anal erotism. *Standard Edition*, 9:167–76. London: Hogarth Press, 1959.
———. (1914), Remembering, repeating and working through. *Standard Edition*, 12:145–56. London: Hogarth Press, 1958.
———. (1916), Some character-types met with in psychoanalytic work. *Standard Edition*, 14:309–36. London: Hogarth Press.
———. (1919), A child is being beaten. *Standard Edition*, 17:175–204. London: Hogarth Press, 1955.
———. (1920), Beyond the pleasure principle. *Standard Edition*, 18:1–64. London: Hogarth Press, 1961.
———. (1923), The ego and the id. *Standard Edition*, 19:1–59. London: Hogarth Press, 1959.
———. (1931), Libidinal types. *Standard Edition*, 21:215–20. London: Hogarth Press, 1961.
Greenacre, P. (1957), The childhood of the artist. *The Psychoanalytic Study of the Child*, 12:47–72. New York: International Universities Press.
Guntrip, H. (1971), *Psychoanalytic Theory, Therapy, and the Self*. New York: Basic Books.
Hartmann, H. (1939), *Ego Psychology and The Problem of Adaptation*. New York: International Universities Press, 1958.
———, Kris, E., & Loewenstein, R. (1964), Papers on psychoanalytic psychology. *Psychological Issues*, Monogr. 4. New York: International Universities Press.
Jones, E. (1955), *The Life and Works of Sigmund Freud*, Vol. 2. New York: Basic Books.
Kardiner, A. (1939), *The Individual and His Society*. New York: Columbia University Press.
———, Linton, R., du Bois, C., & West, J. (1945), *The Psychological Frontiers of Society*. New York: Columbia University Press.
——— & Ovesey, L. (1951), *The Mark of Oppression*. New York: World.
Kernberg, O. (1976), *Object Relations Theory and Clinical Psychoanalysis*. New York: Aronson.

Klein, M. (1935). A contribution to the psychogenesis of manic-depressive states. *Internat J. Psycho-Anal.*, 16:145–74.

———. (1946), Notes on some schizoid mechanisms. In: *Developments in Psycho-Analysis.* ed. J. Riviere. London: Hogarth Press, 1952.

Kohut, H. (1971), *The Analysis of The Self.* New York: International Universities Press.

———. (1977), *The Restoration of The Self.* New York: International Universities Press.

——— & Wolf, E. S. (1978), The disorders of the self and their treatment: An outline. *Internat. J. Psycho-Anal.*, 59:413–26.

Lacan, J. (1966), *Écrits.* Paris: Seuil.

———. (1977), *Écrits: A Selection.* trans. A. Sheridan. New York: W. W. Norton.

Leavy, S. (1978), The significance of Jacques Lacan. In: *Psychoanalysis and Language,* Vol. 3 of *Psychiatry and the Humanities,* ed. J. H. Smith. New Haven: Yale University Press.

Marcus, S. (1982), Psychoanalytic theory and culture. *Partisan Rev.*, 49:224–37.

Meissner, W. W. (1979), Internalization in the psychoanalytic process, *Psychological Issues,* Monogr. 50. New York: International Universities Press.

Moore, B. & Fine, B. (1968), *A Glossary of Psychoanalytic Terms and Concepts.* New York: American Psychoanaly. Assn.

Rapaport, D. (1958). A historical survey of psychoanalytic ego psychology. *Bull. Phila. Assn. Psychoanal.*, 8:105–20.

Reich, W. (1929), The genital character and the neurotic character. In: *The Psychoanalytic Reader,* ed. R. Fliess. New York: International Universities Press, 1948.

———. (1930), Character formation and the phobias of childhood. In: *The Psychoanalytic Reader,* ed. R. Fliess. New York: International Universities Press, 1948.

———. (1933), *Character Analysis.* New York: Noonday Press, 1949.

Reiff, P. (1959), *The Mind of the Moralist.* New York: Viking.

Roheim, G. (1919). *Spiegelzauber.* Leipzig: Internationaler Psychoanalytischer.

Schafer, R. (1968), *Aspects of Internalization.* New York: International Universities Press.

———. (1976), *A New Language For Psychoanalysis.* New Haven: Yale University Press.

———. (1983). *The Analytic Attitude.* New York: Basic Books.

Segal, H. (1974). *Introduction to The Work of Melanie Klein.* New York: Basic Books.

Sullivan, H. S. (1953). *The Interpersonal Theory of Psychiatry.* New York: W. W. Norton.

Sutherland, J. D. (1980). The British object relations theorists: Balint, Winnicott, Fairbairn, Guntrip. *J. Amer. Psychoanal. Assn.*, 28:829–60.

Winnicott, D. W. (1960), *The Maturational Processes and the Facilitating Environment.* New York: International Universities Press, 1965.

PART II

THE FORMATION OF CHARACTER AND OF CHARACTER NEUROSIS

3. On the Problem of Character Neurosis

Maxwell Gitelson

We cannot consider character neurosis without first establishing a basis for this in a concept of character.

The original psychoanalytic view of character took form in the context of the theory of neuroses. According to this, a psychoneurosis, in its overt symptomatic manifestations, is the outcome of a conflict arising and unsolved in childhood. The conflict, to begin with, is transiently external. It arises from the existence of biological drives, the so-called instincts, whose aim is gratification and self-assertion. In their original erotic and aggressive-destructive forms, these clash with standards of the parental environment in which the child is reared and on which it is dependent. Under the influence of the regulating and controlling influences of that environment, the pure form of the drive is first suppressed and then repressed. While the original repression thus occurs under external pressure, it is subsequently maintained by self-regulating forces which derive from this. The drives in their original form thus become unconscious.

However, repression is only more or less successful. In those aspects in which it is complete, we may for practical purposes assume that conflict, though not eliminated, has been stilled. But for the most part the drives survive; consequently, conflict with the regulating functions of the mind remains potential. Ordinarily this is manifested in clinically insignificant manners, habits, and sensory, affective and motor characteristics. Dreams normally provide a buffering and regulating mechanism for this potential. And, as is well known, derivatives of drives, variously adjusted and elaborated, become socially suitable and ego syntonic, and enter into the formation of the so-called "normal" personality. Thus instinctual drainage through diversion, neutralization, and sublimation, reduces the strength of surviving conflictual tension. These factors are supportive of repression.

This does not mean that the drives become innocuous. To the extent to which their management has required the elaboration of more purely defensive psychic structuring and maneuver, the ego remains vulnerable to their

Reprinted from the *Hillside Journal of Clinical Psychiatry* 12 (1963): 3–17 by permission.

irruption and penetration. The symptomatic neurosis is external evidence that the ego has failed defensively. The symptom itself represents an emergency defense which is effective because, in its form, it both conceals the nature of the drive which has been released from repression and gives it, autoplastically, partial gratification. In the first aspect it prevents awareness of the primary conflict; and, as gratification, it reduces the tension of the unconscious impulse and thus protects the ego against more general distortion, as this is seen in the asymptomatic character neurosis or against rupture, as in the case of the psychotic breakdown (13).

We may now attempt a definition of character. I suggest the following: character is the final common pathway for the patterned manifestation of the drives and their specific defenses, as these are imbricated, and interplay with their refined, elaborated, and sublimated derivatives. The identifications which have occurred with significant persons provide a formative matrix for this pattern. The pattern is stable and predictable in social and temporal dimensions. Adaptively, it operates according to the principle of multiple functions (26): at once to satisfy the drives, to spare the ego anxiety and guilt, to preserve harmony with the ego ideal, to provide narcissistic gratification and self-esteem, and, over-all, to ensure reality orientation to the given environment. Thus character is an adaptive synthesis of forces stemming from the biological givens, the quality of the infantile environment, the psychic structure, the character of the identifications, and the mores of the social group in which later maturation and development occurs. It is an action and reaction pattern which has crystallized out of this flux of factors (19). And at the heart of the hypothetically "normal" situation is the fact that the phallic position has been reached psychosexually, and the oedipus complex has been resolved (6).

Psychoneurosis may be looked upon as evidence of a partial disruption of this synthesis due to a failure of defense. The result is a disturbance in the economy of the character structure due to a revival of conflict. The balance is restored through the formation of a symptom. The symptom is a compromise formation between an id impulse which has threatened to irrupt into consciousness or action, and a spastic and unconsciously determined reaction of the ego against this. The result is ego alien and produces secondary reactions of lowered self-esteem and suffering. Nevertheless the symptom serves to bind the irrupting impulse while giving it substitutive gratification, and thus it closes the breach in the defensive system. The conflict involved in such a situation pertains to an aspect of the oedipus complex which has remained unsolved and has been repressed. Subsequent regression to an earlier form of instinct gratification and an internal or external revival of this produces emergency defense in the form of the symptom.

In the classical neurotic character, as it was first described by Alexander (1), the problem also centers on the oedipus complex. Repression and regression also occur though neither of these seem to be as effective as in the psychoneurotic. And the autoplastic modification of the ego involved in symptom formation is not conspicuous. Instead there is a plunge into external reality which is variously exploited to fit the unconscious wish and need. Why this is so—why symptoms appear in one instance and not in the other —we do not really know. It is possible that it is due to a variation in the phase of ego development at which specific psychosexual vicissitudes occurred. It may be that the matter is determined by the constitutional capacity of the ego to oppose the drives or, as Alexander suggested, that it is the unusual strength of the drives themselves which results in *relative* weakness in the ego. On the basis of clinical evidence in some cases it seems possible that specific circumstances surrounding the first appearance of an impulse or wish may produce a fixation to the conflict thus engendered, in its external form, prior to repression and regression. This could be a determining factor in setting the person concerned on a career of repeated and unsuccessful efforts to find a solution in external reality (according to the Zeigarnik principle) (3). However the case may be, it is the quality of compelled and patterned acting out which is the most striking aspect of the neurotic character. It is this which has given vivid cogency to its other designation, "the neurosis of fate" (2).

On the assumption that there will be more detailed attention given to this in the clinical presentations I refer only in passing to Hamlet (21), and to the well-known Don Juan characters (11) as examples. As a matter of fact, in many of these clinical situations we scarcely see the effects of repression and regression. More prominent are the rather easily identified displacements to mother, father and sibling surrogates and the not too deeply concealed though often rather grotesque dramatizations of the oedipus complex. Added to this is the prevalence of actual if disguised instinctual gratification, instead of the substitutive compromise of a symptom. The relationship of such phenomena to the condensation of gratification and defense as we see this in psychoneurotic symptoms is demonstrated in intimate and inevitable sequences of crime and invited punishment, and, in other cases, puzzling combinations of asceticism, self-sacrifice, debauchery, and failure of gratification.

But such instances are for the books. More common, more subtle, and more fateful for the world as well as for the persons concerned are those character patterns which only careful study reveals to be indeed neurotic. The symptomatology is not only apparently ego syntonic but socially useful and even laudable, narcissistically gratifying and even productive of prestige and tangible reward in the goods of this life. Of these "character neuroses" I shall speak now.

In life there are no pure types. In general usage the diagnoses "neurotic character" and "character neurosis" appear interchangeably. But sharp boundaries have heuristic convenience, and I have reversed the order of words in the diagnostic rubric to emphasize an important difference from the previous type. The so-called "character neurosis" (8), in contrast to the so-called "neurotic character" presents, outstandingly, the picture and structure of defense. If we look at this group in terms of its most commonly designated subclasses: obsessional or compulsive character, hysterical character, or schizoid character, we are impressed by the fact that, as in the case of the psychoneuroses, the symptomatology is autoplastic. But it is the personality itself which is shaped by the neurosis into a defensive pattern of socially adapted adjustment. I do not mean by this that these people do not live in the world. But their impact on it and their penetration of it stems, not primarily from libido or aggression, but from defense against these.

The phenomenology of the "character neurosis" ranges from a preponderance of self-centeredness, comparable to an encapsulated hysterical or compulsive symptom, to an imbrication with other persons which is almost as deep, though not so ostentatious, as in the case of the "neurotic characters." However, where the latter are struggling with an unsolved problem, in which the conflict has been externalized, and, it would appear, that for them other people have become libidinal and aggressive transference objects, the "character neurosis" remains largely internalized. What *is* externalized and transferred is the particular pattern of defense which has proven successful during earlier development and in later social accommodation. These are the people whom Wilhelm Reich (24) so graphically described as presenting a "character armor" in analysis and who present a facade in life. Winnicott (27) has referred to the latter as a "false self" because these persons experience themselves in the terms of their defense. Fenichel (8) suggested that the formation of the typical "neurosis of character" and its several traits corresponds to a single massive act of repression which avoids the necessity for the "ad hoc" management of subsequent specific anxiety situations. In any case characterological traits become fixed anchorages for defense against instinct irruption. As such, in various combinations, they are "worked into the ego." This is what produces the relative constancy of the defensive attitude and establishes it as the "sign" of the personality, no matter how diverse may be the stimuli from the unconscious or from reality.

The consequence of this is that the "symptom," whether it be the characterological style as a whole, or its several explicit traits, is ego syntonic. As in the case of the psychoneuroses, the primary gain is preserved in various forms of concealed gratification. In contrast to the psychoneurotic symptom, however, secondary gain is greatly enhanced. This accrues from the approval of the world, whether it be by way of recognition of intellectual qualities, commendation for hard, faithful and sometimes productive labor, the label of "good fellow," or applause for self-assertive achievement. In this way primitive oral, anal, and urethral impulses are made to pay off.

Much of this passes as allegedly "normal" (16) and if taken at face value often gives the impression of really satisfying instincts, even though transformed by passage through the ego. This is particularly the case when counterphobic activity (7) is a part of the defensive structure, as it frequently is. But such activity does not in fact gratify the drives for which it stands. These are themselves inhibited. The expression of one instinct may substitute for the repression of another. In a character neurosis we may see how the ego, seeming to accept genital sexuality explicitly, and presenting the impression of normality in this respect, is actually fobbing off on an unsuspecting public oral or anal impulses which are themselves repressed. On the other hand, oral and anal traits may substitute for sexual impulses. Furthermore, while character traits are deeply rooted in the instincts their formal qualities and configurations are determined to a large extent by the nature of the culture in which they develop and operate. Thus "normal" sexuality, even if libertine, is acceptable to the "modern" ego. The sad fact is, however, that it does not always serve the mature genital impulse but is often a front for omnipotent fantasies, sadistic impulses, and oral greed. And, saddest of all, it may be a reaction formation against affective emptiness and profound isolation.

Finally, we must consider that the distortions and disguises through which the various libidinal and aggressive impulses express themselves in the character defense are supported by the fact of the frequency with which they occur in a given group. The interpersonal usefulness of prevalent defenses not only serves to conceal them from the particular person concerned but from the eyes of the world at large. One might say that the mores of various social segments constitute an unconscious conspiracy of silence. There is a sort of tacit agreement not to acknowledge the forms in which the primitive nature of man continues to express itself.

However, character does not consist exclusively of fixation to an infantile trauma and its repeated re-enactment, as in the case of the first group which I have discussed, nor of transformed instinctual drives, as in the case of the second group. As I have already indicated in general terms, character, as the resultant of a parallelogram of forces, depends also on the relationship and interaction of id, ego, and superego (20). And each of these contributes its particular hallmark.

The direct contribution of the ego derives from its several attributes. The qualities of intelligence, talent, perceptual capacities, body build, motor patterns, reactive rhythms—these, together with the organizing, adaptive, and defensive functions, provide modes and channels of expression for instincts and affects. Directly and indirectly they outline both the external image of the person, and his self-image and self-experience. Thus, for example, oral incorporative, anal sadistic, and phallic aggressive impulses are determined in their expression by variations in the balance among these ego factors. It is not merely instinctual fixation points or psychosexual regression which determine the symptomatology of character. For this reason we see hysterical characters with an obsessional, or if you please, an intellectual façade; or obsessional characters with hysterical or paranoid "features," or investment in truly creative work in the presence of idiosyncratic behavior. Furthermore, the ego's attributes are aspects of reality which confront the ego within its own context and reflexly call on it for adaptation or defense. From this point of view Adlerian theory has some cogency to the facts of life. Organ inferiority does have its real effect in modifying the quality of the ego and may determine a characterological response. But even so it must be remembered that it is not simply a matter of organ inferiority and reactions to it. Inferiority feelings also arise from the castration complex, loss of love, humiliation, and the sense of guilt. Besides which the instincts also exploit the ego's assets and liabilities, while the ego borrows the power of the instincts to implement its purposes. In any case the given attributes of the ego are of supreme importance in determining the shape of the person to the world at large and in his own eyes.

The attributes of the ego are not exclusively inborn, however. The history of the nature of the relationship of the person to the formative people in his environment is of equal or greater significance in determining the ego's role as mediator between the instincts and the external world. It follows that the characters of the significant formative persons are of the essence in the effect they exert. Here we encounter and must consider the phenomenon of identification.

The crucial environmental objects, of course, are the parents, and to begin with, the mother. The relationship with her establishes the most deeply rooted patterns for the nature of the child's subsequent relationships with other people. It may be said that the climate of that first relationship establishes the fundamental and typical "mood" of the person. The intimacy of the symbiosis of mother and child is what makes it so extremely difficult to be certain as to what is constitutionally given and what is acquired through introjection and elaborated in an unconscious identity with the mother's "set." Of course, this is further complicated by subsequent identifications with father and siblings and later on with other significant persons. The latter, including the parents as they are and appear in later years, impose various modifications, for better or for worse, on the original identifications. Still, these are essentially indestructible and retain their effectiveness.

The earliest identifications enter into the formation of what have been referred to as "ego nuclei" (18). Much depends on the extent to which these are in the end miscible, or contrariwise, incompatible and in conflict. In the neuroses of character, that is one of the factors that enter into setting up the peculiar paradoxes which they so often present—"splits" that reach their extreme in the multiple personality. But a more general complication in the normal establishment of identifications is the factor of bisexuality. The psychological determinants of this are more readily discerned clinically than are the determining factors which today we know are based on hormonal distributions. In any case, predisposing feminine tendencies in the male interfere with the normal tendency for the boy to identify finally with the father and other men. The reverse situation obtains in the female. The consequence, depending on still other factors, may be various degrees of psychosexual inversion, or reactive, overcompensatory, and pathologically deformed assertions of masculinity or femininity.

Identification is normally the basis for the withdrawal of primitive erotic and aggressive impulses from the objects toward which they are originally directed. This so-called "inhibition of aim" results in the "taming" of the relationship with the persons concerned while the libidinal and aggressive energy which is thus made available enters into the promotion of psychic development. This released energy charges the ego's talents in the formation of sublimations and shares in the shaping of the ego-syntonic, adaptive, and defensive patterns. Failures in this aspect of the identification process account for the important role played by ambivalence in the personal relations of neurotic characters. Because of such failure they exhibit disturbances in the capacity for love and altruism, oscillations of mood, unsteadiness in thinking and working capacity, and, in grosser forms, overt primitive sensuality and destructiveness.

Most important of all is the part played by identification in the formation of the superego. The primary influence of the parents is thus internalized and made permanent. Aggressive and libidinal energy which is withdrawn from its original focus on the parents becomes available to the superego itself, providing it with powers which are exerted against the forces of the id and its derivatives in the ego. The superego originates in part from the conditionings which occur in the preverbal and pregenital relationship to the mother; it is transiently stabilized in the context of the oedipus complex, in middle childhood; it appears in its ultimate form after puberty, and in this form it is crucial to the definitive molding of character. However, its strength is relative not only to the quality of identifications which have entered into its formation but also to the strength of the id.

The normal superego derives from stable relationships in which there is minimal ambivalence. Love has been preponderant over hate. The instincts have been of ordinary intensity, and the ego has had ordinary capacity for perception, organization, and adaptation to reality. The defective superego may be excessively severe or it may be weak. The former may reflect the harshness of the formative figures, or it may be a spastic response to threat from excessively strong primitive destructive impulses, inborn or responsive to the environment. A weak superego may reflect identification with weak or corrupt parental figures; or it may be only relatively so in the presence of unusually strong drives. The latter could be a consequence of constitutional factors or the outcome of cultivation through spoiling indulgence, or even seduction. Thus the id, in its over-all quality, as well as in terms of its specific elements, contributes explicitly to the characterological picture.

A specific example may be found in Freud's description of the "erotic" character type (14). In these persons, libidinal development has advanced to the genital level; they have a strong orientation toward objects; and the wish for gratification is explicitly centered on love, especially in its anaclitic form. The life goal is pleasure, and this drive is strong enough to overcome or circumvent moral values, and even good sense, so that they are unreliable and irresponsible. In the aggressive form this type of impulse-ridden character has been referred to classically as "psychopathic personality," assumed to be without a sense of guilt. However, we are no longer so sure of this assumption. The fact is that the prime effect of the operation of the superego, the sense of guilt, is still capable of exerting its influence. The ego, exploiting for this purpose the very impulses and drives which are being permitted gratification, is found to be inviting punishment and in other ways working toward securing external controls in lieu of the superego's failure to exercise them internally. The psychopathic recidivists who fill our prisons are evidence of this. More subtle types are ubiquitous. And in the erotic type we see also that despite the preponderant role played by the id, the ego and the superego are insignificant only by comparison. The evidence for this is found in the fact that even though the leading symptomatology takes the form of "acting out," without conscious guilt, nonetheless the erotic types are prone to conversion reactions, phobias, and anxiety.

In addition to (1) the erotic type with which I have illustrated the more overt manifestations of the id in character neuroses, Freud (14) also described two types in which the other psychic structures are dominant. (2) In the *compulsive* type, the fixations and regressions are found at the anal sadistic level of psychosexual development. Persons with this character structure have intense sensitiveness to guilt. Their drives are strongly inhibited even in their "normal" context; they tend to be arid though sometimes kindly in their emotional qualities, lacking in flexibility in their adaptive and adjustive capacities, faithful and self-sacrificing but diffident and ambivalent in their personal relations. They are often dedicated in their social commitments and also productive but at great cost in tension and effort. Their essential conservatism renders them vulnerable to new life situations which expose them to unaccustomed stimulation. They typically react to such stress with depression or psychosomatic disturbances. The "anal character" is a subtype, whose admixture produces the classical phenomena of reaction formations against sadistic and soiling impulses. The dynamic situation is, in general, one of domination by the superego and of rigidity in the adaptive and organizing functions of the ego. (3) The *narcissistic* types are, in common parlance, the egoists. They are oriented towards self-love, self-gratification, and self-interest. Insensitive to others they are highly sensitive to anything suggestive of slight or indifference to themselves. They do not invest themselves deeply in their relations with others excepting as it may serve their own ends. They are not open to influence or persuasion. Oral and phallic characteristics are intermixed and, if prevalent, create subtypes. If the oral history has been gratifying, the resulting optimism and cheerfulness may provide an amelioration of the cold picture of the major type. If the phallic drive is strong, aggressive competitiveness becomes a characteristic. Because in these people there is commonly an underlying early injury to self-esteem, they tend to respond to traumatic frustration with depression and paranoid reactions.

But, nearly always, what we see are mixtures of such so-called characterological "types." The typical ones described by Freud are the erotic-compulsive, the erotic-narcissistic, and the narcissistic-compulsive. Freud (12) described three specifically psychological forms of character: "the exceptions," "those wrecked by success," and "criminals from a sense of guilt." And various other types have been emphasized by subsequent workers (8), for example: the masochistic, the passive-feminine, the urethral characters. However, on the basis of what I have already said it will be clear enough that what we can expect to find in all these forms is a clinical demonstration of the fact that pathological character, like "normal" character, is a synthesis in function and a mosaic in form; a unification and systematization of patterns and traits which are to be traced to instinctual and adaptive elements in the id, ego, and superego, each in varying degrees of fusion and defusion.

No clinical forms demonstrate this more graphically than the so-called borderline cases (17). These patients seem to be peculiar to our times. It is only in the last twenty-five or thirty years that they have been studied analytically. The appellations applied to them are as various as the clinical pictures which they present—"psychotic personality," "prepsychotic," "pseudo-neurotic schizophrenia," "ego deficit," "ego distortion," and the most general designation of all, "character disorder." Phenomenologically, they include among others, eccentrics, "as if" personalities, affectively inhibited people, imposters, fantastic liars, and persons with various manifestations of impaired reality perception and defective judgment. Like the clinical conditions which I have discussed previously, they are nonsymptomatic in the strictly autoplastic sense of the psychoneuroses but there is this difference: the neurotic characters, and the character neuroses, as I have already stated, stem from the vicissitudes encountered in the oedipus complex; in the present group the central conflict germinated in the preoedipal relationship to the mothering person or persons.

The oedipus complex is characterized above all by the triangular situation involving the love of one parent and hostile rivalry with the other. In the pregenital situation the father is not yet a rival but simply another obscure figure of the environment who may be pleasing or displeasing; the mother is the central figure; other persons in the environment are not sexually differentiated and are only additional objects for passive and active polymorphous perverse aims. Freud (15) emphasized the great intensity of the preoedipal libidinal strivings, "greater than anything that comes later," and gave them neurosogenic status in their own right. Fenichel (5), who was less liberal than Freud himself in this regard, nevertheless modified his position to say: "Every single analysis provides fresh evidence of [the fact of the centrality of the oedipus complex] *except* those cases of extreme malformation of character which resemble a life-long psychosis and in which the subject's object relations were destroyed, root and branch, at an early period."

Fenichel goes overboard a bit. "Root and branch" is a little too much. However, it does emphasize the leading importance of the occurrence of severely disturbed relations with primary objects in the pathogenesis of these disorders. This hinges on parental indifference to some extent; but chiefly, it is the unpredictability, the unsteadiness of the milieu, beginning with the mother and recurrent with auxiliary figures and in later life. From this follows serious impairment in that part of ego development which depends on the identification process, failure to integrate the phallic position with the oedipus complex, defective formation of the superego and of the reality principle, and incompleteness of repression and reaction formation. These persons remain open to conscious awareness of primitive fantasies and impulses which they sometimes act upon. Their attitudes are frankly dependent, or this may be denied by omnipotence. Their relationships are preponderantly based on temporary identifications with those who happen to be around them; they live in the presence of others, not with them; they are affectively shallow. On the basis of primary identificatory learning—I refer here to mimicry— some of them conduct themselves with seeming adequacy and, if they are intelligent, and retain some ego autonomy, they may present a facade of seemingly normal ego operations.

With these persons the vicissitudes of development have not turned on the transient defensive anxieties attendant on the usual developmental and adaptive crises. The *actual frustration and precocious stimulation* which we discover them to have lived through is often enormous. These have literally threatened to overwhelm them. But their developmental and maturational arrest is not merely due to weakness. It may be the manifestation of an inherent adaptive strength sufficient to have avoided actual destruction by psychosis or death. Each case represents an idiosyncratic way of life which has been compelled by gravely disordered early environmental conditions. Instinctual and ego development have been grossly out of phase. The ego is immature, that is, it has not moved to its potential distance from the drives and it has not been sufficiently differentiated from them. But, at its level of development, it is intact. We might perhaps think of it as manifesting a capacity for defense in depth. It has survival value by way of facultative accommodation to the id and to external reality (17).

We recognize in this broad clinical sketch that these persons have on one hand the psychological characteristics of the infant, and on the other hand, qualities of the schizophrenic. From the standpoint of psychoanalytic ego psychology it is apparent why they have been referred to in terms of ego defect or weakness. But this is a debatable view. What we see is a broad front of developmental incompleteness resulting from a lack of stable object relations and compatible identifications—central factors in the building of human personality and character.

The borderline case may, strictly speaking, seem irrelevant to our topic. However, you will have noted that throughout my discussion I have been moving back and forth from conceptions of character based on ideas about its "normal" structure and functions, to considerations referring to its pathology. Whichever way we turn we see overlapping. This is an inevitable consequence of the nature of our material. As soon as we look beneath the phenomenological surface we are confronted by the fact, as I have said before, that there are no pure types. Ideally psychosexual development goes on in phase with the maturing powers of the ego to deal with vicissitudes of drives, and in the presence of environmental influences which are attuned to lend the support appropriate to progressively changing cross-sections of this process. But, in fact, this is only more or less the case. It is a question of economics. Given a range of operating formative factors, varying internal and external conditions produce various quantitative and configurational distributions of the derivatives of these factors. As Nunberg (23) has said, "the difference between symptom neurosis and character neurosis (or neurotic character) is not as significant as it seems at first glance." And as for the relevance of the borderline case, we may recall Freud's observation (13) that "every normal person is only approximately normal; his ego resembles that of the psychotic in one point or another, in a greater or lesser degree; and its distance from one end of the scale and proximity to the other may provisionally serve as a measure of [the] 'modification[s] of the ego'." Thus, it may be necessary for us to define the "hypothetical normal ego" and with it the "normal character" largely in negative terms, that is, distinguished by the absence of specialized defenses, attitudes or properties. But that would be pretty dull.

My own preference is to look upon character development, normal or pathological, as being directed, in the over-all, toward the establishment of some kind of systemic balance. The principle involved does not differ from that which operates in organismic structure and function as it has been observed at the biological level. Operationally, or from the standpoint of one or another value system, the upshot may be looked upon as "good" or "bad." The neurotic character may impress us as a hero, a fool, or a victim. The person with the character neurosis may be looked upon as a suitable member for our club, or an inconvenient or annoying presence. The person with the character disorder may be just "strange," or a sometimes charming or creative individualist. And, of course, there are the people with psychoneurotic symptoms. All of them have qualities of the others. And all of us who look upon ourselves as "normal" are only more or less so. Taste and circumstances alter cases.

This brings me to my final statement in this theoretical consideration of the problem of the "neuroses" and "disorders" of character: why are they more prevalent today than the psychoneuroses; why do most of our nonpsychotic patients come to us with complaints of interpersonal unhappiness, feelings of inadequacy and incompleteness, vague tension and anxiety, psychosomatic symptoms, and emptiness in the presence of apparent surfeit? These questions present us with an enormous problem. It would be presumptuous to say more than that we are aware of its existence. I can make only a few generalizations. While I was thinking over what these could be, with complete fortuitousness, I ran into an article by Bruce Mazlish (22), of M.I.T., entitled "Our 'Heraclitean' Period." I think some citations from this article may advance our present purpose.

The title has reference to the philosophical views of Heraclitus, that everything is in a flux and nothing remains fixed except the rational principle in the universe—the logos. Mazlish goes on to say: ". . . ours is . . . a period in which forms and fixity have all but disappeared. We live in a kaleidoscopic world in which forms cannot be smashed because they hardly exist . . . the true iconoclasts have preceded us. Form-smashing in the Western World did occur . . . not in our time, but largely before World War I . . . from about 1830 on.'' Marx, Darwin, Nietzsche, Freud, and others like them have produced the ''Heraclitean'' aspect of our time in the moral field. ''The result has been a widespread denial of faiths, abandonment of traditions, and repudiation of values . . . we no longer believe in forms at all . . . nor are there 'fixed' views, whether of the self or of society. . . . Modern man is a little like the player in Gilbert and Sullivan, engaged in a game, 'On cloth untrue, with a twisted cue, and elliptical billiard balls.' ''

Thus, in the absence of clear goals, we cannot say of ourselves that we are ''on the march.'' But, with uncertain direction and shifting values we *are* ''on the move.'' To use Matthew Arnold's lines, we have been

> Wandering between two worlds, one dead
> The other powerless to be born.

I think that all this is reflected in the psychological climate of the families from which we and our patients come. The sexual status of the parents has become unclear; their hierarchal differentiation and function uncertain. The chief consequence is that repression is no longer the primary and central mechanism of defense and adaptation. For this is dependent for its effective operation on definite structure in the personalities of the formative people, and an established hierarchy of relationships among them in the operations of the family. In the absence of a model towards which to aspire, object relations become relative and conditional; identifications are impaired and conflictful. While the instincts and the mechanisms of defense retain their intrinsic qualities, whatever I have said about them in the context of the classical conceptions of character and neuroses becomes, operationally, a matter of ''more or less,'' contingent on the new factors which now surround them. The secondary ''adjustment'' value of such defenses as identification with the aggressor, altruistic surrender, ego restriction, denial, isolation, and reaction formation makes them more important than outright repression. In effect, what has become important is not repression of the content of the unconscious but the successful deployment of defenses, in the guise of adaptation, but enlisted in the service of social accommodation. Personality thus, to a large extent, has returned to its original Latin meaning in the word ''persona,'' a ''mask.'' This is of the essence of the ''crisis of identity'' to which Erikson (4) has devoted his attention. It is also near the heart of the problem of the neurosis of character, in our time.

REFERENCES

(1) Alexander, F.: The Neurotic Character. *Int. J. Psychoanal.*, 11:292–311, 1930.
(2) Deutsch, H.: Hysterical Fate Neurosis. In: *Psychoanalysis of Neuroses*. London: Hogarth Press, 1932.
(3) English, H. B. & English, A. C.: *Psychological and Psychoanalytical Terms*. New York: Longmans, Green, 1958.
(4) Erikson, E. H.: *Childhood and Society*. New York: Norton, 1950.
(5) Fenichel, O.: The Pregenital Antecedents of the Oedipus Complex. *Int. J. Psychoanal.*, 12:141–166, 1931.
(6) Fenichel, O.: Specific Forms of the Oedipus Complex. *Int. J. Psychoanal.*, 12:412–430, 1931.
(7) Fenichel, O.: The Counterphobic Attitude. *Int. J. Psychoanal.*, 20:263–274, 1939.
(8) Fenichel, O.: *The Psychoanalytic Theory of Neuroses*. New York: Norton, 1945.
(9) Flugel, J. C.: *Man, Morals and Society*. New York: Int. Univ. Press, 1945.
(10) Freud, A.: *The Ego and the Mechanisms of Defense* (1936). New York: Int. Univ. Press, 1946.
(11) Freud, S.: Contributions to the Psychology of Love: A Special Type of Choice of Object (1910). *Collected Papers*, 4:184–191. London: Hogarth Press, 1934.
(12) Freud, S.: Some Character-Types Met with in Psychoanalytic Work (1915). *Collected Papers*, 4:318–344. London: Hogarth Press, 1934.
(13) Freud, S.: Neurosis and Psychosis (1924). *Collected Papers*, 2:250–254. London: Hogarth Press, 1933.
(14) Freud, S.: Libidinal Types (1931). *Collected Papers*, 5:247–251. London: Hogarth Press, 1950.
(15) Freud, S.: Female Sexuality (1931). *Collected Papers*, 5:252–272. London: Hogarth Press, 1950.
(16) Gitelson, M.: Therapeutic Problems in the Analysis of the "Normal" Candidate. *Int. J. Psychoanal.*, 35:174–183, 1954.
(17) Gitelson, M.: On Ego Distortion. *Int. J. Psychoanal.*, 39:245–257, 1958.
(18) Glover, E.: The Concept of Dissociation. *Int. J. Psychoanal.*, 24:7–13, 1943.
(19) Hartmann, H.: *Ego Psychology and the Problem of Adaptation* (1939). New York: Int. Univ. Press, 1958.
(20) Hartmann, H.: Mutual Influences in the Development of Ego and Id. *The Psychoanalytic Study of the Child*, 7:9–30. New York: Int. Univ. Press, 1952.
(21) Jones, E.: *Hamlet and Oedipus*. New York: Norton, 1947.
(22) Mazlish, B.: Our "Heraclitean" Period. *Nation*, 192:336–338, 1961.
(23) Nunberg, H.: *Principles of Psychoanalysis*. New York: Int. Univ. Press, 1955, Chap. X.
(24) Reich, W.: The Characterological Mastery of the Oedipus Complex. *Int. J. Psychoanal.*, 12:452–467, 1931.
(25) Sterba, R.: On Character Neurosis. *Bull. Menninger Clin.*, 17:81–92, 1953.
(26) Waelder, R.: The Principle of Multiple Function: Observations and Overdetermination (1930). *Psychoanal. Quart.*, 5:45–62, 1936.
(27) Winnicott, D. W.: On Transference, *Int. J. Psychoanal.*, 37:386–388, 1956.

PART III

TECHNIQUES OF THERAPY

A. The Classic Position

4. On the Technique of Character-Analysis

Wilhelm Reich

INTRODUCTORY REVIEW

Our therapeutic method is determined by the following basic theoretical concepts. The *topical* standpoint determines the technical principle that the unconscious has to be made conscious. The *dynamic* standpoint determines the rule that this has to take place not directly but by way of resistance analysis. The *economic* standpoint and the psychological structure determine the rule that the resistance analysis has to be carried out in a certain order according to the individual patient.

As long as the topical process, the making conscious of the unconscious, was considered the only task of analytic technique, the formula that the unconscious manifestations should be interpreted *in the sequence in which they appeared* was correct. The dynamics of the analysis, that is, whether or not the making conscious also released the corresponding affect, whether the analysis influenced the patient beyond a merely intellectual understanding, that was more or less left to chance. The inclusion of the dynamic element, that is, the demand that the patient should not only remember things but also experience them, already complicated the simple formula that one had to "make the unconscious conscious." However, the dynamics of the analytic affect do not depend on the contents but on the resistances which the patient puts up against them and on the emotional experience in overcoming them. This makes the analytic task a vastly different one. From the topical stand-point, it is sufficient to bring into the patient's consciousness, one after the other, the manifest elements of the unconscious; in other words, the guiding line is the *content* of the material. If one also considers the dynamic factor one has to relinquish this guiding line in favor of another which comprehends the content of the material as well as the affects: that of the *successive resistances*. In doing so we meet, in most patients, with a difficulty which we have not yet mentioned.

Reprinted from Wilhelm Reich, *Character Analysis* 3d enl. ed., translated by P. Wolfe (New York): Orgone Institute Press, 1949), 39–113. Originally published in 1933.

CHARACTER ARMOR AND CHARACTER RESISTANCE

a) The Inability to Follow the Fundamental Rule

Rarely are our patients immediately accessible to analysis, capable of following the fundamental rule and of really opening up to the analyst. They cannot immediately have full confidence in a strange person; more importantly, years of illness, constant influencing by a neurotic milieu, bad experiences with physicians, in brief, the whole secondary warping of the personality have created a situation unfavorable to analysis. The elimination of this difficulty would not be so hard were it not supported by the character of the patient which is part and parcel of his neurosis. It is a difficulty which has been termed "narcissistic barrier." There are, in principle, two ways of meeting this difficulty, in especial, the rebellion against the fundamental rule.

One, which seems the usual one, is a direct education to analysis by information, reassurance, admonition, talking-to, etc. That is, one attempts to educate the patient to analytic candor by the establishment of some sort of positive transference. This corresponds to the technique proposed by Nunberg. Experience shows, however, that this pedagogical method is very uncertain; it lacks the basis of analytic clarity and is exposed to the constant variations in the transference situation.

The other way is more complicated and as yet not applicable in all patients, but far more certain. It is that of *replacing the pedagogical measures by analytic interpretations*. Instead of inducing the patient into analysis by advice, admonitions and transference manoeuvres, one focuses one's attention on the actual behavior of the patient and its meaning; *why* he doubts, or is late, or talks in a haughty or confused fashion, or communicates only every other or third thought, why he criticizes the analysis or produces exceptionally much material or material from exceptional depths. If, for example, a patient talks in a haughty manner, in technical terms, one may try to convince him that this is not good for the progress of the analysis, that he better give it up and behave less haughtily, for the sake of the analysis. Or, one may relinquish all attempts at persuasion and wait until one understands why the patient behaves in this and no other way. One may then find that his behavior is an attempt to compensate his feeling of inferiority toward the analyst and may influence him by consistent interpretation of the meaning of his behavior. This procedure, in contrast to the first-mentioned, is in full accord with the principle of analysis.

This attempt to replace pedagogical and similar active measures seemingly necessitated by the characteristic behavior of the patient, by purely analytic interpretations led unexpectedly to the analysis of the *character*.

Certain clinical experiences make it necessary to distinguish, among the various resistances we meet, a certain group as *character resistances*. They get their specific stamp not from their content but from the patient's specific way of acting and reacting. The compulsive character develops specifically different resistances than does the hysterical character; the latter different resistances from the impulsive or neurasthenic character. The *form* of the typical reactions which differ from character to character—though the contents may be the same—*is determined by infantile experiences just like the content of the symptoms or phantasies.*

b) Whence the Character Resistances?

Quite some time ago, Glover worked on the problem of differentiating character neuroses from symptom neuroses. Alexander also operated on the basis of this distinction. In my earlier writings, I also followed it. More exact comparison of the cases showed, however, that this distinction makes sense only insofar as there are neuroses with circumscribed symptoms and others without them; the former were called "symptom neuroses," the latter, "character neuroses." In the former, understandably, the symptoms are more obvious, in the latter the neurotic character traits. But, we must ask, are there symptoms without a neurotic reaction basis, in other words, without a neurotic character? The difference between the character neuroses and the symptom neuroses is only that in the latter the neurotic character also produced symptoms, that it became concentrated in them, as it were. If one recognizes the fact that the basis of a symptom neurosis is always a neurotic character, then it is clear that we shall have to deal with character-neurotic resistances in *every* analysis, that every analysis must be a character-analysis.

Another distinction which becomes immaterial from the standpoint of character-analysis is that between chronic neuroses, that is, neuroses which developed in childhood, and acute neuroses, which developed late. For the important thing is not whether the symptoms have made their appearance early or late. The important thing is that the neurotic character, the reaction basis for the symptom neurosis, was, in its essential traits, already formed at the period of the Oedipus phase. It is an old clinical experience that the boundary line which the patient draws between health and the outbreak of the disease becomes always obliterated during the analysis.

Since symptom formation does not serve as a distinguishing criterion we shall have to look for others. There is, first of all, insight into illness, and rationalization.

The lack of insight into illness is not an absolutely reliable but an essential sign of the character neurosis. The neurotic symptom is experienced as a foreign body and creates a feeling of being ill. The neurotic character trait, on the other hand, such as the exaggerated orderliness of the compulsive character or the anxious shyness of the hysterical character, are organically built into the personality. One may complain about being shy but does not feel ill for this reason. It is not until the characterological shyness turns into pathological blushing or the compulsion-neurotic orderliness into a compulsive ceremonial, that is, not until the neurotic character exacerbates symptomatically, that the person feels ill.

True enough, there are also symptoms for which there is no or only slight insight, things that are taken by the patient as bad habits or just peculiarities (chronic constipation, mild ejaculatio praecox, etc.). On the other hand, many character traits are often felt as illness, such as violent outbreaks of rage, tendency to lie, drink, waste money, etc. In spite of this, generally speaking, insight characterizes the neurotic symptom and its lack the neurotic character trait.

The second difference is that the symptom is never as thoroughly rationalized as the character. Neither a hysterical vomiting nor compulsive counting can be rationalized. The symptom appears meaningless, while the neurotic character is sufficiently rationalized not to appear meaningless or pathological. A reason is often given for neurotic character traits which would immediately be rejected as absurd if it were given for symptoms: "he just is that way." That implies that the individual was born that way, that this "happens to be" his character. Analysis shows this interpretation to be wrong; it shows that the character, for definite reasons, had to become that way and no different; that, in principle, it can be analyzed like the symptom and is alterable.

Occasionally, symptoms become part of the personality to such an extent that they resemble character traits. For example, a counting compulsion may appear only as part of general orderliness or a compulsive system only in terms of a compulsive work arrangement. Such modes of behavior are then considered as peculiarities rather than as signs of illness. So we can readily see that the concept of disease is an entirely fluid one, that there are all kinds of transitions from the symptom as an isolated foreign body over the neurotic character and the "bad habit" to rational action.

In comparison to the character trait, the symptom has a very simple construction with regard to its meaning and origin. True, the symptom also has a multiple determination; but the more deeply we penetrate into its determinations, the more we leave the realm of symptoms and the clearer becomes the characterological reaction basis. Thus one can arrive—theoretically—at the characterological reaction basis from any symptom. The symptom has its immediate determination in only a limited number of unconscious attitudes; hysterical vomiting, say, is based on a repressed fellatio phantasy or an oral wish for a child. Either expresses itself also characterologically, in a certain infantilism and maternal attitude. But the hysterical character which forms the basis of the symptom is determined by many—partly antagonistic—strivings and is expressed in a specific attitude or *way of being*. This is not as easy to dissect as the symptom; nevertheless, in principle it is, like the symptom, to be reduced to and understood from infantile strivings and experiences. While the symptom corresponds essentially to a single experience or striving, the character represents the specific way of being of an individual, an expression of his total past. For this reason, a symptom may develop suddenly while each individual character trait takes years to develop. In saying this we should not forget the fact that the symptom also could not have developed suddenly unless its characterological neurotic reaction basis had already been present.

The totality of the neurotic character traits makes itself felt in the analysis as a compact *defense mechanism* against our therapeutic endeavors. Analytic exploration of the development of this character "armor" shows that it also serves a definite economic purpose: on the one hand, it serves as protection against the stimuli from the outer world, on the other hand against the inner libidinous strivings. The character armor can perform this task because libidinous and sadistic energies are consumed in the neurotic reaction formations, compensations and other neurotic attitudes. In the processes which form and maintain this armor, anxiety is constantly being bound up, in the same way as it is, according to Freud's description, in, say, compulsive symptoms. We shall have to say more later about the economy of character formation.

Since the neurotic character, in its economic function of a protecting armor, has established a certain *equilibrium,* albeit a neurotic one, the analysis presents a danger to this equilibrium. This is why the resistances which give the analysis of the individual case its specific imprint originate from this narcissistic protection mechanism. As we have seen, the mode of behavior is the result of the total development and as such can be analyzed and altered; thus it can also be the starting point for evolving the technique of character-analysis.

c) The Technique of Analyzing the Character Resistance

Apart from the dreams, associations, slips and other communications of the patients, their attitude, that is, *the manner* in which they relate their dreams, commit slips, produce their associations and make their communications, deserves special attention.[1] A patient who follows the fundamental rule from the beginning is a rare exception; it takes months of character-analytic work to make the patient halfway sufficiently honest in his communications. The manner in which the patient talks, in which he greets the analyst or looks at him, the way he lies on the couch, the inflection of the voice, the degree of conventional politeness, all these things are valuable criteria for judging the latent resistances against the fundamental rule, and understanding them makes it possible to alter or eliminate them by interpretation. The *how* of saying things is as important "material" for interpretations is *what* the patient says. One often hears analysts complain that the analysis does not go well, that the patient does not produce any "material." By that is usually meant the content of associations and communications. But the manner in which the patient, say, keeps quiet, or his sterile repetitions, are also "material" which can and must be put to use. There is hardly any situation in which the patient brings "no material"; it is our fault if we are unable to utilize the patient's behavior as "material."

That the behavior and the form of the communications have analytic significance is nothing new. What I am going to talk about is the fact that these things present an avenue of approach to the analysis of the character in

1. *Footnote, 1945:* The *form* of expression is far more important than the *ideational content.* Today, in penetrating to the decisively important infantile experiences, we make use of the form of expression *exclusively.* Not the ideational contents but the form of expression is what leads us to the biological reactions which form the basis of the psychic manifestations.

a very definite and almost perfect manner. Past failures with many cases of neurotic characters have taught us that in these cases the form of the communications is, at least in the beginning, always more important than their content. One only has to remember the latent resistances of the affect-lame, the "good," over-polite and ever-correct patients; those who always present a deceptive positive transference or who violently and stereotypically ask for love; those who make a game of the analysis; those who are always "armored," who smile inwardly about everything and everyone. One could continue this enumeration indefinitely; it is easy to see that a great deal of painstaking work will have to be done to master the innumerable individual technical problems.

For the purpose of orientation and of sketching the essential differences between character-analysis and symptom-analysis, let us assume two pairs of patients for comparison. Let us assume we have under treatment at the same time two men suffering from premature ejaculation; one is a passive-feminine, the other a phallic-aggressive character. Also, two women with an eating disturbance; one is a compulsive character, the other a hysteric.

Let us assume further that the premature ejaculation of both men has the same unconscious meaning: the fear of the paternal penis in the woman's vagina. In the analysis, both patients, on the basis of their castration anxiety which is the basis of the symptom, produce a negative father transference. Both hate the analyst (the father) because they see in him the enemy who frustrates their pleasure; both have the unconscious wish to do away with him. In this situation, the phallic-sadistic character will ward off the danger of castration by insults, depreciation and threats, while the passive-feminine character, in the same case, will become steadily more passive, submissive and friendly. In both patients, the character has become a resistance: one fends off the danger aggressively, the other tries to avoid it by a deceptive submission. It goes without saying that the character resistance of the passive-feminine patient is more dangerous because he works with hidden means: he produces a wealth of material, he remembers all kinds of infantile experiences, in short, he seems to cooperate splendidly. Actually, however, he camouflages a secret spitefulness and hatred; as long as he maintains this attitude he does not have the courage to show his real self. If, now, one enters only upon *what* he produces, without paying attention to his way of behavior, then no analytic endeavor will change his condition. He may even remember the hatred of his father, but he will not *experience* it unless one interprets consistently the meaning of his deceptive attitude *before* beginning to interpret the deep meaning of his hatred of the father.

In the case of the second pair, let us assume that an acute positive transference has developed. The central content of this positive transference is, in either patient, the same as that of the symptom, namely, an oral fellatio phantasy. But although the positive transference has the same content in either case, the form of the transference resistance will be quite different: the hysterical patient will, say, show an *anxious* silence and a shy behavior; the compulsive character a *spiteful* silence or a cold, haughty behavior. In one case the positive transference is warded off by aggression, in the other by anxiety. And the form of this defense will always be the same in the same patient: the hysterical patient will always defend herself anxiously, the compulsive patient aggressively, no matter what unconscious content is on the point of breaking through. That is, *in one and the same patient, the character resistance remains always the same and only disappears with the very roots of the neurosis.*

In the character armor, the *narcissistic defense* finds its concrete chronic expression. In addition to the known resistances which are mobilized against every new piece of unconscious material, we have to recognize a constant factor of a *formal* nature which originates from the patient's character. Because of this origin, we call the constant formal resistance factor "character resistance."

In summary, the most important aspects of the character resistance are the following:

The character resistance expresses itself not in the content of the material, but in the formal aspects of the general behavior, the manner of talking, of the gait, facial expression and typical attitudes such as smiling, deriding, haughtiness, over-correctness, the *manner* of the politeness or of the aggression, etc.

What is specific of the character resistance is not *what* the patient says or does, but *how* he talks and acts, not *what* he gives away in a dream but *how* he censors, distorts, etc.

The character resistance remains the same in one and the same patient no matter what the material is against which it is directed. Different characters present the same material in a different manner. For example, a hysteric patient will ward off the positive father transference in an anxious manner, the compulsive woman in an aggressive manner.

The character resistance, which expresses itself formally, can be understood as to its content and can be reduced to infantile experiences and instinctual drives just like the neurotic symptom.[2]

During analysis, the character of a patient soon becomes a resistance. That is, in ordinary life, the character plays the same role as in analysis: that of a psychic protection mechanism. The individual is "characterologically armored" against the outer world and against his unconscious drives.

Study of character formation reveals the fact that the character armor was formed in infancy for the same reasons and purposes which the character resistance serves in the analytic situation. The appearance in the analysis of the character as resistance reflects its infantile genesis. The situations which make the character resistance appear in the analysis are exact duplicates of those situations in infancy which set character formation into motion. For this reason, we find in the character resistance both a defensive function and a transference of infantile relationships with the outer world.

Economically speaking, the character in ordinary life and the character resistance in the analysis serve the same function, that of avoiding unpleasure, of establishing and maintaining a psychic equilibrium—neurotic though it may be—and finally, that of absorbing repressed energies. One of its cardinal functions is that of binding "free-floating" anxiety, or, in other words, that of absorbing dammed-up energy. Just as the historical, infantile element is present and active in the neurotic symptoms, so it is in the character. This is why a consistent dissolving of character resistances provides an infallible and immediate avenue of approach to the central infantile conflict.

What, then, follows from these facts for the technique of character-analysis? Are there essential differences between character-analysis and ordinary resistance analysis? There are. They are related to

a) the selection of the sequence in which the material is interpreted;
b) the technique of resistance interpretation itself.

As to a): If we speak of "selection of material," we have to expect an important objection: some will say that any selection is at variance with basic psychoanalytic principles, that one should let oneself be guided by the patient, that with any kind of selection one runs the danger of following one's personal inclinations. To this we have to say that in this kind of selection it is not a matter of neglecting analytic material; it is merely a

---

2. By the realization of this fact, the formal element becomes included in the sphere of psychoanalysis which, hitherto, was centered primarily on the content.

matter of *safeguarding a logical sequence* of interpretation which corresponds to the structure of the individual neurosis. All the material is finally interpreted; only, in any given situation this or that detail is more important than another. Incidentally, the analyst always makes selections anyhow, for he has already made a selection when he does not interpret a dream in the sequence in which it is presented but selects this or that detail for interpretation. One also has made a selection if one pays attention only to the content of the communications but not to their form. In other words, the very fact that the patient presents material of the most diverse kinds forces one to make a selection; what matters is only that one select *correctly* with regard to the given analytic situation.

In patients who, for character reasons, consistently fail to follow the fundamental rule, and generally where one deals with a character resistance, one will be forced *constantly to lift the character resistance out of the total material* and to dissolve it by the interpretation of its meaning. That does not mean, of course, that one neglects the rest of the material; on the contrary, every bit of material is valuable which gives us information about the meaning and origin of the disturbing character trait; one merely postpones the interpretation of what material does not have an immediate connection with the transference resistance until such time as the character resistance is understood and overcome at least in its essential features. I have already tried to show [See Wilhelm Reich, *Character Analysis,* 3d enl. ed., translated by P. Wolfe (New York: Orgone Institute Press, 1949), Chap. 3] what are the dangers of giving deep-reaching interpretations in the presence of undissolved character resistances.

As to b): We shall now turn to some special problems of character-analytic technique. First of all, we must point out a possible misunderstanding. We said that character-analysis begins with the emphasis on and the consistent analysis of the character resistance. It should be well understood that this does not mean that one asks the patient, say, not to be aggressive, not to deceive, not to talk in a confused manner, etc. Such procedure would be not only un-analytic but altogether sterile. The fact has to be emphasized again and again that what is described here as character-analysis has nothing to do with education, admonition, trying to make the patient behave differently, etc. In character-analysis, we ask ourselves *why* the patient deceives, talks in a confused manner, why he is affect-blocked, etc.; we try to arouse the patient's interest in his character traits in order to be able, with his help, to explore analytically their origin and meaning. All we do is to lift the character trait which presents the cardinal resistance out of the level of the personality and to show the patient, if possible, the superficial connections between character and symptoms; it is left to him whether or not he will utilize his knowledge for an alteration of his character. In principle, the procedure is not different from the analysis of a symptom. What is added in character-analysis is merely that we isolate the character trait and confront the patient with it repeatedly until he begins to look at it objectively and to experience it like a painful symptom; thus, the character trait begins to be experienced as a foreign body which the patient wants to get rid of.

Surprisingly, this process brings about a change—although only a temporary one—in the personality. With progressing character-analysis, that impulse or trait automatically comes to the fore which had given rise to the character resistance in the transference. To go back to the illustration of the passive-feminine character: the more the patient achieves an objective attitude toward his tendency to passive submission, the more aggressive does he become. This is so because his passive-feminine attitude was essentially a reaction to repressed aggressive impulses. But with the aggression we also have a return of the infantile castration anxiety which in infancy had caused the change from aggressive to passive-feminine behavior. In this way the analysis of the character resistance leads directly to the center of the neurosis, the Oedipus complex.

One should not have any illusions, however. The isolation of such a character resistance and its analytic working-through usually takes many months of sustained effort and patient persistence. Once the breakthrough has succeeded, though, the analysis usually proceeds rapidly, with *emotionally* charged analytical experiences. If, on the other hand, one neglects such character resistances and instead simply follows the line of the material, interpreting everything in it, such resistances form a ballast which it is difficult if not impossible to remove. In that case, one gains more and more the impression that every interpretation of meaning was wasted, that the patient continues to doubt everything or only pretends to accept things, or that he meets everything with an inward smile. If the elimination of these resistances was not begun right in the beginning, they confront one with an insuperable obstacle in the later stages of the analysis, at a time when the most important interpretations of the Oedipus complex have already been given.

I have already tried to refute the objection that it is impossible to tackle resistances before one knows their *infantile* determination. The essential thing is first to see through the *present-day* meaning of the character resistance; this is usually possible without the infantile material. The latter is needed for the *dissolution* of the resistance. If at first one does no more than to show the patient the resistance and to interpret its present-day meaning, then the corresponding infantile material with the aid of which we can eliminate the resistance soon makes its appearance.

If we put so much emphasis on the analysis of the *mode* of behavior, this does not imply a neglect of the contents. We only add something that hitherto has been neglected. Experience shows that the analysis of character resistances has to assume first rank. This does not mean, of course, that one would only analyze character resistances up to a certain date and then begin with the interpretation of contents. The two phases—resistance analysis and analysis of early infantile experiences—overlap essentially; only in the beginning, we have a preponderance of character-analysis, that is, "education to analysis *by* analysis," while in the later stages the emphasis is on the contents and the infantile. This is, of course, no rigid rule but depends on the attitudes of the individual patient. In one patient, the interpretation of the infantile material will be begun earlier, in another later. It is a basic rule, however, not to give any deep-reaching interpretations—no matter how clear-cut the material—as long as the patient is not ready to assimilate them. Again, this is nothing new, but it seems that differences in analytic technique are largely determined by what one or the other analyst means by "ready for analytic interpretation." We also have to distinguish those contents which are part and parcel of the character resistance and others which belong to other spheres of experiencing. As a rule, the patient is in the beginning ready to take cognizance of the former, but not of the latter. Generally speaking, our character-analytic endeavors are nothing but an attempt to achieve the greatest possible security in the introduction of the analysis and in the interpretation of the infantile material. This leads us to the important task of studying and systematically describing the various forms of characterological transference resistances. If we understand them, the technique derives automatically from their structure.

d) Derivation of the Situational Technique from the Structure of the Character Resistance (Interpretation Technique of the Defense)

We now turn to the problem of how the situational technique of character-analysis can be derived from the structure of the character resistance in a patient who develops his resistances right in the beginning, the structure of which is, however, completely unintelligible at first. In the following case the character resistance had a very complicated structure; there were a great many coexistent and overlapping determinations. We shall try to describe the reasons which prompted me to begin the interpretation work with one aspect of the resistance and not with any other. Here also we will see that a consistent and logical interpretation of the defenses and of the mechanisms of the "armor" leads directly into the central infantile conflicts.

A Case of Manifest Inferiority Feelings

A man 30 years of age came to analysis because he "didn't get any fun out of life." He did not really think he was sick but, he said, he had heard about psychoanalysis and perhaps it would make things clearer to him. When asked about symptoms, he stated he did not have any. Later it was found that his potency was quite defective. He did not quite dare approach women, had sexual intercourse very infrequently, and then he suffered from premature ejaculation and intercourse left him unsatisfied. He had very little insight into his impotence. He had become reconciled to it; after all, he said, there were a lot of men who "didn't need that sort of thing."

His behavior immediately betrayed a severely inhibited individual. He spoke without looking at one, in a low voice, haltingly, and embarrassedly clearing his throat. At the same time, there was an obvious attempt to suppress his embarrassment and to appear courageous. Nevertheless, his whole appearance gave the impression of severe feelings of inferiority.

Having been informed of the fundamental rule, the patient began to talk hesitatingly and in a low voice. Among the first communications was the recollection of two "terrible" experiences. Once he had run over a woman with an automobile and she had died of her injuries. Another time, as a medical orderly during the war, he had had to do a tracheotomy. The bare recollection of these two experiences filled him with horror. In the course of the first few sessions he then talked, in the same monotonous, low and suppressed manner about his youth. Being next to the youngest of a number of children, he was relegated to an inferior place. His oldest brother, some twenty years his senior, was the parents' favorite; this brother had traveled a good deal, "knew the world," prided himself on his experiences and when he came home from one of his travels "the whole house pivoted around him." Although the content of his story made the envy of his brother and the hatred of him obvious enough, the patient, in response to a cautious query, denied ever having felt anything like that toward his brother. Then he talked about his mother, how good she had been to him and how she had died when he was 7 years of age. At this, he began to cry softly; he became ashamed of this and did not say anything for some time. It seemed clear that his mother had been the only person who had given him some love and attention and that her loss had been a severe shock to him. After her death, he had spent 5 years in the house of his brother. It was not the content but the tone of his story which revealed his enormous bitterness about the unfriendly, cold and domineering behavior of his brother. Then he related in a few brief sentences that now he had a friend who loved and admired him very much. After this, a continuous silence set in. A few days later he related a dream: *He saw himself in a foreign city with his friend; only, the face of his friend was different.* The fact that the patient had left his own city for the purpose of the analysis suggested that the man in the dream represented the analyst. This identification of the analyst with the friend might have been interpreted as a beginning positive transference. In view of the total situation, however, this would have been unwise. He himself recognized the analyst in the friend, but had nothing to add to this. Since he either kept silent or else expressed his doubts that *he* would be able to carry out the analysis, I told him that he had something against me but did not have the courage to come out with it. He denied this categorically, whereupon I told him that he also never had had the courage to express his inimical impulses toward his brother, not even to think them consciously; and that apparently he had established some kind of connection between his older brother and myself. This was true in itself, but I made the mistake of interpreting his resistance at too deep a level. Nor did the interpretation have any success; on the contrary, the inhibition became intensified. So I waited a few days until I should be able to understand, from his behavior, the more important present-day meaning of his resistance. What was clear at this time was that there was a transference not only of the hatred of the brother but also a strong defense against a feminine attitude (*cf.* the dream about the friend). But an interpretation in this direction would have been inadvisable at this time. So I continued to point out that for some reason he defended himself against me and the analysis, that his whole being pointed to his being blocked against the analysis. To this he agreed by saying that, yes, that was the way he was generally in life, rigid, inaccessible and on the defensive. While I demonstrated to him his defense in every session, on every possible occasion, I was struck by the monotonous expression with which he uttered his complaints. Every session began with the same sentences: "I don't feel anything, the analysis doesn't have any influence on me, I don't see how I'll ever achieve it, nothing comes to my mind, the analysis doesn't have any influence on me," etc. I did not understand what he wanted to express with these complaints, and yet it was clear that here was the key to an understanding of his resistance.[3]

Here we have a good opportunity for studying the difference between the character-analytic and the active-suggestive education to analysis. I might have admonished him in a kindly way to tell me more about this and that; I might have been able thus to establish an artificial positive transference; but experience with other cases had shown me that one does not get far with such procedures. Since his whole behavior did not leave any room for doubt that he refuted the analysis in general and me in particular, I could simply stick to this interpretation and wait for further reactions. When, on one occasion, the talk reverted to the dream, he said the best proof for his not refuting me was that he identified me with his friend. I suggested to him that possibly he had expected me to love and admire him as much as his friend did; that he then was disappointed and very much resented my reserve. He had to admit that he had had such thoughts but that he had not dared to tell them to me. He then related how he always only *demanded* love and especially recognition, and that he had a very *defensive* attitude toward men with a particularly masculine appearance. He said he did not feel equal to such men, and in the relationship with his friend he had played the feminine part. Again there was material for interpreting his feminine transference but his total behavior warned against it. The situation was difficult, for the elements of his resistance which I already understood, the transference of hatred from his brother, and the narcissistic-feminine attitude toward his superiors, were strongly warded off; consequently, I had to be very careful or I might have provoked him into breaking off the analysis. In addition, he continued to complain in every session, in the same way, that the analysis did not touch him, etc.; this was something which I still did not understand after about four weeks of analysis, and yet, I felt that it was an essential and acutely active character resistance.

3. *Footnote, 1945:* The explanation given here is insufficient, although it is psychologically correct. Today we know that such complaints are the immediate expression of muscular armoring. The patient complains about affect-lameness because of a block in his plasmatic currents and sensations. The disturbance, then, is primarily of a *biophysical* nature. Orgone therapy eliminates the block in motility not with psychological but with biophysical means.

I fell ill and had to interrupt the analysis for two weeks. The patient sent me a bottle of brandy as a tonic. When I resumed the analysis he seemed to be glad. At the same time, he continued his old complaints and related that he was very much bothered by thoughts about death, that he constantly was afraid that something had happened to some member of his family; and that during my illness he had always been thinking that I might die. It was when this thought bothered him particularly badly one day that he had sent me the brandy. At this point, the temptation was great to interpret his repressed death wishes. The material for doing so was ample, but I felt that such an interpretation would be fruitless because it would bounce back from the wall of his complaints that "nothing touches me, the analysis has no influence on me." In the meantime, the secret double meaning of his complaint, "nothing touches me" ("*nichts dringt in mich ein*") had become clear; it was an expression of his most deeply repressed transference wish for anal intercourse. But would it have been justifiable to point out to him his homosexual love impulse—which, it is true, manifested itself clearly enough—while he, with his whole being, continued to protest against the analysis? First it had to become clear what was the meaning of his complaints about the uselessness of the analysis. True, I could have shown him that he was wrong in his complaints: he dreamed without interruption, the thoughts about death became more intense, and many other things went on in him. But I knew from experience that that would not have helped the situation. Furthermore, I felt distinctly the armor which stood between the unconscious material and the analysis, and had to assume that the existing resistance would not let any interpretation penetrate to the unconscious. For these reasons, I did no more than consistently to show him his attitude, interpreting it as the expression of a violent defense, and telling him that we had to wait until we understood this behavior. He understood already that the death thoughts on the occasion of my illness had not necessarily been the expression of a loving solicitude.

In the course of the next few weeks it became increasingly clear that his inferiority feeling connected with his feminine transference played a considerable role in his behavior and his complaints. Yet, the situation still did not seem ripe for interpretation; the meaning of his behavior was not sufficiently clear. To summarize the essential aspects of the solution as it was found later:

a) He desired recognition and love from me as from all men who appeared masculine to him. That he wanted love and had been disappointed by me had already been interpreted repeatedly, without success.

b) He had a definite attitude of envy and hatred toward me, transferred from his brother. This could, at this time, not be interpreted because the interpretation would have been wasted.

c) He defended himself against his feminine transference. This defense could not be interpreted without touching upon the warded-off femininity.

d) He felt inferior before me, because of his femininity. His eternal complaints could only be the expression of this feeling of inferiority.

Now I interpreted his inferiority feeling toward me. At first, this led nowhere, but after I had consistently held up his behavior to him for several days, he did bring some communications concerning his boundless envy, not of me, but other men of whom he also felt inferior. Now it suddenly occurred to me that his constant complaining could have only one meaning: "The analysis has no influence on me," that is, "It is no good," that is, "the analyst is inferior, is impotent, cannot achieve anything with me." *The complaints were in part a triumph over the analyst, in part a reproach to him.* I told him what I thought of his complaints. The result was astounding. Immediately he brought forth a wealth of examples which showed that he always acted this way when anybody tried to influence him. He could not tolerate the superiority of anybody and always tried to tear them down. He had always done the exact opposite of what any superior had asked him to do. There appeared a wealth of recollections of his spiteful and deprecatory behavior toward teachers.

Here, then, was his suppressed aggression, the most extreme manifestation of which thus far had been his death wishes. But soon the resistance reappeared in the same old form, there were the same complaints, the same reserve, the same silence. But now I knew that my discovery had greatly impressed him, which had *increased* his feminine attitude; this, of course, resulted in an intensified defense against the femininity. In analyzing the resistance, I started again from the inferiority feeling toward me; but now I deepened the interpretation by the statement that he did not only feel inferior but that, because of his inferiority, he felt himself in a female role toward me, which hurt his masculine pride.

Although previously the patient had presented ample material with regard to his feminine attitude toward masculine men and had had full insight for this fact, now he denied it all. This was a new problem. Why should he now refuse to admit what he had previously described himself? I told him that he felt so inferior toward me that he did not want to accept any explanation from me even if that implied his going back on himself. He realized this to be true and now talked about the relationship with his friend in some detail. He had actually played the feminine role and there often had been sexual intercourse between the legs. Now I was able to show him that his defensive attitude in the analysis was nothing but the struggle against the surrender to the analysis which, to his unconscious, was apparently linked up with the idea of surrendering to the analyst in a female fashion. This hurt his pride, and this was the reason for his stubborn resistance against the influence of the analysis. To this he reacted with a confirmatory dream: he lies on a sofa with the analyst, who kisses him. This clear dream provoked a new phase of resistance in the old form of complaints that the analysis did not touch him, that he was cold, etc. Again I interpreted the complaints as a depreciation of the analysis and a defense against surrendering to it. But at the same time I began to explain to him the economic meaning of this defense. I told him that from what he had told thus far about his infancy and adolescence it was obvious that he had closed himself up against all disappointments by the outer world and against the rough and cold treatment by his father, brother and teachers; that this seemed to have been his only salvation even if it demanded great sacrifices in happiness.

This interpretation seemed highly plausible to him and he soon produced memories of his attitude toward his teachers. He always felt they were cold and distant — a clear projection of his own attitude — and although he was aroused when they beat or scolded him he remained indifferent. In this connection he said that he often had wished I had been more severe. This wish did not seem to fit the situation at that time; only much later it became clear that he wished to put me and my prototypes, the teachers, in a bad light with his spite. For a few days the analysis proceeded smoothly, without any resistances; he now remembered that there had been a period in his childhood when he had been very wild and aggressive. At the same time he produced dreams with a strong feminine attitude toward me. I could only assume that the recollection of his aggression had mobilized the guilt feeling which now was expressed in the passive-feminine dreams. I avoided an analysis of these dreams not only because they had no immediate connection with the actual transference situation, but also because it seemed to me that he was not ready to understand the connection between his aggression and the dreams which expressed a guilt feeling. Many analysts will consider this an arbitrary selection of material. Experience shows, however, that the best therapeutic effect is to be expected when an immediate connection is already established between the transference situation and the infantile material. I only ventured the assumption that, to judge from his recollections of his aggressive infantile behavior, he had at one time been quite different, the exact opposite of what he was today, and that the analysis would have to find out at what time and under what circumstances this change in his character had taken place. I told him that his present femininity probably was an avoidance of his aggressive masculinity. To this the patient did not react except by falling back into his old resistance of complaining that he could not achieve it, that the analysis did not touch him, etc.

I interpreted again his inferiority feeling and his recurrent attempt to prove the analysis, or the analyst, to be impotent; but now I also tried to work on the transference from the brother, pointing out that he had said that his brother always played the dominant role. Upon this he entered only with much hesitation, apparently because we were dealing with the central conflict of his infancy; he talked again about how much attention his mother had paid to his brother, without, however, mentioning any subjective attitude toward this. As was shown by a cautious approach to the question, the envy of his brother was completely repressed. Apparently, this envy was so closely associated with intense hatred that not even the envy was allowed to become conscious. The approach to this problem provoked a particularly violent resistance which continued for days in the form of his stereotyped complaints about his inability. Since the resistance did not budge it had to be assumed that here was a particularly acute rejection of the person of the analyst. I asked him again to talk quite freely and without fear about the analysis and, in particular, about the analyst, and to tell me what impression I had made on him on the occasion of the first meeting.[4] After much hesitation he said the analyst had appeared to him so masculine and brutal, like a man who is absolutely ruthless with women. So I asked him about his attitude toward men who gave an impression of being potent.

This was at the end of the fourth month of the analysis. Now for the first time that repressed attitude toward the brother broke through which had the closest connection with his most disturbing transference attitude, the envy of potency. With much affect he now remembered that he had always condemned his brother for always being after women, seducing them and bragging about it afterwards. He said I had immediately reminded him of his brother. I explained to him that obviously he saw in me his potent brother and that he could not open up to me because he condemned me and resented

4. Since then I am in the habit of soon asking the patient to describe my person. This measure always proves useful for the elimination of blocked transference situations.

my assumed superiority just as he used to resent that of his brother; further-more, it was plain now that the basis of his inferiority feeling was a feeling of impotence.

Then occurred what one always sees in a correctly and consistently carried-out analysis: *the central element of the character resistance rose to the surface.* All of a sudden he remembered that he had repeatedly compared his small penis with the big one of his brother and how he had envied his brother.

As might have been expected, a new wave of resistance occurred; again the complaint, "I can't do anything." Now I could go somewhat further in the interpretation and show him that he was acting out his impotence. His reaction to this was wholly unexpected. In connection with my interpretation of his distrust he said for the first time that he had never believed anyone, that he did not believe anything, and probably also not in the analysis. This was, of course, an important step ahead, but the connection of this statement with the analytic situation was not altogether clear. For two hours he talked about all the many disappointments which he had experienced and believed that they were a rational explanation of his distrust. Again the old resistance reappeared; as it was not clear what had precipitated it this time, I kept waiting. The old behavior continued for several days. I only interpreted again those elements of the resistance with which I was already well acquainted. Then, suddenly, a new element of the resistance appeared: he said he was *afraid of the analysis because it might rob him of his ideals.* Now the situation was clear again. He had transferred his castration anxiety from his brother to me. He was afraid of me. Of course, I did not touch upon his castration anxiety but proceeded again from his inferiority feeling and his impotence and asked him whether his high ideals did not make him feel superior and better than everybody else. He admitted this openly; more than that, he said that he was really better than all those who kept running after women and lived sexually like animals. He added, however, that this feeling was all too often disturbed by his feeling of impotence, and that apparently he had not become quite reconciled to his sexual weakness after all. Now I could show him the neurotic manner in which he tried to overcome his feeling of impotence: he was trying to recover a feeling of potency in the realm of ideals. I showed him the mechanism of compensation and pointed out again the resistances against the analysis which originated from his secret feeling of superiority. I told him that not only did he think himself secretly better and cleverer than others; it was for this very reason that he resisted the analysis. For if it succeeded, he would have taken recourse to the aid of somebody else and it would have vanquished his neurosis, the secret pleasure gain of which had just been unearthed. From the standpoint of the neurosis this would be a defeat which, furthermore, to his unconscious, would mean becoming a woman. In this way, by progressing from the ego and its defense mechanisms, I prepared the soil for an interpretation of the castration complex and of the feminine fixation.

The character-analysis had succeeded, then, in penetrating from his mode of behavior directly to the center of his neurosis, his castration anxiety, the envy of his brother because of his mother's favoritism, and the disappointment in his mother. What is important here is not that these unconscious elements rose to the surface; that often occurs spontaneously. What is important is the logical sequence and the close contact with the ego-defense and the transference in which they came up; further, that this took place without any urging, purely as the result of analytic interpretation of the behavior; further, that it took place with the corresponding affects. This is what constitutes a consistent character-analysis; it is a thorough working through of the conflicts assimilated by the ego.

In contrast, let us consider what probably would have happened without a consistent emphasis on the defenses. Right at the beginning, there was the possibility of interpreting the passive-homosexual attitude toward the brother, and the death wishes. Undoubtedly, dreams and associations would have provided further relevant material for interpretation. But without a previous systematic and detailed working through of his ego-defense, no interpretation would have affectively penetrated; the result would have been an intellectual knowledge of his passive desires alongside with a violent affective defense against them. The affects belonging to the passivity and the murderous impulses would have continued to remain in the defense function. The final result would have been a chaotic situation, the typical hopeless picture of an analysis rich in interpretations and poor in results.

A few months' patient and persistent work on his ego-defense, particularly its form (complaints, manner of speech, etc.) raised the ego to that level which was necessary for the assimilation of the repressed, it loosened the affects and brought about their displacement in the direction of the repressed ideas. One cannot say, therefore, that in this case two different techniques would have been feasible; there was only one possibility if one was to alter the patient *dynamically*. I trust that this case makes clear the different concept of the application of theory to technique. The most important criterion of an orderly analysis is the giving of *few* interpretations which are to the point and consistent, instead of a great many which are unsystematic and do not take into consideration the dynamic and economic element. If one does not let oneself be led astray by the material, if, instead, one evaluates correctly its dynamic position and economic role, then one gets the material later, it is true, but more thoroughly and more charged with affect. The second criterion is a continuous connection between present-day situation and infantile situation. While in the beginning the various elements of the content coexist side by side without any order, this changes into a logical sequence of resistances and contents, a sequence determined by the dynamics and structure of the individual neurosis. With unsystematic interpretation, one has to make one new start after another, guessing rather than knowing one's way; in the case of character-analytic work on the resistances, on the other hand, the analytic process develops as if by itself. In the former case, the analysis will run smoothly in the beginning only to get progressively into more and more difficulties; in the latter case, the greatest difficulties are met in the first few weeks and months of the treatment, to give way progressively to smooth work even on the most deeply repressed material. The fate of every analysis depends on its introduction, that is, the correct or incorrect handling of the resistances. The third criterion, then, is that of tackling the case not in this or that spot which happens to be tangible but at the spot which hides the most essential ego-defense; and the systematic enlarging of the breach which has been made into the unconscious; and the working out of that infantile fixation which is affectively most important at any given time. A certain unconscious position which manifests itself in a dream or an association may have a central significance for the neurosis and yet may at any given time be quite unimportant with regard to its technical significance. In our patient, the feminine attitude toward the brother was of central pathogenic significance; yet in the first few months the technical problem was the fear of the loss of the compensation for the impotence by high ideals. The mistake which is usually made is that of attacking the central pathogenic point of the neurosis which commonly manifests itself somehow right at the beginning. What has to be attacked instead are the respective important present-day positions which, if worked on systematically, one after the other, lead of *necessity* to the central pathogenic situation. It is important, therefore, and in many cases decisive, *how*, *when* and from which side one proceeds toward the central point of the neurosis.

What we have described here as character-analysis fits without difficulty into Freud's theory of resistances, their formation and dissolution. We know that every resistance consists of an id-impulse which is warded off and an ego-impulse which wards it off. Both impulses are unconscious. In principle, then, one would seem to be free to interpret first either the id-impulse or the ego-impulse. For example: If a homosexual resistance in the form of keeping silent appears right at the beginning of the analysis, one can approach the id-impulse by telling the patient that he is occupied with thoughts about loving the analyst or being loved by him; one has interpreted his positive transference, and if he does not take flight it will, at best, take a long time before he can come to terms with such a forbidden idea. The better way, then, is to approach first the *defense of the ego* which is more closely related to the conscious ego. One will tell the patient at first only that he is keeping silent because — *"for one reason or another,"* that is, without touching upon the id-impulse — he is defending himself against the analysis, presumably because it has become somehow dangerous to him. In the first case one has tackled the id aspect, in the latter case the ego aspect of the resistance, the defense.

Proceeding in this manner, we comprehend the negative transference in which every defense finally results, as well as the character, the armor of the ego. The superficial, more nearly conscious layer of *every* resistance must of necessity be a negative attitude toward the analyst, no matter whether the warded-off id-impulse is hatred or love. The ego projects its defense against the id-impulse to the analyst who has become a dangerous enemy because, by his insistence on the fundamental rule, he has provoked id-impulses and has disturbed the neurotic equilibrium. In its defense, the ego makes use of very old forms of negative attitudes; it utilizes hate impulses from the id even if it is warding off love impulses.

If we adhere to the rule of tackling resistances from the ego side, we always dissolve, at the same time, a certain amount of negative transference, of hatred. This obviates the danger of overlooking the destructive tendencies which often are extremely well hidden; it also strengthens the positive transference. The patient also comprehends the ego interpretation more easily because it is more in accordance with conscious experience than the id interpretation; this makes him better prepared for the latter which follows at a later time.

The ego defense has always the same form, corresponding to the character of the patient, whatever the repressed id-impulse may be. Conversely, the same id-impulse is warded off in different ways in different individuals. If we interpret only the id-impulse, we leave the character untouched. If, on the other hand, we always approach the resistances from the defense, from the ego side, we include the neurotic character in the analysis. In the first case, we say immediately *what* the patient wards off. In the latter case. we first make clear to him *that* he wards off "something," then, *how* he does it, what are the means of defense (character-analysis); only at last, when the analysis of the resistance has progressed far enough, is he told — or finds out for himself — what it is he is warding off. On this long detour to the interpretation of the id-impulses, all corresponding attitudes of the ego have been analyzed. This obviates the danger that the patient learns something too early or that he remains affectless and without participation.

Analyses in which so much analytic attention is centered upon the attitudes take a more orderly and logical course while the theoretical research does not suffer in the least. One obtains the important infantile experiences later, it is true; but this is more than compensated for by the emotional aliveness with which the infantile material comes up *after* the analytic work on the character resistances.

On the other hand, we should not fail to mention certain unpleasant aspects of a consistent character-analysis. It is a far heavier burden for the patient; he suffers much more than when one leaves the character out of consideration. True, this has the advantage of a selective process: those who cannot stand it would not have achieved success anyhow, and it is better to find that out after a few months than after a few years. Experience shows that if the character resistance does not give way a satisfactory result cannot be expected. The overcoming of the character resistance does *not* mean that the character is altered; that, of course, is possible only after the analysis of its infantile sources. It only means that the patient has gained an objective view of his character and an analytic interest in it; once this has been achieved a favorable progress of the analysis is probable.*

The difficulties in the cases presented in the Seminar were of a very similar nature: It was always the same underestimation or the complete neglect of the behavior as interpretable material; again and again the attempt to remove the resistance from the id side instead of by analysis of the ego defense; and finally, almost always, the idea — which was used as an alibi — that the patient simply did not want to get well or that he was "all too narcissistic."

* [Pages 67–73 from the original article have been deleted.]

In principle, the loosening of the narcissistic defense is not different in other types than in the one described. If, say, a patient is always affectless and indifferent, no matter what material he may be presenting, then one is dealing with the dangerous affect-block. Unless one works on this before anything else one runs the danger of seeing all the material and all the interpretations go to waste and of seeing the patient become a good analytical theorist while otherwise he remains the same. Unless one prefers in such a case to give up the analysis because of "too strong narcissism" one can make an agreement with the patient to the effect that one will continue to confront him with his affect-lameness but that, of course, he can stop whenever he wants to. In the course of time — usually many months, in one case it took a year and a half — the patient begins to experience the continued pointing out of his affect-lameness and its reasons as painful, for in the meantime one has acquired sufficient means of undermining the protection against anxiety which the affect-lameness presents. Finally the patient rebels against the danger which threatens from the analysis, the danger of losing the protective psychic armor and of being confronted with his impulses, particularly with his aggression. This rebellion activates his aggressivity and before long the first emotional outburst in the sense of a negative transference occurs, in the form of an attack of hatred. That achieved, the road becomes clear. When the aggressive impulses make their appearance, the affect-block is breached and the patient becomes capable of being analyzed. The difficulty consists in bringing out the aggressivity.

The same is true when narcissistic patients express their character resistance in their way of talking; they will talk, for example, always in a haughty manner, in technical terms, always highly correctly or else confusedly. Such modes of talking form an impenetrable barrier and there is no real experiencing until one analyzes the mode of expression itself. Here also, the consistent interpretation of the behavior results in narcissistic indignation, for the patient does not like to be told that he talks so haughtily, or in technical terms, in order to camouflage his feeling of inferiority before himself and the analyst, or that he talks so confusedly because he wants to appear particularly clever and is unable to put his thoughts into simple words. In this manner, one makes an important breach in the neurotic character and creates an avenue of approach to the infantile origin of the character and the neurosis. Of course, it is insufficient to point out the nature of the resistance at one time or another; the more stubborn the resistance, the more consistently does it have to be interpreted. If the negative attitudes against the analyst which are thus provoked are analyzed at the same time the risk of the patient's breaking off the analysis is negligible.

The immediate effect of the analytic loosening of the character armor and the narcissistic protection mechanism is twofold: First, the loosening of the affects from their reactive anchoring and hiding places; second, the creation of an avenue of approach to the central infantile conflicts, the Oedipus complex and the castration anxiety. An enormous advantage of this procedure is that one not only reaches the infantile experiences as such, but that one analyzes them in the specific manner in which they have been assimilated by the ego. One sees again and again that one and the same piece of repressed material is of different dynamic importance according to the stage which has been reached in the loosening of the resistances. In many cases, the affect of the infantile experiences is absorbed in character defenses; with simple interpretation of the contents, therefore, one may be able to elicit the memories but not the corresponding affects. In such cases, interpretation of the infantile material without *previous* loosening of the affect energies which are absorbed in the character is a serious mistake. It is responsible, for example, for the hopelessly long and relatively useless analyses of compulsive characters.[5] If, one the other hand, one first frees the affects from the defense formations of the character, a new cathexis of the infantile impulses takes place automatically. If the line of character-analytic resistance interpretation is followed, remembering without affect is practically out of the question; the disturbance of the neurotic equilibrium which goes with the analysis of the character from the very beginning makes it practically impossible.

In other cases, the character has been built up as a solid protective wall against the experiencing of infantile anxiety and has served well in this function, although at the expense of much happiness. If such an individual comes to analysis because of some symptom, this protective wall serves

5. The following case illustrates the decisive importance of the neglect of a mode of behavior. A compulsive character who had been in analysis for twelve years without any appreciable result and knew all about his infantile conflicts, such as his central father conflict, talked in the analysis in a peculiarly monotonous, sing-song intonation and kept wringing his hands. I asked him whether this behavior had ever been analyzed, which was not the case. One day it struck me that he talked as if he were praying, and I told him so. He then told me that as a child he had been forced by his father to go to the synagogue and to pray. He had prayed, but only under protest. In the same manner he had also prayed — for twelve long years — before the analyst: "Please, I'll do it if you ask me to, but only under protest." The uncovering of this seemingly incidental detail of his behavior opened the way to the analysis and led to the most strongly hidden affects.

equally well as character resistance and one realizes soon that nothing can be done unless this character armor which covers up and absorbs the infantile anxiety is destroyed. This is the case, for example, in "moral insanity" and in many manic, narcissistic-sadistic characters. In such cases one is often confronted with the difficult question whether the symptom justifies a deep-reaching character-analysis. For one must realize that the character-analytic destruction of the characterological compensation temporarily creates a condition which equals a breakdown of the personality. More than that, in many extreme cases such a breakdown is inevitable before a new, rational personality structure can develop. One may say, of course, that sooner or later the breakdown would have occurred anyhow, the development of the symptom being the first sign. Nevertheless, one will hesitate about undertaking an operation which involves so great a responsibility unless there is an urgent indication.

In this connection another fact must be mentioned: character-analysis creates in every case violent emotional outbursts and often dangerous situations, so that it is important always to be master of the situation, technically. For this reason, many analysts will refuse to use the method of character-analysis; in that case, they will have to relinquish the hope for success in a great many cases. A great many neuroses cannot be overcome by mild means. The means of character-analysis, the consistent emphasis on the character resistance and the persistent interpretation of its forms, ways and motives, are as potent as they are unpleasant for the patient. This has nothing to do with education; rather, it is a strict analytic principle. It is a good thing, however, to point out to the patient in the beginning the foreseeable difficulties and unpleasantness.

e) On the Optimal Conditions for the Analytic Reduction of the Present-Day Material to the Infantile

Since the consistent interpretation of the behavior spontaneously opens the way to the infantile sources of the neurosis, a new question arises: Are there criteria to indicate *when* the reduction of the present-day modes of behavior to their infantile prototypes should take place? This reduction, we know, is one of the cardinal tasks of analysis, but this formulation is too general to be applied in everyday practice. Should it be done as soon as the first signs of the corresponding infantile material appear, or are there reasons for postponing it until a certain later time? First of all it must be pointed out that in many cases the purpose of the reduction — dissolution of the resistance and elimination of the amnesia — is not fulfilled: either there is no more than an intellectual understanding, or the reduction is refuted by doubts. This is explained by the fact that — as is the case with the making conscious of unconscious ideas — the topical process is complete only if combined with the *dynamic-affective* process of the becoming conscious. This requires the fulfilment of two conditions: first, the main resistances must be at least loosened up; second, the idea which is to become conscious — or, in the case of the reduction, is to enter a new association — must become charged with a certain minimum of affect. Now, we know that the affects are usually split off from the repressed ideas, and bound up in the acute transference conflicts and resistances. If, now, one reduces the resistance to the infantile situation before it has fully developed, as soon as there is only a trace of its infantile origin, then one has not fully utilized its affective energies; one has interpreted the content of the resistance without also having mobilized the corresponding affect. That is, dynamic considerations make it necessary not to nip the resistance in the bud, but, on the contrary, to bring it to full development in the transference situation. In the case of chronic, torpid character incrustations there is no other way at all. Freud's rule that the patient has to be brought from acting out to remembering, from the present day to the infantile, has to be complemented by the further rule that *first* that which has become chronically rigid must be brought to new life in the actual transference situation, just as chronic inflammations are treated by first changing them into acute ones. With character resistances this is always necessary. In later stages of the analysis, when one is certain of the patient's cooperation, it becomes less necessary. One gains the impression that with many analysts the immediate reduction of as yet completely immature transference situations is due to the fear of strong and stormy transference resistances; this fits in with the fact that — in spite of better theoretical knowledge — resistances are very often considered something highly unwelcome and only disturbing. Hence the tendency to circumvent the resistance instead of bringing it to full development and then treating it. One should not forget the fact that the neurosis itself is contained in the resistance, that with the dissolution of every resistance we dissolve a piece of the neurosis.

There is another reason why it is necessary to bring the resistance to full development. Because of the complicated structure of each resistance, one comprehends all its determinations and meanings only gradually; the more completely one has comprehended a resistance situation, the more successful is its later interpretation. Also, the double nature of the resistance — present-day and historical — makes it necessary first to make fully conscious the forms of ego defense it contains; only after its present-day meaning has become clear should its infantile origin be interpreted. This is true of the cases who have already produced the infantile material necessary for an understanding of the resistance *which follows*. In the other, more numerous cases, the resistance must be brought to full development for no other reason than that otherwise one does not obtain enough infantile material.

The resistance technique, then, has two aspects: *First, the comprehension of the resistance from the present-day situation through interpretation of its present-day meaning; second, the dissolution of the resistance through association of the ensuing infantile material with the present-day material*. In this way, one can easily avoid the flight into the present-day as well as into the infantile, because equal attention is paid to both in the interpretation work. Thus the resistance turns from an impediment of the analysis into its most potent expedient.

f) Character-Analysis in the Case of Amply Flowing Material

In cases where the character impedes the process of recollection from the beginning, there can be no doubt about the indication of character-analysis as the only legitimate way of introducing the analysis. But what about the cases whose character admits of the production of ample memory material in the beginning? Do they, also, require character-analysis as here described? This question could be answered in the negative if there were cases without a character armor. But since there are no such cases, since the narcissistic protection mechanism always turns into a character resistance — sooner or later, in varying intensity and depth — there is no fundamental difference between the cases. The practical difference, though, is this: In cases such as described above, the narcissistic protection mechanism is at the surface and appears as resistance immediately, while in other cases it is in deeper layers of the personality so that it does not strike one at first. But it is precisely these cases that are dangerous. In the former case one knows what one is up against. In the latter case, one often believes for a long period of time that the analysis proceeds satisfactorily, because the patient seems to accept everything very readily, shows prompt reactions to one's interpretations, and even improvements. But it is just in these patients that one experiences the worst disappointments. The analysis has been carried out, but the final success fails to materialize. One has shot all one's interpretations, one seems to have made completely conscious the primal scene and all infantile conflicts; finally the analysis bogs down in an empty, monotonous repetition of the old material, and the patient does not get well. Worse still, a transference success may deceive one as to the real state of affairs, and the patient may return with a full relapse soon after his discharge.

A wealth of bad experiences with such cases suggested as a rather self-evident conclusion that one had overlooked something. This oversight could not refer to the contents, for in that respect these analyses left little to be desired; it could only be an unrecognized latent resistance which nullified all therapeutic endeavor. It was soon found that these latent resistances consisted precisely in the great willingness of the patients, in the lack of manifest resistances. In comparing them with successful cases, one was struck by the fact that these analyses had shown a constantly even flow, never interrupted by violent emotional outbursts; more importantly, they had taken place in almost constant "positive" transference; rarely, if ever, had there been violent negative impulses toward the analyst. This does not mean that the hate impulses had not been analyzed; only, they did not appear in the transference, or they had been remembered without affect. The prototypes of these cases are the narcissistic affect-lame and the passive-feminine characters. The former show a lukewarm and even, the latter an exaggerated "positive" transference.

These cases had been considered "going well" because they procured infantile material, that is, again because of a one-sided overestimation of the contents of the material. Nevertheless, all through the analysis, the character had acted as a severe resistance in a form which remained hidden. Very often, such cases are considered incurable or at least extremely difficult to handle. Before I was familiar with the latent resistances of these cases, I used to agree with this judgment; since then, I can count them among my most gratifying cases.

The character-analytic introduction of such cases differs from others in that one does not interrupt the flow of communications and does not begin the analysis of the character resistance until such time as the flood of communications and the behavior itself has unequivocally become a resistance. The following case will illustrate this as it will again show how character-analysis leads of itself into the most deeply repressed infantile conflicts. We shall follow this analysis farther along than those previously described, in order to show the logical development of the neurosis in the transference resistances.

A Case of Passive-Feminine Character

Anamnesis

A 24-year-old bank employee came to analysis because of his anxiety states; these had set in a year previously on the occasion of his going to a hygiene exhibit. Even before that he had had *hypochondriac* fears: he thought he had a *hereditary* taint, he would go *crazy* and would *perish in a mental institution*. For these fears, he seemed to have rational grounds: his father had acquired syphilis and gonorrhea ten years previous to his marriage. The paternal grandfather also was supposed to have had syphilis. A paternal uncle was very nervous and suffered from insomnia. The maternal heredity was even more serious: the mother's father committed suicide, as did one of her brothers. A great-aunt was "mentally abnormal." The patient's mother was an anxious and nervous woman.

This double "heredity" (syphilis on the paternal, suicide and psychosis on the maternal side) made the case all the more interesting in that psychoanalysis — in contradistinction to orthodox psychiatry — considers heredity only one of many etiological factors. As we shall see, the patient's idea about his heredity had also an irrational basis. He was cured in spite of his heredity and did not relapse during a follow-up period of five years.

This presentation covers only the first seven months of the treatment which were taken up with the analysis of the character resistances. The last seven months are presented only very briefly because, from the standpoint of resistance and character-analysis, they presented little which would be of interest. What is to be presented here is chiefly the introduction of the treatment, the course of the resistance analysis, and the way it established the contact with the infantile material. We shall follow the red thread of the resistances and their analysis. In reality, of course, the analysis was not as simple as it may appear here.

The patient's anxiety attacks were accompanied by palpitations and a paralysis of all initiative. Even in the intervals between the attacks he was never free of a feeling of malaise. The anxiety attacks often occurred spontaneously but also were precipitated by his reading about mental diseases or suicides in the newspaper. In the course of the past year his working capacity had begun to suffer and he was afraid that he might be discharged because of inefficiency.

Sexually he was severely disturbed. Shortly before the visit to the hygiene exhibit, he had attempted coitus with a prostitute and had failed. He said that this had not bothered him particularly. There was very little conscious sexual desire: he said he did not suffer from his sexual abstinence. A few years earlier, he had succeeded in carrying out the sexual act, although he had suffered from a premature and pleasureless ejaculation.

Asked whether his anxiety states had not had any precursors, he related that already as a child he had been very apprehensive, and particularly during puberty he had been *afraid of world catastrophes*. Thus he was very much afraid when in 1910 the end of the world through a collision with a comet was predicted; he was surprised that his parents could talk about it so calmly. This "fear of catastrophe" gradually subsided, being completely replaced by his fear of the hereditary taint. He had had severe anxiety states since childhood, although less frequently.

Apart from the hypochondriac idea of the hereditary taint, the anxiety states and the sexual weakness, there were no symptoms. Awareness of illness was at first present only with regard to the anxiety states which was the symptom which bothered him most. The idea of the hereditary taint was too well rationalized and the sexual weakness produced too little suffering to produce insight into their pathological character. Symptomatologically speaking, then, we were dealing with the hypochondriac form of anxiety hysteria with a particularly marked actual-neurotic core (stasis neurosis).

The diagnosis was hysterical character with hypochondriac anxiety hysteria. The diagnosis "hysterical character" is based on the analytic findings concerning his fixations. Phenomenologically, he was a typical passive-feminine character: he was always over-friendly and humble; he kept apologizing for the most trifling things; on arriving and on leaving he made several deep bows. In addition, he was *awkward, shy and circumstantial*. If he was asked, for example, whether his hour could be changed, he did not simply say, Yes, but assured me at length that he was completely at my disposal, that he was agreeable to any change I wished to make, etc. When he asked for something, he would stroke the analyst's arm. When I first mentioned the possibility of a distrust of the analysis, he returned on the same day, highly perturbed, saying that he could not stand the thought of my thinking him distrustful; he asked repeatedly for forgiveness in case he should have said thing that could have given me any such impression.

The Development and Analysis of the Character Resistance

The analysis developed according to the resistances which were determined by this kind of character, as follows:

After being told the fundamental rule, he talked rather fluently about his family and the hereditary taint. He asserted that he loved both his parents equally well but had more respect for his father whom he described as an energetic, clear-thinking person. The father had always *warned him against masturbation and extramarital sexual intercourse*. He had told him about his own bad experiences, his syphilis and gonorrhea, of his relationships with women which had come to a bad end; all this with the intention of saving the patient from similar experiences. The father had never beaten him but had always gotten his way by telling him, "I'm not forcing you, I only advise you to . . ."; this, however, had been done very forcefully. The patient described the relationship with his father as very good and his father as his very best friend in whom he had the greatest confidence.

Soon he switched to an extensive description of the relationship with his mother. She was always very solicitous and kind. He was also very kind to her; on the other hand he let her wait on him hand and foot. She took care of his laundry, brought breakfast to his bed, sat beside him until he went to sleep, even now, she combed his hair, in a word, he led the life of a pampered mother's boy.

After six weeks, he was *close to becoming conscious of the wish for coitus*. Apart from this, he had been fully conscious of the tender relationship with his mother, in part he had known it even before the analysis: he had often thrown his mother on his bed to which she had reacted with "bright eyes and flushed cheeks." When she would come in her nightgown to say good night to him, he would embrace her and press her against him. Though he always tried to emphasize the sexual excitation on the part of his mother — undoubtedly in order to give away less of his own intentions — he mentioned several times, parenthetically as it were, that he himself had definitely felt sexual excitation.

A very cautious attempt to make him understand the real significance of these things, however, led to a violent resistance: he could assure me, he said, that he felt exactly the same thing with other women. I had made this attempt by no means in order to interpret the incest phantasy to him but only in order to see whether I was correct in surmising that this straight advance of his in the direction of the historically important incest love was actually a manoeuvre to divert attention from something that *at present* was much more important. The material about his mother was unequivocal; it really appeared as if he needed only one more step to arrive at the core. But something militated against the interpretation of this material: the content of his communications was in striking contrast to the content of his dreams and to his over-friendly behavior.

For this reason, I centered my attention more and more on his behavior and on his dream material. He produced no associations to his dreams. During the session, he enthused about the analysis and the analyst, while outside he was very much concerned about his future and ruminated about his hereditary taint.

The content of the dreams was of a twofold nature: On the one hand, they also contained incest phantasies; what he did not express during the day he expressed in the manifest dream content. For example, in one dream he went after his mother with a knife, or crept through a hole before which his mother was standing. On the other hand, there was often some obscure *murder story,* the hereditary taint, a crime which somebody committed or *derisive remarks made by somebody,* or *distrust* expressed by somebody.

During the first 4 to 6 weeks of the analysis, we had obtained the following material: his statements regarding the relationship with his mother; his anxiety states and the heredity idea; his over-friendly, submissive behavior; his dreams, those which continued the incest phantasy and those of murder and distrust; and certain indications of a positive mother transference.

Confronted with the choice of interpreting his clear-cut incest material or to emphasize the signs of his distrust, I chose the latter. For there could be no doubt that here was a *latent resistance* which for many weeks did not become manifest because it consisted precisely in that the patient presented too much and was too little inhibited. As was shown later, it was also the first important transference resistance the specific form of which was determined by the patient's character. *He was deceiving:* by offering up all the material on his experiences, which was therapeutically useless, by his over-friendly behavior, by his many clear-cut dreams, by his seeming confidence in the analyst. He tried *to please* the analyst, as he had tried to please his father all along, and for the same reason: because he was *afraid of him.* If this had been my first case of this nature I could not possibly have known that such behavior was a decisive and dangerous resistance. Previous experience in such cases had shown, however, that such patients are incapable of producing a manifest resistance, over periods of months or even years; and further, that they do not react therapeutically in the least to the interpretations which, prompted by the clear-cut material, one gives them. One cannot say, therefore, that in such cases one should wait until the transference resistance makes its appearance; it is, in fact, present from the very first moment in a fully developed, but typically *hidden* form.

Clearly, the presented heterosexual incest material could not really be material which had broken through from the depths. If one pays any attention to the actual function of the presented material one often finds that deeply repressed impulses are temporarily used for the purpose of warding off *other* contents, without any change in the state of repression taking place. This is a peculiar fact, not easily understood depth-psychologically. It is obvious that from this fact, though, that the direct interpretation of such material is a definite mistake. Such interpretation not only has no therapeutic effect; more than that, it interferes with the maturing of the respective repressed contents for later interpretation. Theoretically one might say that psychic contents appear in consciousness under two totally different conditions: either born by the affects which specifically belong to them, or born by extraneous interests. In the first case, it is the result of the inner pressure of dammed-up excitation, in the latter case it occurs in the service of defense. It is the same difference as that between freely flowing love and manifestations of love which serve to compensate for hatred, that is, reactive love.

In our patient, the handling of the resistance was, of course, far more difficult than it is in the case of manifest resistances. The meaning of the resistance could not be deduced from the patient's communications, but it could be deduced from his behavior and from the seemingly incidental details of many of his dreams. From these it was evident that, for fear of rebelling against his father, he had camouflaged his spite and distrust by reactive love and had escaped anxiety by being submissive.

The first resistance interpretation was given on the fifth day on the occasion of the following dream:

My handwriting is submitted to a graphologist for an opinion. His opinion was: "This man belongs in a mental institution." My mother is completely desperate. I want to commit suicide. Then I wake up.

To the graphologist, he associated Professor Freud. He added that the Professor had told him that analysis cured such diseases as his with "absolute certainty." I called his attention to the following contradiction: since in the dream he was afraid of having to be committed to a mental institution, he apparently did not believe that the analysis would help him. This he could not see; he refused to accept the interpretation and kept insisting that he had the fullest confidence in the analysis.

Until the end of the second month he dreamt much, though little that would have lent itself to interpretation, and continued talking about his mother. I let him talk, without urging him on and without giving interpretations, being careful all the time not to miss any indication of distrust. After the first resistance interpretation, however, he had camouflaged his secret distrust even more thoroughly, until finally he produced the following dream:

> A crime, possibly *a murder, has been committed.* Somehow and against my will, I have been implicated in it. *I am afraid of discovery and punishment.* One of my fellow employees, who impresses me with his courage and decision, is there. I am keenly aware of his superiority.

I emphasized only the fear of discovery and related it to the analytic situation, telling him that his whole attitude indicated that he was hiding something. As early as the following night, he had the following confirmatory dream:

> A crime is going to be committed in our apartment. It is night and I am on the dark stairs. I know that *my father* is in the apartment. I want to go to his aid but *I am afraid of falling into the hands of the enemies.* I want to call the police. I have a roll of paper with me which has all the details of the intended crime on it. I need *a disguise,* otherwise *the leader of the gang,* who has placed a lot of spies, will prevent me. I take a large cape and a false beard and leave the house, bent over like an old man. The leader of the gang stops me and asks one of his men to search me. He finds the roll of paper. I feel that I am going to be lost if he reads its contents. *I act as innocently as possible* and tell him that they are notes which don't mean anything. He says he'll have to look anyhow. There is a moment of painful tension, then, in desperation, a look for a weapon. I find a revolver in my pocket and fire it. The man has disappeared, and suddenly I feel myself very strong. The leader of the gang has changed into a woman. I am seized by a desire for this woman. I pick her up and carry her into the house. I am overcome by a pleasurable feeling, and wake up.

At the end of the dream, we have the whole incest motif before us, but earlier in the dream unmistakable allusions to the patient's masquerading in the analysis. I entered only upon the latter because the patient would have to give up his attitude of deceit before deeper interpretations could be given. This time, however, I went a step further in the resistance interpretation. I told him that not only was he distrustful of the analysis; that, furthermore, by his behavior, he pretended the exact opposite. Upon this, the patient became highly excited, and through six sessions he produced three different hysterical actions:

1. He thrashed around with arms and legs, yelling: "Let me alone, don't come near me, I'm going to kill you, I'm going to squash you!" This action often changed into another:
2. He grabbed his throat and whined in a rattling voice: "Please let me alone, please, I'm not going to do anything any more!"
3. He behaved not like one who is violently attacked but like a girl who is sexually attacked: "Let me alone, let me alone." This, however, was said without the rattling voice and, while during the action of the second type he pulled up his legs, he now spread them apart.

During these six days he was in a manifest resistance, and continued to talk about his hereditary taint, from time to time falling back into the actions just described. Peculiarly enough, as soon as the actions would cease he would continue to talk calmly as if nothing had happened. He only remarked, "Certainly something queer goes on in me, Doctor."

Without entering upon the content I merely told him that apparently he was acting something in front of me which earlier in his life he had experienced or at least fantasied. This explanation pleased him evidently and from now on he acted out much more frequently than before. My resistance interpretation, then, had stirred up an important part of his unconscious which now expressed itself in the form of these actions. The patient, however, was far from understanding these actions analytically; rather, he utilized them in the sense of his resistance: he thought he would please me particularly if he produced these actions very frequently. Later I found out that in his nightly anxiety attacks he behaved just as he did in the second and third action. Although I understood the meaning of the actions and could have told him the meaning in connection with the murder dream, I stuck consistently to the analysis of his character resistance which his actions had made so much more intelligible.

The following picture presented itself of the *layering of the contents of his characterological transference resistance:*

The first action represented his murderous impulses toward his father and, in transference, toward me (deepest layer).

The second action contained the fear of the father because of the murderous impulse (middle layer).

The third action represented his hidden, grossly sexual feminine attitude, the identification with the (violated) woman, and at the same time the passive-feminine defense against the murderous impulses.

He gave himself, then, in order to keep the father from carrying out the punishment (castration).

But even the interpretation of the actions of the most superficial layer was as yet not admissible. The patient might have *seemingly* accepted each and every interpretation, in order to "please" the analyst, but they would have had no therapeutic effect. For the real understanding of the presented unconscious material would have been made impossible by the *transferred feminine defense against a similarly transferred fear of me*. This fear in turn was due to a *hatred* and distrust transferred to me from the father. That is, hatred, fear and distrust were hidden behind his submissive, trusting attitude, a wall from which every interpretation of unconscious material would have bounced back.

For this reason, I continued to interpret only his unconscious deception, telling him that he was producing his actions so frequently in order to please me. I added, however, that in themselves the actions were highly significant, but that we could not get closer to understanding them until he had gained insight into the meaning of his behavior. He objected less to the resistance interpretation but he could still not agree with me. The following night, however, he dreamed for the first time *openly* about his distrust of the analysis:

Dissatisfied because of the failure of the analysis thus far, I go to Professor Freud. As a means of curing my illness, he gives me a long rod in the shape of an ear-spoon. I feel gratified.

During the analysis of this dream he admitted for the first time that he had been somewhat distrustful of the Professor's prognostic optimism and that, on coming to me, he had been disagreeably surprised to find such a young man. I told him I was struck by two things: first, that he had told me this again in order to please me, and second, that he was suppressing something. Somewhat later I found out that he had cheated me in the question of the fee.

During this consistent work on his character resistance, on his deception through obedience and submission, there flowed increasingly rich material from different age periods, about his infantile relationship with his mother, his relationships with young men, his infantile anxiety, the pleasure he had found as a child in being sick, etc. Of all this, nothing was interpreted except what had an immediate connection with his character resistance.

The dreams about his distrust and his hidden derisive attitude became more frequent. A few weeks later, for example, he had the following dream:

My father remarks that he never dreams. I say to him that certainly is not true, that obviously he forgets his dreams because they consist largely of forbidden wishes. *He laughs scornfully.* I get excited, saying that this is the theory of no less a man than Professor Freud. But while I say this I am somehow worried.

I showed him that he let his father laugh scornfully because he himself did not dare do so and pointed out the worry in the dream which I interpreted as the sign of a bad conscience.

He accepted this interpretation, and during the next 10 days the question of the fee was discussed. It turned out that during the initial interview he had consciously lied to me, "in order to protect himself," that is, because he distrusted my honesty. Without being asked about it, he mentioned the amount of money which he had at his disposal, a lower amount than what he actually had. As usual, I had told him my average fee and my minimum fee. On the basis of his statements, I took him at the minimum fee. He was perfectly able to pay more, however; not only because he had more savings and a better salary than he had said but also because his father defrayed half the expense of the analysis.

The Reduction of the Present-Day Material to the Infantile

During the discussion of the "money affair," always in connection with his character resistance, his secret fear and distrust, he once made a slip of the tongue, saying, "I had wished my money in the bank to become steadily bigger" [instead of "more"]. With that, he betrayed the connection between money and penis and *the fear of losing the money and the fear of losing his penis.* I did not interpret the slip because I did not want to interpret the castration anxiety as such too early; I only remarked that his tendency to economize must have something to do with his fear of catastrophe, that apparently he felt more secure when he had more money. He accepted this with real understanding and brought confirming associations from childhood: Very early, he had begun to save up pennies. He had never forgiven his father for having once taken his savings, without asking him, and having spent them. *For the first time he uttered spontaneously a reproach to the father;* this reproach referred consciously to the money, unconsciously, of course, to the castration danger. In this connection I said that his father, in suppressing the patient's sexuality as he did, had acted with the best intentions, but unwisely. The patient admitted that he had often had thoughts along this line but had never dared to contradict his father who, he thought, acted only in the patient's best interests. It was yet too early to tell him that this acquiescence of his was based on a deep guilt feeling and a fear of the father.

From now on the analysis of the transference resistance proceeded hand in hand with the analysis of the hidden negative attitude toward the father. Every aspect of the transference situation was related to the father and was understood by the patient who at the same time produced a wealth of material about his real attitude toward him. True, all his productions were still strongly censored, not yet accessible to deep interpretation, but the analysis of his childhood was correctly begun. He no longer produced the material as a fence in order to evade other things, but, as a result of the analysis of the character defense, in the growing conviction that his relationship with his father had not been what he had believed it to be, and that it had had a harmful influence on his development.

Every time he came close to the murder phantasy his anxiety increased. The dreams became shorter and less frequent but clearer and the connection with the analytic situation closer. The material which previously had been used as a fence no longer appeared. Everything else was in close connection with his father complex: his phantasy of being a woman, and his incest wish. In the course of the next six weeks, undisguised castration dreams appeared for the first time, without any corresponding interpretation or hint on my part:

1. I am lying in my bed, suddenly get scared and see that my former school principal sits on me. I wrestle with him and get him under me, but he gets one hand free and *threatens my penis.*

2. My older brother climbs through a window into our apartment. He tells somebody to bring him a sword because *he wants to kill me. But I get the start of him and kill him.*

We see, then, how the basic conflict with the father unfolds more and more clearly, without any specific effort on my part, merely as the result of correct resistance analysis.

In this phase, there were repeated blocks and definite manifestations of distrusting the analysis. The resistance was now connected with the fee question: he distrusted my honesty. The doubts and the distrust always appeared when he came closer to the hatred of his father, the castration complex and the murder phantasy. True, the resistances were still sometimes masked by feminine surrender, but now it was no longer difficult to get behind this mask.

After a five weeks' vacation, the analysis was resumed. The patient, who had not taken a vacation, had lived with a friend during this time, because his parents had been out of town and he had been afraid of being alone. His anxiety states had not subsided; on the contrary, they had become more intense after my leaving. In this connection he told me that as a child he was always afraid when his mother left, that he always wanted to have her around, and that he was angry with his father when he took her to a concert or the theatre.

It was rather clear, then, that besides his negative father transference he had developed a strong tender mother transference. This had existed from the very beginning, alongside with the reactive, passive-feminine attitude; the patient, comparing the vacation period with the preceding months, stated that he had felt very secure with me. He found out for himself that with me he felt as safe and secure as with his mother. I did not enter upon this, for the tender mother transference was as yet no interference; on the other hand, it was too early for an analysis of the mother transference, and his reactive-feminine father transference, as a result of the interruption, was again as strong as before. He talked again in a humble and submissive manner as he had done in the beginning of the analysis, and largely about his relationship with his mother.

On the third and fourth day after the resumption of the analysis he had two dreams about the *incest wish, his infantile attitude toward his mother, and the phantasy of the maternal womb.* In connection with these dreams, he remembered bathroom scenes with his mother. She had washed him until he was 12 years old, and he could never understand why his pals teased him about it. Then he remembered his childhood fear of criminals who might break into the apartment and kill him. In other words, the analysis already revived the infantile anxiety hysteria, without any corresponding interpretations or hints having been given. A deep-reaching analysis of these dreams was avoided because his whole attitude was again a deceptive one. A dream of the next night was still more explicit:

1. I am hiking through the Arnbrechtthal, where I spent my summer vacations when I was five or six, with the intention of reviving childhood impressions. Suddenly I get to a place one cannot get out of except through a castle. The doorkeeper opens the gate and says that I cannot visit the castle at this time. I say that this was not my

intention; I merely wanted to get into the open through the castle. The proprietress of the castle appears, an elderly lady who seeks to win me with her coquettish behavior. I want to retire, but suddenly notice that I have forgotten my key (which opens my trunks and seems to be otherwise of great importance to me) in the private box of the castle lady. I have a feeling of discomfort which disappears when the box is opened and the key is returned to me.

2. My mother calls me from upstairs. I grab a newspaper, roll it into the shape of a penis, and go to my mother.

3. I am in a large room with my cousin and her mother. My cousin, whose looks please me, is dressed only in a shirt, and so am I. I embrace her. Suddenly I find that I am much smaller than she, for my penis is halfway between her knees and her genital. I have an ejaculation and am very much embarrassed because there might be stains on my shirt which would give me away.

In the cousin, he himself recognized his mother. In connection with being undressed, he mentioned that he never took off his clothes on the occasions of his attempts at coitus, that he had some vague fear of doing so.

In this dream, the incest phantasy (in part 2 and 3) and the castration anxiety (part 1) were clearly expressed. Why did he censor so little? In view of his obvious deception manoeuvres I avoided interpretations or making attempts to get further associations. I first wanted the theme to unfold itself more; more importantly, it should not be discussed *before the next transference resistance had become manifest and had been eliminated.*

This resistance was not long in coming. It came in connection with a remark about the second dream part which I had let slip against my better knowledge. I had called his attention to the fact that once before he had dreamt about a paper penis. This remark was unnecessary, and he reacted to it—in spite of the clear-cut manifest dream content—with one of his typical resistances: "Yes, surely, but . . ." That night, he had a violent anxiety attack and two dreams. One concerned his "money resistance" (transferred castration anxiety), the other brought forth, *for the first time, the primal scene,* which, in the last analysis, motivated the money resistance:

1. I am in a crowd in the Prater, standing in front of an amusement stand. Suddenly I notice that a man behind me tries to steal my wallet from my hip pocket. I reach for it, and at the last moment prevent the theft.

2. I am in the last car of a train in the region south of the Wörthersee. In a curve, I suddenly notice that on the one-track line another train comes toward us. The catastrophe seems inevitable; in order to save myself, I jump off.

Here it was shown that I had done well not to interpret his incest dreams, for a strong latent resistance was in the way. We also see that the resistance dream had a close connection with his infantile anxiety (fear of castration—fear of the primal scene). Between his third and sixth year, he used to spend his summer vacation at the Wörthersee.

He had no associations to the dream. Relating the man in the first dream to myself, I brought up again his whole attitude, his secret fear of me and his hidden distrust in the money matter, without, for the time being, mentioning the connection with the fear of catastrophes. From the second dream, I emphasized only the "inevitable catastrophe" and reminded him that to him money meant a protection against catastrophes, that he was afraid I might rob him of this protection.

He did not quite agree, seeming rather horrified at the idea of seeing a robber in me; but he also did not refute the interpretation. In the next few days he produced dreams in which he assured me of his attachment and his trust; I also appeared as his mother. In addition, there was a new element: *his mother as a man.* She appeared as a Japanese. This we did not understand until many months later when the significance of his infantile phantasies about the Russo-Japanese War became clear. The Russian was the father, the Japanese—because of his smallness—the mother. Furthermore, his mother had at that time worn Japanese pyjamas: the mother in pants. Repeatedly, he made a slip of the tongue, speaking of "mother's penis." The "school pal" in many dreams also represented the cousin who resembled his mother.

The clear-cut incest dreams had been resistance dreams: they were to hide his fear of the woman, the woman with the penis.

From then on, for about six weeks, the analysis took a peculiar zigzag-like course: Dreams and communications regarding his money resistance alternated with others about his desire for his mother, about the mother as man, the dangerous father and the castration anxiety in its various forms. In the interpretation work, I always took the money resistance (= castration anxiety) as the starting point, and kept deepening the analysis of the infantile situation from there, every day. This was not difficult because *the infantile material was always in closest connection with the transference situation.* Not all the infantile fears and desires which came up now, however, also appeared in the transference; rather, the transference revolved completely about the castration anxiety which became more and more acute. Only the core of the infantile situation had appeared in the transference resistance. Since I was certain that the analysis proceeded in order, I could postpone deep interpretations until the proper time; all I did was to work consistently on the fear of me, by constantly relating it with the fear of the father.

What I was trying to do was to penetrate to the infantile incest phantasies by eliminating the transferred father resistance as thoroughly as possible in order to obtain them as free of resistance as possible. This would avert the danger of wasting the most important interpretations. Thus I did not yet interpret the incest material which came to the fore increasingly clearly and consistently.

Schematically, the topical layering of the resistance and the material at the beginning of this phase was the following:

1. The foreground was occupied by his castration anxiety in the form of his money resistance.
2. This he tried continually to ward off by means of a feminine attitude toward me; this was, however, much less successful than at the beginning.
3. The feminine attitude covered up a sadistic-aggressive attitude toward me (i.e., the father) and was accompanied by
4. a deep tender mother attachment which also was transferred to me.
5. With these ambivalent attitudes which were centered in the transference resistance were connected the incest wishes which had appeared in dreams, the masturbation anxiety, his longing for the maternal womb and the violent fear originating from the primal scene. Of all this, nothing had been interpreted except his deception and its motives, and the fear and hatred of the father.

During the fifth month of the analysis he had his first incestuous masturbation anxiety dream:

I am in a room. A young woman with a round face sits at the piano. I can see only the upper part of her body, the rest is hidden by the piano. I hear the voice of the analyst beside me: "You see, that's the cause of your neurosis." I feel more close to the woman but then I suddenly get frightened and yell out loudly.

On the previous day, in the course of a dream interpretation, I had said to him, "You see, this is one of the causes of your neurosis." I had been referring to his infantile attitude, his desire to be loved and to be taken care of. As if the patient had known the true cause of his neurosis, he connected this remark with his repressed *masturbation anxiety*. The subject of masturbation came up again in connection with the incest motif. He woke up with anxiety. The fact that the lower part of the woman's body in the dream was not visible expressed his fear of the female genital. Nevertheless, I left the subject alone because he was still at the height of his resistance, and had no associations to the dream.

Then the patient had a dream in which "a naked family" consisting of father, mother and child were enveloped by a gigantic snake. Another dream was the following:

1. I am lying in bed, the analyst sitting beside me. He says: "Now I'm going to show you the cause of your neurosis." I yell with fear—but there is also a pleasurable sensation—and I almost faint. He goes on saying that he is going to analyze me in our bathroom. This idea seems pleasant to me. As we open the door to the bathroom, it is dark inside.

2. I walk through the woods with my mother. I notice that we are being followed by a robber. I notice a revolver in my mother's dress and take it in order to shoot the robber. Walking fast, we reach an inn. As we mount the steps, the robber is on our heels. I fire a shot at him. The bullet, however, *changes into a money bill.* For the time being we are safe but the robber, who sits in the anteroom, may still be planning something bad. *In order to win his favor, I give him another bill.*

That I was correct in not interpreting those dreams—clear-cut as they were —was shown in the fact that the patient, apart from not having any associations, did not refer with one word to the person of the robber. Instead he kept silent or talked excitedly about "all the money" which he had to pay and expressed his doubts as to whether the analysis would help him.

No doubt, this resistance was also directed against a discussion of the incest material. But such an interpretation would not have done any good; I had to wait for the proper opportunity of interpreting his money anxiety as castration anxiety.

In the first part of the "robber dream" the analysis is going to take place in the bathroom. Later we found that, in masturbating, he had felt safest in the bathroom. In the second part of the dream I (the father) appear as robber (= castrator). *His present-day resistance* (distrust in money matters), then, *had the closest connection with his old masturbation anxiety* (castration anxiety).

With regard to the second part of the dream I told him that he was afraid I might do him harm but that this fear really referred to his father. After some hesitation, he accepted this interpretation and began spontaneously to talk about his exaggerated friendliness. He recognized his exaggerated friendliness toward his superiors to be an expression of a vague fear that he might do something wrong; they also should be kept from noticing that secretly he ridiculed them. To the extent to which he took an objective view of his character and began to look through it, he became freer, more candid and open, in the analysis as well as outside. He dared to express criticism and began to be ashamed of his previous behavior. *For the first time, the neurotic character became a foreign-body-like symptom.* With that, the character-analysis had achieved its first success: the character began to be analyzed.

The money resistance continued to exist, and in the dreams, in connection with the primal scene, the fear for his penis came more and more to the fore; this *without the slightest help on my part.*

This fact deserves special emphasis. With systematic and consistent analysis of the character resistance, one need not make any effort to obtain the infantile material. It flows spontaneously, increasingly clear-cut and closely associated with the actual resistance—provided, of course, that one has not disturbed this process by premature interpretations of the infantile material. The less one tries to penetrate into childhood, the more correctly one works on the resistances, the faster does one get there.

This was again exemplified after the interpretation that he was afraid of being harmed. The following night he dreamed that he passed a chickenyard and saw a chicken killed. A woman was stretched out on the ground and another woman repeatedly stuck a big fork into her. Then he embraced a girl; his penis was *halfway between her knees and her genital,* and he had an ejaculation.

Since the money resistance had somewhat subsided, an attempt was made to interpret the dream. To the chickenyard he associated that as a child, during the summer in the country, he had often watched animals having sexual intercourse. At that time, we had as yet no idea how important the detail "summer in the country" was. In the first woman he recognized his mother, without, however, being able to explain her position. Only about the dream with the ejaculation he had more to say. In the dream, he had appeared as a child; he remembered that he used to press against women until he had an ejaculation.

It seemed a good sign that the patient, in spite of the undisguised material, did not offer any interpretations. If I had interpreted symbols or important unconscious contents *before* the analysis of his resistances, he would have immediately accepted the interpretations for reasons of resistance, and we would have gone from one chaotic situation to the other.

My interpretation of his fear of being harmed had set the analysis of his character in full motion. For days, the money resistance was absent, he constantly discussed his infantile behavior and brought example after example of situations in his life in which he had acted "cowardly" and "slyly," modes of behavior which he now honestly condemned. I tried to convince him that such behavior had been largely the result of his father's influence.

This attempt, however, provoked the most violent resistance. *He did not yet dare to reproach his father.*

After a longer interval he dreamed again of that theme behind which I surmised the primal scene:

I am standing at the seashore. Some polar bears tumble about in the water. Suddenly they become anxious, and I see the back of an enormous fish emerge from the water. He chases a bear and injures him with frightful bites. Finally he lets go of the mortally wounded bear. The fish himself, however, is severely wounded; a stream of blood gushes from his gills.

I pointed out that his dreams were always of a cruel nature. For several sessions he related his masturbation phantasies and various cruel acts he used to indulge in before puberty. Most of these were determined by the "sadistic concept of the sexual act." After analysis, I had him write them down:

3rd to 5th year: During summer vacation, I happen to witness the butchering of pigs. I hear the groaning of the animals and see the blood spurt from them. I feel a deep pleasure.

4th to 6th year: The idea of the butchering of animals, especially horses, fills me with pleasure.

5th to 11th year: I like to play with tin soldiers. I arrange battles in which there is always hand-to-hand fighting. I press the bodies of the soldiers against each other; the favored soldiers get the others down.

6th to 12th year: I press two ants together so that they grab each other with their tweezers. Biting into each other, they fight for their lives. I scatter sugar between two ant colonies which then engage in regular battles. I also found pleasure in putting a wasp and a fly together in a waterglass; after a while, the wasp would bear down on the fly and bite off its wings, legs and head.

12th to 14th year: I keep a terrarium and like to watch the animals having sexual intercourse. I also observe this in the chickenyard where I like to see how the stronger cocks chase away the weaker ones.

8th to 16th year: I like to wrestle with the chambermaids. In later years, I used to pick them up, carry them to a bed and throw them down on it.

5th to 12th year: I like to play with railroads, running the train through the whole apartment, making tunnels of boxes, chairs, etc. I also try to imitate the noise of the locomotive.

15th year, *masturbation phantasies:* Regularly, I am only an *onlooker.* The woman tries to fight off the man *who usually is considerably smaller than she.* After a long struggle, the woman is *overpowered.* The man brutally grabs her breasts, loins or thighs. *I never think of a male or female genital and never of the sexual act itself.* In the moment in which the woman ceases her resistance I have an orgasm.

The situation at this time was the following: He was ashamed of his cowardice and remembered the sadism in his past. The analysis of the phantasies and actions just summarized lasted until the end of the treatment. It made him much freer in the analysis, and more courageous and aggressive generally, but for the time being there was still an apprehensive note in his behavior. His anxiety states had become less frequent but kept recurring again and again in connection with the money resistance.

We see here again that the production of the genital incest material served mainly the purpose of covering up his infantile sadism, although, of course, it was at the same time an attempt to progress toward a genital object cathexis. His genital striving, however, was intermixed with sadistic strivings; the therapeutic task, therefore, was that of crystallizing it out of this intermixture.

Early in the sixth month of the analysis came the first opportunity of interpreting his *fear for his penis,* on the occasion of the following dreams:

1. I am lying on a sofa in an open field on summer vacation. A girl I know comes toward me and lies on top of me. I get her under me and attempt intercourse. Though I am getting an erection, I notice that *my penis is too short* to have intercourse. This makes me very sad.
2. I am reading a drama. The people in it are 3 Japanese, father, mother and a child of four. I feel that the piece will come to a *tragic ending.* What moves me most is *the fate of the child.*

For the first time, an attempt at coitus appeared in the manifest dream content. The second part, in which there was an allusion to the primal scene (age 4) was not analyzed at this time. In uninterrupted discussion of his cowardice and apprehensiveness, he himself came to talk of his penis. Now I told him that his fear of being harmed or cheated really related to his genital. The question why and of whom he was afraid was not yet discussed, nor was the real meaning of the fear interpreted. The interpretation seemed plausible to him, but now he developed a resistance which lasted for six weeks and which was based on *a passive-feminine, homosexual defense against the castration anxiety.*

That the patient was in a resistant phase could be seen from the following indications: He did not openly rebel or express any doubts; instead, he became again exaggeratedly polite, friendly and submissive. His dreams, which in the course of the resistance analysis had become less frequent, shorter and clearer, because again long and confused. His anxiety states became as frequent and intense as ever; in spite of this, he did not express any distrust of the analysis. The heredity idea also cropped up again; here, his doubt about the outcome of the analysis found a disguised expression. As in the beginning of the analysis, he began again to act a woman who is being raped. In his dreams also, the passive-feminine attitude was predominant. There were no longer any dreams about coitus or ejaculation. We see, then, how—in spite of the fact that the analysis of his character had progressed quite far—the old character resistance reappeared in its full force when a new layer of the unconscious came to be analyzed. This layer was that which was most decisive for his character: his castration anxiety.

Consequently, the subject of the resistance analysis was not the castration anxiety which had provoked the resistance but again his total behavior. For full six weeks, hardly anything was done but exclusive interpretation of his behavior as a protection against dangers. Every detail of his behavior was scrutinized in this light and brought to his attention; with this, we gradually progressed to the core of his behavior, the fear for his penis.

The patient kept trying to evade me by "offering up" infantile material, but the meaning of this was also constantly interpreted to him. Gradually he began to realize that he felt a woman also toward me and said this in so many words, adding that he felt sexual excitation in the perineum. I explained this transference phenomenon: He felt my attempts at explaining his behavior to be reproaches, *felt guilty and tried to expiate his guilt by feminine submission.* The deeper meaning of this behavior—identification with the mother because he was afraid to be a man (the father)—I left untouched for the present. Then he produced among other things, the following confirmatory dream:

I'm in the Prater and get to talking with a young fellow. It seems he misunderstands a remark of mine and says that he is willing to give himself to me. In the meantime, we have arrived at our apartment and the fellow gets into my father's bed. His underwear seems to be dirty.

In analyzing this dream I was able again to reduce the feminine transference to the father. Now he remembered for the first time that in his masturbation phantasies he used to imagine himself to be a woman. The dirty underwear led to the analysis of his anal activities and habits (bathroom ceremonials). Another character trait, his circumstantiality, was clarified here.

In resolving the resistance, not only its old form but also its erogenous, anal basis had been discussed. Now I went a step further in the analysis of his character. I explained to him the connection between his submissive behavior and the phantasy of being a woman: his behavior was feminine, that is, exaggeratedly kind, submissive and trusting because he was afraid of being a man. I added that we would have to find out for what reason he was afraid of being a man, that is, in his sense, courageous, open, and honest instead of crawling. Almost as an answer to this question he produced a dream in which the castration anxiety and the primal scene again stood out:

I am at my cousin's, a young, pretty woman [the mother, W.R.]. All of a sudden I have the feeling of being *my own grandfather*. I get terribly depressed. At the same time I feel somehow that I am *the center of a planetary system* and that planets revolve around me. Simultaneously I suppress—still in the dream—my anxiety and am annoyed by my weakness.

The most important detail of this incest dream was his being his own grandfather. There was no doubt that here his fear of a hereditary taint played an important role. It was also clear that he fantasied of creating himself, in identification with his father, that is, of having intercourse with his mother; this, however, was not discussed at this time.

As to the planetary system, he said, it referred to his egotism: "everything revolved around him." I surmised an additional, deeper meaning, namely the primal scene, but did not mention it. For some days he talked almost exclusively about his egotism, his desire of being a child loved by everyone, and realized that he himself neither wanted to love nor was able to love. I showed him the connection between his egotism and his fear for his beloved self and his penis.[6] His next dreams brought out the infantile background:

1. I am undressed and look at my penis which bleeds at the tip. Two girls walk away and I am sad because I assume that they will *despise me because of the smallness of my penis*.
2. I am smoking a cigarette through a cigarette holder. I take it off and realize to my surprise that is a cigar holder. As I put the cigarette back into my mouth, *the tip breaks off*. I have an unpleasant sensation.

Thus, without my doing anything about it, the castration idea began to take definite forms. The patient now interpreted the dreams without my aid and produced a wealth of material concerning his fear of the female genital and his fear of touching his penis or having somebody else touch it. In the second dream, an oral ideal is obvious (cigarette holder). He was struck by the fact that in a woman he desired everything *except* the genital; but what he

6. This, taken in its total setting, should show to some individual psychologists why we psychoanalysts cannot recognize the inferiority feeling as an ultimate factor: because the real problem, and the real work, starts precisely where for Alfred Adler it stops.

desired most was the breast; with that, he began to talk about the oral fixation to his mother.

I told him it was not sufficient to know about his fear of the genital; that one had to find out why he had this fear. In response to this, he dreamed again of the primal scene, without an inkling that he had entered upon my question:

I am behind the last car of a stationary railroad train, just at a switch. A second train goes by and I get *caught between the two trains*.

Before continuing the presentation of the analysis, I should mention the fact that during the seventh month of the treatment, after the resolution of his passive-homosexual resistance, the patient made a courageous move in the direction of a woman. This took place without my knowledge; he mentioned it later more or less in passing. He made the acquaintance of a girl in the park. His mode of sexual activity was this: He pressed himself against the girl, had a strong erection and an ejaculation. The anxiety states gradually subsided. It did not occur to him to have sexual intercourse. Calling this to his attention, I said that apparently he was afraid of sexual intercourse. This he did not admit, using the lack of opportunity as an excuse, until finally he was struck by the infantile manner of his sexual activity. It had occurred in many of his dreams, and now he remembered that as a child he used to press himself against his mother in this manner.

The subject of his incest love with which—deceptively—he had started the analysis came up again; this time, however, with little resistance, certainly without the previous ulterior motive. Thus the analysis of his attitudes took place corresponding to his experiences.

Again and again he rejected the interpretation that he really had desired his mother. The corresponding material which he had produced in the course of seven months was so clear, and the connections, as he himself admitted, so evident, that I did not try to convince him but started to investigate why he was afraid of admitting the fact to himself.

This question had been discussed together with his fear for his penis; thus there were two problems to be solved:

1. What was the origin of his castration anxiety?
2. Why, in spite of conscious agreement, did he not accept the fact of sexual incest love?

The analysis now progressed rapidly in the direction of the primal scene. This phase was ushered in by the following dream:

I am in the hall of a castle where the king and his entourage are assembled. *I deride the king*. His people pounce on me. I'm being thrown down and I feel that they are inflicting deadly cuts on me. My dead body is being dragged away. Suddenly I feel that I'm still alive, *but I keep very still in order to make the gravediggers believe that I'm dead*. There is a thin layer of soil over me and my breath is impeded. *I keep absolutely still and thus keep from being found out*. A little later, I am free. I go again into the palace, a terrible weapon in each hand, perhaps thunderbolts. Whoever opposes me is killed by me.

He thought that the idea of the gravediggers had something to do with his fear of catastrophes. I was able to show him now that this fear, the fear of heredity and the fear for his penis were one and the same thing. I ventured the assumption that the dream contained that scene in his childhood from which the fear for the penis originated.

He was struck by the fact that he "played dead," in order not to be found out. In this connection, he remembered that in his masturbation phantasies he was always the onlooker and he himself brought up the question whether perhaps he had experiences "something like that" with his parents. However, he rejected the idea immediately, saying that he had never slept in his parents' bedroom. This was disappointing, for I was convinced, on the basis of his dream material, that he had actually experienced the primal scene. I pointed out the contradiction and said one should not give up too readily, the analysis would solve it in time. Still in the same session the patient thought he must have seen a certain maid with her friend. Then he remembered two occasions on which he might have watched his parents. He remembered that his bed used to be moved to his parents' bedroom when they had guests. Also, in his preschool years, he had slept in one room with his parents *during summer vacations*. In this connection he recalled the various dreams about the summers in the country and the representation in one of them of the primal scene in the killing of chickens.

In this connection he came back to the acting-out in the beginning of the analysis and his night terrors in childhood. A detail of these fears was now explained: he was afraid of a white female figure coming out from between curtains. Now he remembered that when he used to cry at night his mother would come to his bed, in her nightgown.

Apparently, we had gone too far in this hour, for during the next night he had a definitely derisive resistance dream:

I am standing on a wharf and am about to get on a large boat, as *companion of a mental patient*. Suddenly the whole thing appears to me to be *a play* in which a certain role has been assigned to me. On the gangplank *I have to say the same thing three times,* which I do.

He himself interpreted the getting-on-the-boat as wish for coitus, but I led him to the more important thing, the "play-acting." That he had to say the same thing three times was a derisive allusion to my consistent interpretations. He had to admit that he had often smiled inside about my efforts. He said further that he intended to look up a woman and to have intercourse three times. "To please me," I added. But I also explained to him that this resistance had another, deeper meaning, his avoiding attempts at coitus because of fear of the sexual act.

The following night he had again dreams of homosexual surrender on the one hand and fear of coitus on the other:

1. I meet a young fellow in the street who belongs to the lower classes but looks very healthy and strong. I feel that he is stronger than I and *try to gain his favor.*
2. I am on a skiing tour with the husband of one of my cousins. Going down a steep slope, I find that the snow is sticky and say that this is bad terrain for skiing because *in going down one is bound to fall down frequently.* We come to a road leading along the slope of a mountain. In a sharp curve *I lose a ski which drops into the abyss.*

He did not enter upon the dream at all. Instead, he began with the theme of the fee: he had to pay so much and did not know whether it was going to help at all, he was dissatisfied, was suffering from anxiety again, and so forth.

Now it was possible to reduce the money resistance to the still unresolved genital anxiety and fear of coitus. Now I could show him the deeper motive of his feminine surrender: *When he approached a woman, he became afraid of the consequences and became a woman himself, that is, homosexual and passive in his character.* The fact that he had made himself into a woman he understood very well, but he could not understand why and of what he was so afraid. It was perfectly clear to him that he was afraid of sexual intercourse. But what, was the question, could happen to him?

He was now constantly occupied with this question, but instead of discussing the fear of the father he discussed the fear of the woman. As we know, in his infantile anxiety hysteria he had also been afraid of the woman; he used to say, "the penis of the woman." Up until puberty he had believed that the woman also had a penis. He himself connected this idea with the primal scene the reality of which he was now convinced of.

At the end of the seventh month he dreamed that he saw how a girl lifted her skirt so that her underwear became visible. He turned away like somebody "who sees something that he shouldn't." Now I told him that he was afraid of the female genital because it looked like an injury, a wound, and that he must have been frightened by the first sight of it. This interpretation seemed plausible to him inasfar as he felt the female genital to be not only disgusting but frightening. However, he could not recall an actual experience.

The situation at this time was the following: The core of his symptoms, the castration anxiety, had been worked through but not yet resolved in its deepest and ultimate significance because the close individual connections with the primal scene were still lacking and because the latter had been only deduced but not analytically handled.

One time when these things were again discussed in a period free of resistance and there was nothing tangible to work with, the patient said in a low voice, as to himself: "I must have been caught at one time." He said he had the feeling as if he had done something once in a sly manner and had been caught in doing it. Now the patient remembered that even as a small boy he had secretly rebelled against his father. He had made fun of him behind his back while openly playing the obedient son. In puberty, the rebellion against the father had ceased entirely. That is, the patient had repressed the hatred of his father because he feared him.

His idea of the hereditary taint, also, proved to be a reproach to his father. It meant, "my father has damaged me when he made me." Analysis of the phantasies about the primal scene revealed that the patient imagined himself in the maternal womb while his father had intercourse with his mother. The phantasy of being harmed at the genital combined with the phantasy of the womb into the phantasy that *he was castrated by his father in his mother's womb.*

The remaining part of the analysis can be described briefly. It was relatively free of resistance and consisted plainly of two parts.

The first part was taken up by the working through of his infantile masturbation phantasies and his masturbation anxiety. His castration anxiety manifested itself for a long time in the fear of the female genital. The "injury," the "wound," seemed to prove the reality of castration. Finally, the patient dared masturbate. With that, the anxiety states disappeared completely; this shows that they were due to libido stasis and not to the castration anxiety, for the latter continued to exist. Further analysis of infantile material reduced it sufficiently so that he undertook an attempt at coitus in which he was erectively potent. Subsequent sexual acts revealed two disturbances: he was orgastically impotent, that is, he experienced less pleasure than in masturbation, and his attitude toward the woman was one of indifference and contempt. His genitality was still dissociated into tender and sensual components.

The second part was taken up with the analysis of his orgastic impotence and his infantile narcissism. As always before, he wanted to get everything from the woman, the mother, without having to give anything himself. With great understanding, the patient worked himself on his disturbances. He began to experience his narcissism as painful and finally overcame it, when the last remnant of his castration anxiety, which was anchored in his orgastic impotence, was analytically resolved. He was *afraid of the orgasm* because he thought that the excitation connected with it was harmful. The following dream shows this fear:

I visit a picture gallery. I am struck by a picture called "Drunken Tommy." It is of a young, pretty English soldier in the mountains. It storms, he seems to have lost his way. The hand of a skeleton has taken his arm and seems to be leading him, apparently a symbol that he is *going to meet with disaster*. Another picture is called "Hard Profession." It is also in the mountains. A man and a boy fall down a precipice. At the same time, a knapsack empties: the boy is surrounded by a whitish mass.

The fall represented the orgasm,[7] the whitish mass the sperm. The patient talked about the fears he had experienced during puberty with ejaculation and orgasm. His sadistic phantasies about women also were worked through more thoroughly. A few months later, during the summer, he began a relationship with a young girl; the disturbances were now much milder.

The resolution of the transference created no difficulties because it had been worked on systematically from the very beginning, in its positive as well as its negative aspects. He left the analysis full of hope. In the course of the ensuing five years, I saw the patient five times. His apprehensiveness and anxiety states had entirely disappeared. He considered himself completely healthy and expressed his satisfaction about having lost his crawling and sly traits and was now able to meet difficulties courageously. His potency had still increased since the termination of the treatment.

7. *Cf.* the symbolism of the orgasm in Die Funktion des Orgasmus, 1927.
Translator's note: Cf. also The Function of the Orgasm, Orgone Institute Press, 1942, 1948.

Summary

Arrived at the conclusion of this history, we are keenly aware of the difficulty of putting analytic processes into words. But that should not keep us from sketching at least the rough outlines, in order to bring about an understanding in the problems of character-analysis. To summarize:

1. Our case is the prototype of the passive-feminine character who—no matter what symptoms make him seek analytic help—always presents us with the same type of character resistance. It also demonstrates to us the typical mechanisms of the latent negative transference.

2. Technically, the main emphasis was on the analysis of the passive-feminine character resistance, on the deceiving through exaggerated friendliness and submissive behavior. This procedure made the infantile material develop in the transference neurosis according to its own inner laws. This prevented the patient from gaining mere intellectual insight into his unconscious, for reasons of feminine surrender (in order "to please"), which would have had no therapeutic effect.

3. The case history shows that with systematic and consistent emphasis on the character resistance and with avoidance of premature interpretations, the corresponding infantile material appears increasingly clearly and unequivocally *of itself*. This makes the subsequent interpretations of meaning and of symptoms incontrovertible and therapeutically effective.

4. The case history shows that one can begin to work on the character resistance as soon as one has recognized its present-day meaning and function, that is, without knowing the corresponding infantile material. The emphasis on and the interpretation of its present-day meaning brought the infantile material to the fore, without any necessity for symptom interpretations or suggestions. When the connection with the infantile material was established *the resolution of the character resistance began*. The subsequent symptom interpretations took place under conditions of full cooperation on the part of the patient. The resistance analysis consisted of two typical phases: first, the *emphasis* on its form and present-day meaning, and second, its *resolution* with the aid of the infantile material thus brought to the fore. In this case, the difference between a character resistance and a simple resistance consisted in the difference between politeness and submissiveness on the one hand, and simple doubt and distrust in the analysis on the other. It was only the former which belonged to his character; they were the *form* in which his distrust was expressed.

5. Consistent interpretation of the latent negative transference resulted in the liberation of his repressed and masked aggressivity toward the analyst, superiors and the father. This eliminated the passive-feminine attitude which, of course, was nothing but a reaction formation against the repressed aggressivity.

6. The repression of his aggression against the father brought with it the repression of his genital urge for the woman. Conversely, under analysis, the masculine genital striving reappeared, together with the aggressivity; this led to the cure of the impotence.

7. The apprehensiveness in his character disappeared with the castration anxiety, when the aggressivity became conscious, and the anxiety states disappeared when he gave up his sexual abstinence. The orgastic discharge of the energy which had manifested itself as stasis anxiety resulted in the elimination of the "somatic core of the neurosis."

In conclusion, I trust that the presentation of these cases will shake the opinion of some of my opponents who contend that I impose a "ready-made schema" on every patient. It will make clear the meaning of the contention which I have made for years: that for each and every case there is only *one* technique which has to be derived from its individual structure.

B. Criticisms of Reich's Position

5. Problems of Therapy[1]

Herman Nunberg

The need for a technique of psychoanalysis, that is, for precise directions on how mentally ill persons are to be treated, is self-evident. This need has always existed; however, in the course of time it increased to such an extent that it produced a series of proceedings which, allegedly, had only to be followed conscientiously in order to achieve certain success. The failure bound to result from such procedures is based, I think, on the one-sidedness, and in a sense, preconceived opinion, with which the patient is approached. It is certainly tempting to overestimate a real or presumed discovery and to make use of it immediately in therapy.

Jung was most impressed by the mythological formations, and now believes that the human mind is a myth. Adler found feelings of inferiority and he believes that man consists exclusively of feelings of inferiority. Rank saw in neurosis a reaction to birth anxiety. Reik and Alexander are of the opinion that punishment is the most important motive force for neurosis. Reich bases his theory on the character changes appearing in the reaction-formations of the compulsive neurosis, believes that character consists of resistances only, and wants to unroll the entire analysis from a single so-called character trait.

Aside from the fact that all of these so-called discoveries are not new and that they had long before found their proper place in the psychoanalytic system, it is impossible to set in motion an apparatus as complicated as the human psyche from one single point.

If one wants to discuss practical advice for treatment, i.e., the technique of psychoanalysis, one first has to try to take account of the theoretical bases of therapy. Therefore I do not intend here to discuss technique, but rather shall attempt to clarify the changes that occur in the human being by means of the present method of treatment, as recommended by Freud.

Before undertaking a description of the process of recovery one must in the first place be clear about the nature of the illness. Psychic illness is by no means a simple process. We distinguish between a primary and a secondary process of illness. The *primary* process, thus the core of the neurosis, is

Originally published in the *International Zeitschrift für Psychoanalyse* 14 (1928). Originally published in English in 1961.

formed by anxiety in relation to an instinctual danger and by the neurotic conflict closely connected with it. The conflict may be either cause or result of the anxiety, according to stratification. The *secondary* process of illness is formed by the symptoms in the broadest meaning of the word; the ego indeed introduces all the complicated processes of repression and other defense measures in order to withdraw from the danger situation, to *avoid the unpleasure and to ban the anxiety*. And the entire symptomatology results from this defensive struggle. But at the same time the success of the defensive struggle means to the ego a solution of the neurotic conflict. The final result of this attempt at a solution is inhibition and modification of the course followed by the instincts, i.e., the barring of the ideational content from consciousness and of the affectivity from motor discharge.[2]

Consequently one might assume that the first therapeutic task is to help the instincts to discharge and to procure access to consciousness for them. Aside from the anxiety felt by the ego at such a direct attempt, there are other reasons for which this fails in most cases. The longer the neurosis lasts, the more the personality loses contact with reality. There are cases, indeed, in which the slightest contact with the external world results in an even more violent rejection of the world. The neurotic is *over-sensitive* to external and internal stimuli. The patient becomes *asocial* through his illness, he is self-sufficient, and he satisfies his needs not through changes of the outside world but through auto-plastic changes of his own organization. Certain parts of the ego are split off in the neurosis; the ego becomes more primitive in its reactions, especially more infantile in relation to danger situations. It clings to infantile reactions and considers as dangerous stimuli that are no longer so; on the other hand, the actual conditions that demand adequate adaptation to reality have thoroughly changed since the first fixations took place. Hence there is little prospect of success in the attempt to influence this *split-off ego*. Aside from this estrangement from reality, there is another difficulty that stems from the ego. The ego has repressed the instinctual demands, and erected various dams against them in the shape of reaction-formations. The ego does not affirm, but rejects the strivings of the id, and thus is deprived of its synthetic function, of its part as mediator between the contrasting impulses within the id on the one hand, and between these impulses and the outside world on the other. Even more: by virtue of their continuous nature the instincts cannot be banned by carrying out a defense measure just one time. Rather, the ego has to expend defensive forces constantly in order to maintain the first repressions. We call this permanent expenditure *resistance;* it manifests itself as a protector of repression. If one is clear about this nature of the resistances one will not consider it likely that an ego that expends so much energy for protection from instinct danger, an ego that has prepared itself for the rejection of instinctual life and opposes any weakening of this rejection, is going to abandon these resistances without a struggle. Certainly the power of holding out is not the same in each of these "resistances." Some of them increase the capacity of the ego to oppose the external influence and veil the connections to the point of utter obscurity, others yield more easily. However, it is impossible to state a priori how obstinate the expected resistance is going to be. One might assume that those resistances that develop last in the course of the neurosis, as for instance, the secondary gain from illness, will be destroyed most easily through direct influence. But not even that is always true. An excellent example is the accident-neurosis. Yet in other forms of illness also, such as obsessional neurosis, it may take the patient a very long time to give up his secondarily erected ideal of a hypermoral person; and in paranoia a similar narcissistic resistance, such as pride in the intellectual achievement of the delusional system, is altogether unassailable. The actual situation is that certain resistances may be influenced directly at one time, and at another time only by being undermined from the depths. Resistance due to the sense of guilt, i.e., that which develops under the influence of the superego might, in the same way, appear easily assailable. But the feeling of guilt has an unconscious root, and in the form of the unconscious need for punishment it energetically opposes any external influence. This powerful resistance not only serves the superego, but in its deepest layer also gratifies the instinctual needs; thus it forms an insurmountable obstacle against any attempt to attack from the surface the behaviour which it determines.

Direct access to the third ego resistance, *the resistance due to repression,* is bound to be more difficult: indeed, it stands at the cradle of the process of illness, introduces the defense, and is in most cases the actual cause for all later resistances which have the task of reinforcing it and of insuring its success.

This enumeration does not exhaust the series of resistances. Still another resistance appears during treatment, the "resistance due to transference" which results from the psychoanalytic situation. Thus it does not seldom happen, for example, that the "love" of a woman patient for her male analyst is conscious to her, but she cannot admit it to herself for reasons of self-esteem (narcissistic protection). Or else the instinct, which is under the pressure of defense, is revived in analysis, comes to be related to the person of the analyst, and under the influence of the repetition-compulsion is expressed through acting out rather than through a memory; in which case, as in the feeling of guilt, an ego tendency combines with an id tendency to form a joint resistance. Moreover, since this resistance serves to gratify a repressed instinctual impulse, it will try to maintain itself under all circumstances.

The true repetition compulsion, as a resistance of the unconscious, is independent of any transference. Its power is shown in the attraction of the unconscious models for the course of the repressed instincts. This resistance unconsciously repeats the defense; apparently it takes its course automatically. Since we know, moreover, that the path from the outside world to the repressed id must lead through the ego, direct access to the symptoms by way of the unconscious id is even less conceivable.

Thus we see that it is just as impossible directly to influence the resistances through the id as through the ego.

These resistances are thoroughly familiar to us. Some of them represent in a sense a narcissistic protection. But it is too simple to consider them as an integral part of character, as Reich does, and to give them the designation "narcissistic shield." Character is more than a conglomerate of resistances.

The neurosis develops from the rift between the strivings of the id and the demands of the ego. The ego always desires to resolve this conflict in some way or other by the introduction of repressions. At first, however, the defense measures of the ego prove to be too weak, and fail. Finally, the ego gains mastery and represses the instincts, *thereby harming them and in turn being harmed.* The therapeutic task may therefore, in principle, consist of making peace between the two parts of the personality, the ego and the id, in the sense that the instincts no longer continue to lead a separate existence excluded from the organization of the ego, and the ego recovers its synthetic power. *To influence the ego as well as the id thus becomes the goal of the therapeutic task.*

Considering that the neurotic person surrounds himself with so many protective measures it seems a problem why he seeks treatment at all, and especially psychoanalytic treatment, for he must suspect that his various resistances will be fought. Certainly it is a fact that, in spite of what has been said before, these resistances can sometimes be attacked directly for a short time by taking the patient by surprise. But one pays a heavy toll for this, for the patient learns in analysis to camouflage his resistances even better. The small opening soon closes. The surgeon, too, has to prepare as broad a field of operation as possible in order to be able to work with technical precision.

However, the problem of therapy is not so hopeless. It is a fact that psychoanalysis shows successes. How then, is treatment set in motion, and recovery eventually accomplished?

In most organic illnesses there are certain tendencies toward recovery that are present either from the very beginning or that arise with the onset of the illness as an automatic reaction. It is therefore the physician's foremost task to create favorable conditions for the normal course of the process of illness by a reinforcement of the "natural" recuperative forces. What then, are the natural tendencies towards cure on which the analyst may count?

We cannot treat a person in a twilight state, nor a severe melancholic, a catatonic, and so on; in short, we cannot treat persons who have *completely* lost contact with their surroundings. It is a necessary pre-condition for treatment that a part of the personality has remained intact, i.e., there must be basic possibility for mutual understanding: the most primitive function of the ego, the capacity of perception and expression, must have been preserved. We cannot influence a person who is deaf or mute. Indeed the word is the most important expedient in analysis. Social relations must not have been completely dissolved. Briefly, some free object libido is essential for any treatment. This, however, is not all that is necessary. Insight into one's illness must also be present, that is to say, a feeling of rejection or strangeness in relation to the neurotic symptoms. Furthermore, there must be an incentive causing the patient to seek treatment. This incentive is provided by the neurotic suffering from which the patient is to be liberated by treatment, and thus is a wish for recovery. It owes its origin to the secondary unpleasure brought on by the illness. However, this wish is not so simple, for it is released by two motives that seem mutually exclusive.

The first motive is the following: every suffering and sick human being is helpless. In his helplessness he is inclined, like a child or a primitive person, to overestimate the power of the one who promises help. He will perhaps look upon the physician as a magician, in the broadest meaning of the word. Indeed, every physician utilizes this "superstition" more or less consciously. The psychoanalyst does not behave any differently when he promises the patient at the introduction of the treatment to cure him, under the condition, it is true, that the patient follow certain rules of the treatment. Incidentally, the importance of the physician's personality for the favorable course of the process of healing becomes apparent right here. If a favorable relationship has been established by the helpless and superstitious patient to his psychoanalyst, whom he has equipped with magic power, much has been gained for the beginning, because the unconscious part of the patient's personality now sides with the physician. The patient thinks, indeed, that the psychoanalyst has nothing else to do but what he himself has done unconsciously for years, that is, to protect him by magic means (as for instance in compulsion neurosis) from the dangers presented by the instincts; thus, to liberate him from his suffering. The patient has outwitted the physician in a sense, but also himself: and yet, in doing so, he has found in his ego some points of contact with the physician. He can thus identify himself with the analyst in the endeavor to procure help for himself. In spite of all resistance he becomes the analyst's helper and begins collaborating with him. In most cases, however, this collaboration is at first misunderstood. The obsessive neurotic, for instance, considers the psychoanalytic rules as magic formulae which he has to comply with conscientiously to the letter. Even where this is not the case, psychoanalysis is sacred to most patients, and the analytic hour is an hour of devotion. Every patient has some kind of ceremonial with which he surrounds the analysis.

However these details may vary, if we appeal to the patient's intact ego by promising help, we meet with unconscious advances from a helpless ego looking for support, even though this support is of an entirely different kind from that which we are willing to give. At any rate, the patient's anxiety is thereby mitigated.

Just as the patient understands the term "help" in a different sense from the physician, that is, he wants to borrow magic powers from the physician for the fight against the unconscious instinct dangers, so the wish for recovery contains still another motive, which likewise leads to a misunderstanding, as I have tried to demonstrate in another context.[3] By "health," too, the patient means something different from what the physician does, namely, the *gratification* of all kinds of desires, impulses, expectations, hopes, and so on. To mention just one example, the impotent patient expects of the cure not merely normal adequate potency but a hyper-potency corresponding to the overcompensation for his castration complex. Thus the wish for recovery contains, in the unconscious, two contrasting roots, one that emanates from the ego and hopes to gain control over the instincts, and the other coming from the id, which hopes for gratification of the instincts. Although so self-contradictory, the wish for recovery has one advantage indispensable for analysis: it begins to establish the transference and even becomes its mainstay. And out of the positive transference, out of love for the analyst, the patient starts collaborating with him—which at first means fighting off the resistances.

What gratification does he find in the transference? What means does he use to set the work in motion? In favorable cases the patient gains gratification from realization of the motives contained in the wish for recovery. He fulfills conscientiously his first task of giving free associations. Analysis becomes rich in content right in the beginning and steers toward its goal without much difficulty. No patient, however, obeys the basic rule exactly, and most patients submit to it only in form. The pleasure derived from speaking becomes evident from the manner in which the speech is brought forth. In analysis the word regains its ancient magic power. The patient believes he delights and dazzles the analyst by his words. This way of speaking veils the old resistances. The patient is able to keep his secret in spite of his apparent obedience to the fundamental psychoanalytic rule. The first gratification derived from the treatment is thus a narcissistic one: to fascinate through speech and not to yield secrets. Not speaking may have exactly the same double meaning. The second direct gratification is derived from the fact that the analyst gives his attention to the patient, listens to him, and is occupied with his troubles. The patient concludes from this that it is love that the analyst feels for him. Disappointment comes later. The necessity to become absorbed in himself, to look into himself, offers a *similar narcissistic gratification*. The same is true of the *intellectual achievement* if at an early stage the patient succeeds in discovering psychological connections. This gratification increases with the progress of the analysis as soon as the patient has gained intellectual interest in it. All of these gratifications may become initial resistances as well, but certainly they are not the only early resistances encountered, nor does each patient raise the same difficulties in the beginning.

This introductory phase, which may vary in duration, does not promote the treatment. It is at best agreeable to the patient. However, something else is now added which, although often disagreeable to the conscious ego, yet brings relief.

We know that any process started in the Unconscious has a progressive tendency. It endeavors to reach the system Pcpt-Cs: to become conscious and to find affective and motor discharge. In neurosis, where direct instinct expansion is inhibited, i.e., repressed, the pressure from below, from the unconscious, is stronger a priori; *therefore the need for discharge is more powerful than it is with instinct energy that is not blocked.* Because of this the neurotic involuntarily unmasks his repressed Unconscious constantly. One may plainly speak of a *self-unmasking tendency* dominating every neurotic. If in addition the patient suffers from a strong sense of guilt, this tendency assumes the character of the *compulsive confession* (Reik), by which the unconscious need for punishment is gratified. But just as the sinner in the Catholic confession expects absolution and clemency in return for his confessions, so does the patient hope for the same from his analyst.

The relation to the analyst is deepened by all these circumstances and the *transference is established.* The weak and helpless ego submits to the analyst, finds support in him and allows itself to be guided by him in the struggle against the resistances. The transference now becomes the bearer of the will to recovery, and substitutes for it, and is placed in the services of the real psychoanalytic task.

In the beginning we stressed that the neurotic patient cannot be influenced in a direct way to give up his resistance. However, insofar as it is a question of helplessness and ungratified instinctual needs, of object hunger, the analyst is able to steal into the patient's ego and there start the breakdown of the resistances. The analyst is not only identified with the patient's magic ego, he is even raised to the ideal. He replaces the patient's ego-ideal. Since the analyst is surrounded by libido in the patient's ego, he neutralizes the severity of the superego. The superego becomes more indulgent and milder through the libidinal absorption of the analyst. The ego need not fear the superego as much as before, just as it needs no longer fear the instinctual demands, because it is protected by the analyst on both fronts. Combining in his person the strivings of the patient's ego and id, the analyst is predestined, so to say, to mediate in the neurotic conflict and to reconcile the conflicting parts of the neurotic personality. Furthermore, since the analyst is benevolent toward the repressed instinctual components, the patient's ego successively abandons its resistances that are due to repression; the patient feels allied with the analyst, in accord with him, protected by him, and therefore need not fear danger situations which, moreover, have long ceased to be real. This explains also why the most severe states of anxiety frequently disappear right after analysis has begun.

To repeat briefly: the patient raises the analyst to his ideal, identifies with him after the fashion of the hypnotized, finds protection in him, and finally transfers the strivings of the id upon him. Under these circumstances influence from within can be achieved: the slow breakdown of the resistances due to repression may be undertaken.

My own experience has taught me that in cases where this relationship could not be established, treatment has had to be stopped sooner or later.

We know that the resistances due to repression show their power mainly in keeping from consciousness the preconscious ideational material. Although it is true that in most of the phobias or obsessive neuroses pathogenic ideas are largely contained in consciousness, they are nevertheless always substitutive ideas, quite removed from the original ones. Therefore the first task of every analysis is to obtain the repressed ideational material in the form of recollections. If the patient has reached the state where he feels protected by alliance with the analyst, he will drop his aversion to remembering and give up all resistances pertaining to it. Even more: he will give up not only the amnesias, as does the hysteric, but also the taboo against contact, as does the obsessive neurotic (for whom remembering is generally easier); and he will connect the remembered experiences in time and space. Connection is established between preconscious and unconscious memory material through recollecting, and thus the repressed object-presentation is enabled to reenter consciousness. Here it is recognized as no longer an actual menace and so is tolerated with a minimum development of anxiety. The real traumatic situation is then reproduced through as close a recollection as possible. A comparison of that situation with the present one shows its non-actual and unreal character. As a result, not only is less anxiety developed, but also can reality-testing be introduced. Since through the work of remembering the patient is brought back to an unpleasurable situation, which he now relives without anxiety, *he learns, moreover, to tolerate unpleasure.* Indeed, the oversensitivity to unpleasure and the closely connected anxiety-readiness, the incapability of tolerating major need-tensions, is the characteristic trait of the neurotic person.

Two factors facilitate the work of remembering. The object-relationship has been disturbed by repression. In obsessional neurosis there is even danger of the loss of the object. In order to evade this danger, the obsessional neurotic forms substitutive ideas. Analysis therefore supports a natural process, with this difference, however: it penetrates through the substitutive images to the primary ones, thus to the real objects.

The second factor is of a more general nature and applies also to hysteria. We spoke of the progressive tendency of the Unconscious. This progression is interrupted by repression; the instincts are under high energy tension due to the blocking of the channels of discharge, and being continuous they cause incessant unrest for the psychic apparatus. This instinctual tension is the *second* factor that impels the unconscious strivings on towards cathecting the system Pcpt.-Cs: towards discharge through the act of becoming conscious and through affectivity. This tendency is disturbed by the repression, and the patient feels relieved when analysis offers him an opportunity for discharge, even though it is under resistances.

It can easily be understood that discharge in affectivity may bring relief. However, it cannot without further consideration be understood why the act of becoming conscious should have a similar result. We know how uncomfortable it is when we try to remember something and cannot, and with what a sigh of relief we greet the sought-for recollection when it emerges. The relief felt by a patient when he succeeds in remembering an important part of forgotten material is even more striking. However it is noteworthy that the relief is felt but one time, that is, at the moment when the forgotten material reappears in consciousness as though illuminated by a searchlight. In order to understand this we have to realize the function of the apparatus of consciousness. Perception of external as well as of internal stimuli is the main task of this apparatus. It has no memory, that is, it cannot preserve memory-traces. An experience becomes conscious only when a preconscious idea combines with an unconscious one and enters consciousness by means of the special act of hyper-cathexis. Therefore the moment of becoming conscious is fleeting: consciousness cannot lastingly maintain its susceptibility to the same idea. Since the system Cs. does not preserve traces of stimuli (recollections), since the ego gets relief through the act of becoming conscious, and since, furthermore, this act occurs but once (though it may be repeated indefinitely), it frees the psychic system of tensions. This relief may be understood in the following way: the psychic energy bound to the repressed ideas is discharged in the act of remembering. According to Freud, *energy thus freed is spent in the act of becoming conscious.* Indeed, it happens that a patient may forget the recollections brought to light through his analysis and yet stay well.

The old theory of abreacting remains valid. However, we understand by it not merely the discharge of affects, but also the discharge involved in the act of becoming conscious. But we know that abreacting does not always eliminate the symptoms, although it gives momentary relief; something else must be added in order to complete the process of healing.

Free association, which must finally lead to the emergence of repressed memories, never proceeds smoothly. It is almost a rule that resistances increase with the deepening of the analysis; it can be observed over and over again that at a certain point during the chain of associations a feeling of discomfort—often an uncanny feeling—of variable intensity, arises, and may increase to the point of anxiety. These feelings can be overcome only with the help of the analyst, but still the patient's *active collaboration* is absolutely necessary. We have stressed before that the patient turns his active interest to inner processes, inner experiences composed of memories, not only out of love for his analyst but also because he feels *protected* by him. This protection enables him to drop his fear of recollecting and to permit the other affects uniting the memories to take their course freely. Thus, for love of the analyst and in the knowledge of protection by him, the ego starts to work actively toward lifting the memories from the unconscious; at the same time it causes discharge of the instincts through "abreacting" and thus brings about an unintentional gain, as it were.

We have to consider still another factor. The further the neurosis has developed, the more the patient loses contact with reality. He withdraws, and renounces real gratification. He becomes more or less indifferent and passive toward the outside world.

Complete harmony reigns for some time between patient and analyst. The patient relies completely upon the analyst, he accepts all his interpretations, and if it were possible he would ask the analyst to do the work of recollecting for him. The time soon comes, however, when this harmony is disturbed. As mentioned before, the resistances become ever stronger the deeper the analysis penetrates, i.e., the more the original pathogenic situation is approached. Added to these difficulties, there is the moment of frustration that is bound to appear in the transference sooner or later. Most patients react to the frustration with slackening in their work, with spite, and with "acting out", i.e., reenacting previous experiences. The patient leaves a part of the active work to the analyst: to guess what the patient wants to express but is unable to say. As a rule this concerns fantasies of being loved. The omnipotence of the patient's own means of expression (which may be mute) and the physician's omnipotence (his magic) are tested to the utmost. In part, the analyst succeeds in unmasking these resistances; in part, it is impossible for him to guess what the patient hides. The conflict now is no longer an inner one, but one between the patient and the analyst and it reaches an apex. The analysis is threatened with failure, i.e., the patient is confronted with the choice between losing the analyst and his love, or resuming active work. The patient becomes fearful of this loss if the transference is sufficiently firm, i.e., if a minimum amount of object-libido has been loosened from its fixations and is again at his disposal.

Frequently in such cases the analysis takes a remarkable turn. When the analyst has given up all hope of a successful conclusion of the analysis and lost interest in the case, the patient suddenly begins to yield a wealth of material, that promises a speedy conclusion of the analysis. This reminds us of those situations where some patients bring interesting material only at the end of the hour in the hope of extending the time they spend with their analyst. The only way in which I can explain this behaviour is: the patient becomes aware that the analyst is losing interest in him and consequently develops fear of losing the analyst's love. To avoid this he tolerates the unpleasure springing from the frustration and from the reproduction of the pathogenic traumatic situation, submits to active collaboration, and raises the last repressed memories from the unconscious. The inertia of instinct life, which found its expression in the repetition compulsion, is now overcome by activity of the ego. The fear of loss of love, which is mobilized object-libido, is the motive power bringing about the transformation of the passivity of instinct life (in the shape of the repetition compulsion) into the activity of the ego.

The activity of the ego serves not only to loosen the last fixations of the instincts and to create the best conditions for their abreacting, but also to facilitate the reality-testing. This testing is prepared for in the analysis in that it is there proved, through conscious recollection, that the infantile strivings are psychic and historical formations corresponding to nothing in present reality. The transference likewise offers increasing opportunity for learning to distinguish between psychic and external reality. In this connection I should like to mention one example that is very instructive. When after many months analysis had succeeded in uncovering an important part of a patient's attachment to her father, she started the following hour with a question concerning my teeth. Puzzled, I tried to obtain some information about this question. The patient related that the day before, when taking leave of me, she had been struck by the appearance of my teeth. Until then she had been convinced that my front teeth had spaces between them. Now she noticed that this was not the case. She could not understand her error until suddenly, while she was discussing this illusion with me, she recalled that her father's teeth had spaces between them.

It is almost self-evident that the greater precision of reality-testing acquired through analysis must lead to the abandonment of omnipotence and magic, just as it is evident that the recovered activity may bring about real changes in the external world which serve to create conditions for actual gratification of those instinctual needs that have just been released from repression.

Were this the final result, analysis at best would create a human being obedient to his instincts, capable of abreacting his erotic and destructive strivings on suitable objects. However, this is not the case; nor would it be possible in a civilized community. On the contrary, people after successful analysis are not only freer in their instinctual life but also better able to tolerate unpleasure and to control themselves; they are more able to endure instinct tensions, to sublimate, and to adapt to reality; and yet they do not fall ill from neurotic conflicts. Of course not even the best analysis can save them from actual conflicts.

We know that the ego is disorganized by the process of symptom-formation; the repressed part of instinct life is expelled from the ego-organization, subjected to the laws of the Unconscious, and inaccessible to the influence of the ego. The repressed part leads a separate existence. Briefly, in neurosis the ego has more or less lost its synthetic function.

Conscious thinking is a synthetic process which in neurosis is partly disturbed. Restitution of the synthetic function of the ego is introduced with the first act of recollecting. Indeed, remembering in analysis is accompanied by making connections and by uniting the repressed ideational elements with the actual ego, by mediating between the two, i.e., by assimilating what has been repressed. In this process analysis merely makes use of an already existing tendency of the ego: it is amazing with what tenacity even the most primitive person clings to his need for causality. The patient obeys the analyst's request to search for the hidden "causes" of his sufferings perhaps more readily and understandingly than he does any other request. The need for causality is in a sense gratified the very first day of analysis, and the last phases of analysis proceed entirely under this stimulus. Remembering then becomes the most important means of finding the "cause." To have found it means to unite what had been estranged, expelled, and repressed from the actual ego. It is through such assimilation that the continuity of the personality is restored and the real entrance of a psychic act into consciousness brought about. In some instances, such as in obsessional neurosis, remembering alone is not sufficient for entrance into consciousness. For this purpose seemingly heterogeneous elements have to be connected with each other. In analysis a process takes place similar to that in the spontaneous attempt at recovery in paranoia—though with different material and on a different level. Thus here too is manifested the power of Eros whose derivatives, in the form of desexualized libido of the ego, exercise their mediating and binding influence in the process of healing.

I intend to discuss this topic in greater detail on another occasion. At this time I should like only to indicate that it is at this point, that some other psychotherapeutic methods begin treatment—whether or not they are called "psychoanalysis." The basic difference between those methods and ours consists in the fact that in their case patients assimilate something foreign imposed upon them from outside, whereas our patients have to assimilate with painful self-conquest, what was *originally their own.*

The various resistances are gradually recognized during the psychoanalytic work and the ego rejects them as unsuitable ways of working. Simultaneous with the unmasking of resistances and the removal of repressions, major changes take place within the structure of the personality itself. The repressed libido is released and the representatives of the instincts are able to enter consciousness at any time and to discharge themselves in affects and actions. As the ego has absorbed the beloved and benign analyst, the severity of the superego is reduced. Since, furthermore, the ego has become freer of anxiety as a result of identification with the helping analyst, it admits and accepts the previously repressed instinctual impulses, and what has been repressed is once again absorbed by the ego. The ego recovers its synthetic function by regaining its capacity to mediate between the superego and the id on the one had and between the id and objects of the external world on the other. It is now capable of establishing harmony between objects of the external world and the strivings of the id.

The description of the process of recovery is not yet ended. The ego, no longer having to spend energy in accomplishing the work of repression, becomes more adequate in its foremost task, that of reality-testing. Consequently, it becomes able to distinguish between real and psychic danger, between external and internal processes. Having gained ability to tolerate unpleasure, it also acquires better capacity to master non-ego-syntonic instinctual demands, i.e., those demands that are accompanied by external danger, and to direct them to other aims, as for instance, sublimation. In doing so it does not harm itself too much. It can procure gratification for other ego-syntonic instincts by useful changes of the external world. Through consideration of and regard for the objects of the external world the patient becomes more social and more resistant to instinct-tensions, i.e., to unpleasure.

Thus the psychoanalytic method of treatment makes use of "natural" recuperative forces which arise with the outbreak of the illness itself. They stem partly from the ego, partly from the id. The method frees the instincts from their fixations but at the same time aids the ego in its struggle against them.

In the ideal case the changes brought about by these recuperative forces involve the entire personality and are therefore as follows: *the energies of the id become more mobile, the superego more tolerant, the ego freer of anxiety and the synthetic function of the ego is restored.* Analysis is therefore *actually a synthesis.*

It should be emphasized that I do not say that the ego becomes free of anxiety, the id mobile, and the superego tolerant: I wish to indicate that analysis can bring about *relative* changes only; that *quantitative differences,* which at best can only be estimated, not measured, are involved here.

I am aware that I have not given a full account of the course of analysis here. That, however, was not my intention. I wanted to select from the almost inexhaustible wealth of problems only those that forced themselves upon my attention through my need for a better understanding of them. My presentation, while referring to an ideal case, is in general a composite of impressions gathered during many years of experience, which, however, I have been able to formulate only since Freud's latest works were published. In this description, I believe that I have come fairly close to the *actual* course of an analysis.

The implications for technique are self-evident: to permit the process of healing to go on undisturbed, but to make use of the natural and concomitant recuperative tendencies. Nevertheless, when the analysis reaches deeper levels it cannot be avoided that the resolution of one resistance is immediately followed by a new one, which arises as a reaction. Indeed, analysis takes an undulating course. In view of the present stage of our theoretic knowledge I should not venture to set up strict rules nor to give precise advice.

REFERENCES

1. Nunberg, H. 1928. *Internationale Zeitschrift für Psychoanalyse* 14.
2. Freud, S. 1926. *S.E.*, 20:77–123.
3. ———.1928. *S.E.*, 21:175–98.

6. Concerning the Theory of Psychoanalytic Technique[1]

Otto Fenichel

I

In discussing the "theory of technique" it is unfortunately still necessary to discuss the justification of this concept. There exist some views about the "irrational" nature of psychoanalytic technique which oppose any attempt at constructing a theory of its technical principles. One of these views, for instance, was expressed recently by Reik.[2] Since the instrument of psychoanalytic technique is the unconscious of the analyst (the "relay" conception), and since intuition is indispensable for apprehending what goes on in the patient, he wants to leave everything in that technique to the unconscious and to intuition. But in view of the fact that the subject matter of psychoanalysis is the irrational, such conceptions must in the final analysis lead to that method itself being regarded as irrational, losing every characteristic of science and becoming pure art.

Per contra, we argue as follows. We have a dynamic-economic conception of psychic life. Our technique, too, which aims at a dynamic-economic change in the patient, must follow dynamic-economic principles. It must always remain true to the mode of thinking underlying psychoanalysis, and must order our behaviour issuing from intuition (which is of course indispensable) according to rational directives.

Freud was the originator of the concepts "dynamics" and "economics" in psychic life. His whole method of studying neurotic phenomena, as well as his papers on technique,[3] leaves no doubt that he considered analytic interpretation, as well as the procedure of the analyst in general, as an intervention in the dynamics and economics of the patient's mind, and thus he demanded of interpretations more than that they should be correct as to content. It was he who asserted that only a procedure which used *resistances* and *transference* could be called psychoanalysis;[4] that is, only a procedure which intervened in the dynamics and did not merely give "translations" of the patient's allusions, as soon as the analyst understood to what they alluded. The formula that the analyst should make the unconscious conscious might lead to such a misunderstanding. Indeed, it is possible that the statement of a symptom's meaning will at times make it disappear; but it need not. Mere topological conceptions do not suffice to explain what determines whether an interpretation does or does not have this effect. Whether it does or not is determined by whether or not a repression (more correctly, an instinctual defense implying continued expenditure of energy) is actually eliminated. But what eliminates a repression? The dynamic conception views the psyche as a continuous struggle between mental trends which seek discharge and the defensive and selective forces of the ego, between the instinctual cathexes and the anti-cathexes of the ego. That the latter too arose from the former does not interest us here. In reviewing an already existing neurotic conflict, we see that it takes place between an unconscious instinctual demand and the defensive forces of the ego, which are supplied with "anti-cathexes," and which manifest themselves in the treatment as resistances. (Kaiser's designation of the energy used by the forces defending against drives as "narcissistic libido," is *per se* correct, but apt to be misleading. To avoid discussions about the genesis of this libido, it is probably better to use for these energies the term "anti-cathexis" introduced by Freud.) What we have to do is to intervene in this interplay between drive and resistance. In so intervening, we need not, and even cannot, reinforce the drive. The repressed drive is our ally in our work; it strives of itself toward consciousness and motility. Our task is only to see that no resistances bar its way. Were it possible to brush aside the resistances, the repressed would appear on its own. This *dynamic* conception of interpretation—that our task is to seek out resistances and to uncover them so that the repressed manifests itself—must be supplemented by the economic conception that our task is to tackle the economically most important and strongest resistance in order to achieve an actual and economically decisive liberation of libido, so that what was tied up so far in the struggle of repression shall be available to real gratification. The infantile sexual impulses which have been repressed then find contact with the ego and change, for the greater part, into genitality capable of orgasm, the rest becoming capable of sublimation.

The "theory of technique" is but a commentary on these propositions. These propositions should be taken seriously; and it cannot be denied that there are many factors in the analytic situation which tempt the analyst not to take them seriously, but, sooner or later, to "drift" and to use the only-an-art conception of analytic technique, making the inevitability of a certain lack of system in the analysis an excuse for letting himself float along in a planless way—that is, letting himself interpret purely intuitively what occurs to him, or at best, to his patient.

II

It is Reich's merit to have especially warned us against this procedure. His proposals for the reform of the technique derive mostly from a serious view of the *economic* conception, namely, from an insight into the fact that our task is to liberate the energy tied up in the repressive struggle and to change repressed infantile sexuality into adult sexuality capable of orgasm, by eliminating repression.[5]

There are a number of "technical formulas" transmitted by tradition from Freud, inspection of which shows that what Reich's proposals on technique are saying is, "Consider whether you are really always applying the true Freudian technique." One of these formulas is, "Work always where the patient's affect lies at the moment." To the thoughtful analyst this clearly does not mean: "Work where the patient *believes* his affects lie." The analyst must always *seek out* the points where at the moment the conflict is decisively centered. Another example: "Interpretation begins always at what is on the surface at the moment." Taken correctly, this can only mean that it makes no sense to give "deep interpretations" (however correct they might be as to content) as long as superficial matters are in the way. For this reason one cannot, as Melanie Klein wants,[6] "get into direct contact with the unconscious of the patient," because to analyze means precisely to come to terms with the patient's *ego*, to compel the patient's ego to face its own conflicts. If we, for instance, know that a compulsion neurosis has regressed, out of castration anxiety, from the genital oedipus conflict to the anal-sadistic stage, we cannot use this knowledge for discussing "immediately" the genital oedipus conflict; the only way to it is by working through the anal-sadistic conflicts. This is obvious. But it is also necessary always to keep in view the hundreds of analogies of everyday life. The defensive attitudes of the ego are *always* more superficial than the instinctual attitudes of the id.

Therefore, before throwing the patient's instincts at his head we have first to interpret to him that he is afraid of them and is defending himself against them, and why he does so.

Here is another formula: "Interpretation of resistance goes before interpretation of content." Every resistance hinders the patient from digesting a contentual interpretation, that is, an utterance of his unconscious trends so that it effects a dynamic change. Thus there is no point in trying to do this before the obstacle is out of the way. Since not all resistances are manifest, however, the analyst must continuously seek out and work on the momentarily acute resistances, first, by separating the patient's judging ego from his resistance-determined behavior; secondly, by getting the patient to experience the latter as arising from his resistance; thirdly, by finding the occasions of the resistance; fourthly, by explaining why the resistance takes precisely this form; and fifthly and lastly, by telling him against what it is directed. Freud has, moreover, repeatedly discussed and demonstrated by examples that not only the content of what the patient says but his modes of behavior, his "accidental" actions, and his manner and bearing are all also the subject matter of the analysis.

There are, it is true, some other traditional formulas as well, which at first sight seem to contradict Reich's views. There is, for instance, Freud's warning against making a kind of "stock-taking" of the situation from time to time during the course of the analysis, in order to clarify the structure of the case for oneself, because in this way one only gets a biased view of it; one should rather respond to the patient's unconscious with one's own unconscious and wait until a structural picture arises of itself.[7] Again, there is his comparison of analysis with a jig-saw puzzle in which one piece after another is observed at random as each presents itself "by accident," until one finds how they fit together.[8] Then, too, there is the formula: "The patient determines the theme of the session."

The apparent contradictions of such formulas are resolved if we keep in mind that the psychoanalytic technique is a *living art,* in which rules never have more than a relative validity. Surely Freud's views, if represented correctly, mean that the analytic technique must guard against two extremes, both equally incorrect: on the one hand, one must not analyze too much according to a rational plan, by intellect alone (the concept of "relay," the analyst's own unconscious as his instrument—"he who wants to analyze must be analyzed"); and on the other hand, one must not be too irrational, because to analyze means to subject the irrational in man to reason. (Otherwise psychoanalytic technique would be unteachable. The frequently used comparison between analytic and surgical technique is here indeed in place; for analytic technique, too, one needs endowment and intuition, but these, without training, do not suffice in surgery either.)

Reich's view is that interpretation has never been as yet consistently thought through and followed out as a dynamic-economic process. Instead of using their insight into the dynamics and economics of psychic processes to build up their technique in a planned and systematic way, analysts succumb to indolence and lack any system. In their work, despite their better knowledge they take the task of interpreting resistances to mean that they are to interpret whatever the patient is talking about. In Reich's opinion, the reason why the analyst usually fails to work "where the affect really is" is that it simply does not occur to him to look for the affect where it should be sought —namely, in characterological behavior. Characterological behavior acts as a kind of armor-plating which covers the real conflicts, and this aspect of it is not taken seriously enough. Indeed, were one to take the rule "to work where the affect actually lies" seriously, it would mean that as long as the leading characterological resistance was unbroken, one would work on no other subject matter, and discuss no other theme with the patient but this. The more "the affect" is "frozen" into an "attitude," the less does the patient know about it, and the more important it is to work on this *first*, so that the contentual interpretations which the analyst will make later on shall not be wasted beforehand. Though the comparison with the jig-saw puzzle is correct, that game too can be played systematically and according to a plan, by not examining the pieces as they accidentally present themselves, but looking every time for the pieces which would fit. The psychic material of the patient has a certain stratification. His resistance attempts to conceal this stratification. The analyst, nevertheless, must discover this stratification and follow it exactly in his interpretations, and he must recognize when material whose content belongs to a deeper stratum emerges only in order to ward off more superficial material. Otherwise, he will be confronted with the dreaded "chaotic situation," in which material from every stratum of the mind is produced in disordered comminglement. Thus Reich thinks the principle "begin always at the surface," too, should be taken more seriously and carried out more consistently than hitherto. Such a consistent procedure demands primarily that material—including dreams—which does not serve the momentary purpose should be left untouched, in order not to "fire away" uselessly the work of interpretation. "The patient determines the theme of the session," not by what he says, but by showing the analyst where his economically crucial resistance lies. This theme the analyst must then compel the patient to work through, even if the latter would rather talk about something else.

I should like to insert a few critical comments at this point. With those principles of the so-called "Reichian technique" which I have attempted to represent here, I am in complete agreement—qua *principles*. I consider them as correctly deduced from Freud's theoretical and technical views.[9] I also agree with Reich that in our everyday work all of us often infringe on these principles, and that in this respect no amount of self-control is too much. The contradictory judgments which have been made in analytic circles about the so-called "Reichian technique"—some saying, "It is nothing new, but only exactly what Freud does," and others saying "It is so different from Freud's analysis, that it ought not to be called psychoanalysis"—can be explained in this way: In so far as these principles are merely elaborations of Freud's views, they are "nothing new"; in so far as they are *consistent elaborations* of it, they *are* something new.

The agreement in principle with Reich which I have just expressed is only limited, on the one hand, by two minor theoretical objections, and on the other, by objections, not against the essence of his views and principles, but simply against the manner of their application on particular points.

The two minor theoretical objections are:

(1) The psychic material in the patient does not have an orderly stratification. Reich's assertion to the contrary is schematic and disregards complicating details. The regularity of the stratification is just as regularly broken through—in different people to different degrees—even when there have been no incorrect analytic interpretations. The phenomenon which geology calls "dislocation" is a general one and consists in materials originally layered over, or side by side with each other, being mixed into each other by various natural events; consequently, the sequence in which the material presents itself to the geologist who drills into the earth is not identical with the age of the layers in question. The material is only "relatively" ordered. In the same way, to my mind, the relatively correct views of Reich on the "consistency" of interpretation must not be taken for absolute either. For there are *spontaneous chaotic situations* too; indeed, there are people whose character neurosis presents a picture which cannot be diagnosed by any other

term but "chaotic situation." Moreover, "dislocation" continues to take place during psychoanalytic treatment. And the fluctuations of everyday life, which cannot be disregarded, also lessen this "consistency" to some extent.

(2) If we are to pay particular attention to "frozen resistances," to habitual actions and attitudes, we must not only know that they express resistance, but get to understand their meaning. Naturally, even only to call the patient's attention to his resistive attitude is better than to overlook it completely. But there is no doubt that we shall succeed the more easily, the more completely we understand the concrete meaning of such a resistive attitude. The discovery of this meaning in turn will be facilitated by every piece of knowledge we gain about the individual patient's past history. We are thus faced with a vicious circle: His past history becomes accessible only through resolving these attitudes—and resolving these attitudes requires knowledge of that history. In my opinion, this vicious circle is best resolved by the analyst's setting out from the beginning to learn for his own information (without major "interpretations") as much as possible about the patient's past. I think that it is always a good thing to use the first period of analysis for *collecting material*. The more *information* one has, the better armed one goes into the actual struggle with the resistances. We do not always succeed in such an initial collection of material; nor is such failure any reason for giving up an analysis. I believe, however, that we should not deliberately by-pass occasions for collecting such material. It seems to me that Reich, in the intention of doing nothing else but work consistently upon the point around which for the moment everything turns, often leaves aside material which, if he had regarded it, would precisely have helped him to understand the point in question. I have especially often had this impression in connection with "by-passed dream analyses." In free associations, we often have the experience to which Freud has called attention,[10] viz., that what the patient says becomes comprehensible only from what follows after it. Therefore, until what is to come after *has* come after, we cannot, I think, know what material we ought to leave aside.

Naturally, there are many situations in which absolutely *every* interpretation of a dream is contraindicated, namely, when "dream interpretation" *per se* has some other unconscious meaning for the patient which the analysis has not yet apprehended. But where this is not the case, I believe that it is precisely through correct dream interpretation that an attitude of the patient can often be understood. After all, the dream is a commentary on the patient's ego-attitudes of the previous day. Among the latent dream thoughts there are always some which are close to the conscious attitude but yet contain an additional element or show the attitude in a relationship which the patient has not thought of on account of his repressions. To interpret a dream does not mean telling the patient, "You want to sleep with your mother"; it may also be "to infer latent dream thoughts and by means of them to show the patient the actual nature of his present behavior and its intentions." Latent dream thoughts, however, cannot be inferred without getting the patient's associations to the elements of the manifest dream. If the patient does not associate, we give up the attempt at interpreting and try to apprehend this resistance. If, however, he does associate, his attention is thereby not necessarily fatefully diverted from consideration of his characterological behavior of the moment; it should rather be possible to use his associations precisely to lead him to that point.

I have called these two objections "minor objections," because they do not undermine Reich's principles, but only make them less absolute. The question now is how these principles are applied. This will vary with each case, and particularly with the personality of the analyst. In spite of Reich's assertions that there is no such danger, I believe that the "shattering of the armor-plating" could be done in a very aggressive way, but that both the aggression and the consequent disintegration of the armor can be *dosed,* and indeed, that it is the task of the physician to make this procedure as little unpleasurable as possible for the patient. The first thing we must be clear about is that the consistent tackling of the patient's character traits wounds his narcissism much more than any other analytic technique. Not only does the degree to which patients can tolerate such wounds vary, but also the degree to which analysts can or should inflict them. As analysts we should in principle certainly not be afraid of "crises" (the surgeon isn't afraid of blood either when he cuts); but that is no reason for inviting such "crises" in every case. On the contrary, I believe that our aim ought to be the *gradual* reduction of the existing insufficient neurotic equilibrium. We are familiar with the resistance of some patients, who long for a "trauma" and expect cure not from a difficult analysis, but from the magic effect of a sudden explosion. There is an analogous longing for a trauma on the part of the analyst also. Let us beware of it!

The conviction that a consistent working through of character resistance is the one and only correct method may make one overlook the fact that experiencing this kind of analysis may itself become for the patient a *transference resistance*. This would naturally be an even more superficial one than the "character resistance" and would have to be dealt with first. In one case, a patient, who in his fear of experiencing sexual excitation, always fell away, at a certain height of excitation, from his active masculinity into a receptive orality ("at this point I dare go no further, you do it for me"), experienced and enjoyed the "activity" with which the analyst pursued his current "attitudes," etc., as the fulfillment of his receptive longing, and this he did without the analyst noticing it. In another case the unconscious content of the neurosis of a woman patient was her rebellion against her father, who throughout her childhood reproached her for her traits and mimicked them. To have begun her treatment with an attempt at a "consistent attitude analysis"—a procedure which became highly necessary later on—would have led to an immediate breaking off by her of the analysis.

NOTES

1. Discussion of H. Kaiser's "Probleme der Technik," *Int. Z. Psa.*, Vol. 20, 1934. First published in *Int. Z. Psa.*, Vol. 21, 1935, pp. 78–95.
2. See T. Reik, "New Ways in Psycho-Analytic Technique," *Int. J. Psa.*, Vol. 14, 1933.
3. S. Freud, "Papers on Technique," *Coll. Pap.*, Vol. II, London, Hogarth, 1948.
4. S. Freud, "The History of the Psychoanalytic Movement," *The Basic Writings*, New York, Random House, 1938.
5. See W. Reich's *Character Analysis*, New York, Orgone Institute Press, 1949.
6. M. Klein, *The Psychoanalysis of Children*, New York, Norton, 1932.
7. S. Freud, "Recommendations for Physicians on the Psycho-Analytic Method of Treatment," *Coll. Pap.*, Vol. II.
8. S. Freud, "The Etiology of Hysteria," *Coll. Pap.*, Vol. I, London, Hogarth, 1948.
9. They have been excellently formulated already by W. Reich in his study "On the Technique of Interpretation and of Resistance Analysis," Chapter 3 of *Character Analysis*.
10. S. Freud, "Recommendations for Physicians on the Psycho-Analytic Method of Treatment," *Coll. Pap.*, Vol. II.

7. Psychoanalysis of Character

Otto Fenichel

As is well known, psychoanalysis started as a therapy of neuroses; therefore, the neurotic symptom was its first main subject. In a neurotic symptom something happens which the subject experiences as strange and unexplainable—either involuntary movements, or other changes of bodily functions and various sensations, as in a hysterical symptom; or an overwhelming and unjustified emotion or mood, as in attacks of anxiety or depression; or queer impulses or thoughts, as in compulsions and obsessions. It is always something which seems to break in from without upon the personality and which disturbs the continuity of the personality and appears like an invasion from something outside the usual habits of the subject, coming as a vivid proof of the limits of the conscious will. It cannot be controlled by means of the usual controlling apparatus of the mind.

Before psychoanalysis undertook to study the essence of "personality," it had to investigate the disturbances of personality and the disruptions of its continuity. It was the study of the insufficiencies of conscious control and those habitual patterns of behavior which we call "character," which enabled us later to attack the problems of character itself. The result of those preliminary studies showed that the impression that the neurotic symptoms represent an invasion from another country was correct. Their ego-alien nature can be explained by the fact that they break in from a region of the mind which the subject had previously purposefully alienated from it—viz., the unconscious. Neurotic symptoms are the outcome of forces which are always at work but which are usually prohibited from expressing themselves. The essence of the psychology of the neuroses is the explanation of how this normal prohibition became insufficient. For repressed instinctual forces which are striving for discharge are to a certain extent present in everybody. The first proof of this fact was given by the interpretation of dreams. Dreams,

"Psychoanalysis of Character" is reprinted from The Collected Papers of Otto Fenichel, Second Series, Collected and Edited by Dr. Hanna Fenichel and Dr. David Rapaport, by permission of W. W. Norton & Company, Inc. Copyright © 1954 by W. W. Norton & Company, Inc. Copyright © renewed 1982 by Peter E. Lippet, Executor of the author, Hanna Fenichel. Originally published in 1941.

like symptoms, are disguised expressions of the repressed, and that is the reason why they appear to the coherent and reasonable ego to be strange, as neurotic (or even more, psychotic) symptoms do. Normal persons may dream, too. And so we see that the unconscious is operative in normal people also. We can understand that it is the state of sleep itself which, with the suspension of consciousness, weakens the suppressing forces of the higher levels of personality, and so enables the deeper parts of the mind to make their appearance. In the case of neuroses, however, the insufficiency of the prohibiting forces proceeds from other causes than the state of sleep. It is a consequence of a too far-reaching suppression of the instinctual satisfactions. That is not of much interest for us today. What matters is the fact that the human mind seems to consist of two principal parts: the so-called "continuous personality," the activities of which seem at least to be of a suppressing nature; and unconscious instinctual forces which usually are suppressed, but which make their appearance in neurotic symptoms and dreams, and also— we hasten to add—in other sudden acts, emotional feelings, or attitudes which are experienced as strange and which have always an impulsive and instinctual character, opposed to intellect and reason. The situation is really very analogous to brain physiology, where it was also ascertained that the activity of the higher centers, the cortex, partly consists in suppression of activities of deeper and more archaic centers, and that the latter find expression whenever the higher suppressing forces become insufficient. Sometimes it looked, therefore, as if the two parts of the human mind might have to be represented by two different psychologies. It has been thought that psychoanalysis, as a "depth psychology," has to study the unconscious and the instincts, but that other, non-analytic psychologies, would have to study the "surface," the personality which suppresses the instincts and which governs the mind of the normal person during the day—the "character."

But such a viewpoint is wrong. It is the genetic point of view which shows us that the relationship of the deep instincts and the unconscious, which are studied by psychoanalysis, and the ego and the so-called character, is more complicated. We certainly do not assume that there are no other phenomena in the human mind than instinctual phenomena, but we do assume that the non-instinctual phenomena can be explained as derivatives of instinctual ones, which took shape under the influence of the outer world. Just as the cellular theory is not contradicted by the existence of bones and nerves, and bones and nerves may be studied by means of the same principles as the cells, as long as it is possible to demonstrate that the bones and nerves are derivatives of cells—so, in the same way, does psychoanalysis, which first studied the unconscious and the instincts, remain competent for the whole human mind as long as it succeeds in demonstrating that the conscious and non-instinctual phenomena are derivatives of unconscious and instinctual ones.

What the "ego" undertakes with the deep unconscious forces is certainly not only their suppression. It is their organization and guidance as well. And so it becomes understandable that an apparatus whose function is suppression, guidance, and organization cannot be understood before the material which is suppressed, organized, and guided is thoroughly known. First comes the psychology of what is comprehended, then the psychology of comprehension. In the so-called "ego psychology," psychoanalysis approaches the same subject as other psychologies, but it approaches it in a different way, namely genetically. I have already anticipated that it can be shown that the whole "daytime personality" which we call the ego is to be regarded basically as being a result of conflicts between primitive instincts and inhibiting outer forces.

By taking symptoms and dreams as its first objects, psychoanalysis has succeeded in studying the nature and genesis of the unconscious instincts which find their distorted expression in them. It is not my task today to talk about this part of psychoanalytic research. I remind you only of the fact that the immense field of infantile sexuality was not known before Freud.

There are three reasons why psychoanalysis could not fail to be extended to ego psychology. To begin with, there were theoretical reasons: The repressing forces are also an object for psychological study and the preliminary study of the repressed forces enabled psychoanalysis to make the next step. In addition, there were two other, practical, reasons, the importance of which has to be estimated still higher. In the first place, when the psychoanalyst tried to get at the hidden meaning of the neurotic symptoms he met the suppressing—or, as I might say in this connection, the repressing—force of the ego in the form of what we know as "resistances." To overcome these resistances became his main practical task. How was it to be done? Everything was tried in this respect, and Freud has said in his *Introductory Lectures* that every means of suggestion is justified for the purpose of overcoming resistances. But if, for example, a patient did not obey the basic rule which tells him to say everything which occurs to him, a scientific mind was tempted not only to influence this unreasonable behavior by means of suggestion, but to get to understand this ego, which had hitherto figured as a reasonable ego, but which in such cases seemed not to be reasonable at all. Consciously, the man was trying to do everything to co-operate; but unconsciously a "suppressing" part of his ego was antagonistic. Here was a conflict at work inside the ego; other material, associations or dreams or sleeping states of the patient, had to be used to analyze this conflict, to make the patient aware *that* he had the resistance, *why* he had the resistance, and why he had it in that form. The principle is that this is always done by the discovery that the patient, even if he does not feel any fear today, was once afraid (or ashamed or disgusted or full of bad conscience) about certain instinctual experience, and that this fear is unconsciously still working in him, so that he develops resistances against utterances which might be connected with the instincts in question. Thus it was the necessity for analyzing the resistance which in practice started psychoanalytic ego psychology. Moreover, in this way two other things were discovered: first, that certain attitudes of the patient's which always recurred when similar instinctual dangers were mobilized served the purpose of resistances, and second that not only was that purpose fulfilled by them in the psychoanalytic treatment, but that the same behavior patterns were also used by the patient in his ordinary life, either to prevent his expressions of certain instincts or to prevent his becoming aware of them. This discovery opened the way to the first "psychoanalysis of character"—that is, to the analysis of the purpose and the historical genesis of certain characterological attitudes as repressions. In the second place, it is an interesting fact that the neuroses themselves, which the analyst had to deal with, have changed. We began today with the statement that in the classical neurosis a continuous personality was suddenly disturbed at certain points by inappropriate actions, impulses, or thoughts. In modern neuroses that is no longer the case. Here the personality does not appear to be uniform, but open, torn, or deformed, and in any case so involved in the illness that one cannot say at what point the "personality" ends and the "symptom" begins. There is a very gradual transition from neurotics to those "psychopaths" and persons with "characterological anomalies," who themselves feel their need for treatment less than do the people around them. I know that you here are especially interested in so-called "criminals," a term which I do not like as a description for psychological facts, because "criminality" is a juridical and not a psychological term. But certainly "criminals" are among such "characterologically deformed" people.

It would be a fascinating task to investigate the cause of the changes in form of neurosis. I merely wish to suggest where I should look for the answer to this question. The method and manner in which the ego admits, repels, or modifies instinctual claims depend to a large extent on the way in which it has been taught to regard them by the surrounding world. During the last decades' morality, this educational attitude toward the instincts has changed very much in our European and American cultures. Classical hysteria works chiefly with the defensive mechanism of genuine repression, which, however, presupposes a simple prohibition of talk concerning the objectionable instincts, chiefly sexual, which upbringing has consistently represented as bad. The inconsistency of present-day education, itself undecided as to which instinctual claims to allow and which to suppress, results in initial license and subsequent sudden, unexpected, and therefore more cruel, deprivation. The inconsistency of the neurotic personality corresponds to this inconsistency in education. The change in the neuroses, it seems to me, reflects the change in morality. In order to understand this, however, one would have to investigate the social changes which have taken place in our culture in the last decades. In any case, the present-day neurotic characters appear to us to possess egos that are restricted by defensive measures, and psychoanalysis has had to adapt itself to this new object—and that might be the decisive reason for the interest in "psychoanalysis of character" and the recent progress which psychoanalytic characterology has made.

Now to the next question: what have "character anomalies" and "neurotic symptoms" in common, and in what respect do they differ from each other? A neurotic symptom is, in general, as you know, a distorted expression of a repressed instinct. But sometimes it is more an expression of the repressing forces—of what safeguards an executed repression. Think, for example, of neurotic impotence or frigidity; this may perhaps occasionally express some masochistic or sadistic instincts too, but it is certainly to a much greater extent, and in all cases, a method of insuring that the subject shall not give in to sexuality, which he unconsciously holds to be dangerous. Or think of the compulsive symptom which reassures the patient against unconscious death wishes. The degree in which repressed instinct and repressing forces participate in the structure of the sympton may vary; but in principle we can say that every symptom is an expression of a conflict between an instinct and counter-forces (anxiety, feelings of guilt, shame, or disgust). The same is true for dreams—cannot the same formula be applied to attitudes or patterns of behavior?

There are some attitudes in which the possibilities for instinctual satisfaction are so obvious to the observer that it does not need psychoanalysis to discover it. Consider, for instance, the amount of sadism which can be satisfied provided the subject thinks that he does it for a higher aim. There are many more attitudes still in which the purpose to repress some instincts, or to defend the subject against an instinctual danger, is obvious. Take, for example, all attitudes of the type of "reaction formation"—that is, over-strained and rigid attitudes that hinder the expression of contrary instinctual attitudes—which nevertheless may sometimes break through in various ways. Thus it seems that in principle these attitudes which a person's ego develops toward his objects as well as his own instincts are also compromises between the instincts and the anxiety which opposes them, just as symptom and dream are. The problems which, after this discovery, are now of more interest, are:

1. What are the differences between dreams and symptoms on the one hand and ego attitudes on the other, and why are those attitudes of an "ego" nature, while dreams and symptoms are alien to the ego?

2. Are all attitudes and behavior patterns such results of instinctual conflicts, or are only a certain type of them of this sort, so that besides them there may exist attitudes which are psychologically of an entirely different character?

We can divide the "attitudes" of an individual into those which are occasional and those which are habitual. The habitual ones may be summarized as "character." Character traits may once more be subdivided into those which appear only in certain situations and those which are comparatively constantly present, suggesting that the instinctual temptation which must be repressed is continually present too. There are people who are impudent, polite, indifferent, ready to prove others at fault, etc., in all situations and to all people. Such attitudes may be called "character defenses" in the narrower sense, in contrast to other types of defense.

It would, of course, be incorrect to consider the word "character" as synonymous with the expression "defensive character attitude." The way in which a person behaves in relation to instinctual actions, how he combines his various tasks in order to find a satisfactory solution—all that too goes to make up "character." In all probability psychoanalytic characterology will have to make a fundamental distinction between character traits in which— most likely after an alliance between them and the object—the original instinctual energy is discharged, and those traits in which psychoanalysis as an "unmasking" psychology can prove that the original instinctual attitude which is contrary to the manifest attitude still exists in the unconscious. We can call the first the "sublimatory" type of character trait, and the second the "reactive formation" type. This second type is betrayed, as already mentioned, either by its forced and rigid nature, or by the occasional breaking through of that which has been repressed.

It can easily be understood why the reactive type is much better understood than the sublimatory type. It is the reactive type which forms characterological anomalies and resistances whose investigation was required of psychoanalysis for practical reasons. They show themselves as frozen residues of former vivid instinctual conflicts. Freud once wrote that "it is always possible for the ego to avoid a rupture in any of its relations by deforming itself, submitting to forfeit something of its unity, or in the long run even to being gashed and rent. Thus the illogicalities, eccentricities and follies of mankind would fall into a category similar to their sexual perversions, for by accepting them they spare themselves repressions." Since the maintenance of these eccentricities must surely correspond to the reactive type and demand an expenditure of energy, it would perhaps be more correct to say that their formation corresponds to a single definite act of repression, so that the necessity for subsequent separate repressions, which would require more energy, and for separate anxiety situations, is avoided. In this way, the ego-restricting attitudes, which act as chronic anchorages of instinctual defense, are not experienced as ego-alien but are worked into the ego. Their constant operation prevents the instinct from becoming manifest, so that we see no living conflict between instinct and defense but something rigid which does not necessarily appear to the patient himself as questionable. The problem for us lies in the relative constancy of the defensive attitude assumed by the ego when faced by different demands both from the external world and from instinctual contents.

This relative constancy could also be understood for certain kinds of attitudes of the reactive type. The special quality of those attitudes seems to depend on a number of factors. It depends partly on the hereditary constitution of the ego, partly on the nature of the instincts against which the defense is directed. (As an example of this, I may quote the classical triad of the anal character: sense of order, parsimony, and obstinacy.) It depends partly, too, on the age at which the child experienced the instinctual conflict in question. At a certain age certain defensive mechanisms and attitudes are more in the foreground than others. In most cases, however, the analysis succeeds in showing that the special attitude was forced on the individual by the external world: either it was the most suitable attitude in a given situation, or all other possible attitudes were blocked in a given situation, or this attitude was promoted by similar modes of behavior in the child's personal environment with which the child identified itself; or else the attitude was exactly the opposite of these modes, which the child was trying *not* to assimilate. In this way the ego which develops a character of a defensive type becomes more and more rigid and unelastic, reproducing the same pattern of behavior instead of reacting individually to individ··al stimuli. Such an ego becomes increasingly poor and loses more and more possibilities of behavior—till analysis succeeds in reawakening the old conflicts and enabling the individual to reach a better solution.

Certainly you will not expect to find that if the analysis succeeds in remobilizing the old conflicts, the once-repressed infantile instincts will come into the open immediately. The child was once afraid of those instinctual impulses, and as a rule its anxiety was actually manifest in the form of an infantile anxiety neurosis. It took time to develop the character attitude of the defensive type with which the individual, as we have seen, escaped from subsequent repressions and anxieties. Thus we can say that in the defensive attitudes anxiety has been *bound*—and we find the proof for this in the fact that in remobilizing the old conflicts the first thing we usually see is that the patient develops more or less severe attacks of anxiety. The analysis of this anxiety which follows, however, brings the instinct in question to the surface. A layer of anxiety has been laid down between the original instinct and the ensuing defensive attitude.

This view that such character attitudes serve the purpose of binding anxiety is not contradicted by what Mrs. Deri has recently said when she stressed the fact that probably of all the attitudes which an individual has developed, those are selected to build up the character—i.e., to become chronic— which are suited to provide satisfactions as well, though it may be in a distorted form. This apparent contradiction can be overcome if two circumstances are borne in mind. First, the defensive attitudes which we are discussing are only one half of the characterological attitudes. There are also the attitudes of the sublimatory type. These have been as yet less inquired into. It may be that the reactive type represents more anxiety, the sublimatory type more satisfaction. The other circumstance which we have to consider is that "satisfaction" does not necessarily only mean "satisfaction of genuine instinctual desires." There exists also a "satisfaction" in the sense of "security"; and the defensive character attitudes certainly are selected because they seem to give to the individual a maximum of security, namely, an avoidance of anxiety situations.

It must be admitted that this whole discussion of character traits as results of conflicts between instincts and the judgment that giving in to the instinct might be a danger, presupposes the existence of a psychic function of judgment or of a psychic instance which is able to experience fear. The question of how the function of judgment develops and how there is gradually established in the infant an apparatus which serves the purpose of communication between the individual and his surroundings, certainly goes beyond the subject of "character analysis." But it was undoubtedly the progress of character analysis which made it possible to see more clearly into that field as well, so that it can be said that the basic functions also of the ego— perception and action—can in principle be explained by the inner actions of outer influences and primitive biological needs. Mention must be made, however, of another complication in the structure of the so-called ego—a complication which occurs much later in life, say from the second to the seventh year of age. I refer to what is known as the "superego." The new elements which are brought into the picture by this agency are of special practical and theoretical importance for character analysis.

I am presuming that you are acquainted with the Freudian conception of the superego as the psychic agency which turns fear into a feeling of guilt. We have said that the first reason why the organism, which is interested in the satisfaction of its instincts, sometimes paradoxically turns against its instincts and tries to defend itself against them—the first reason is fear, based on the judgment that the instincts are dangerous. Some of the feared dangers are real and natural—as when the child gives in to the instinctual demand to grasp at the beautiful fire and burns itself. Some are real and artificial—as when the educating adults punish the child for certain instinctual acts, or threaten to withdraw their affection from the child when it behaves in certain ways (and the child needs this affection urgently), or promise premiums of higher supplies of affection if the child suppresses certain instincts. Others of the feared dangers are imaginary, in so far as the child judges its surroundings according to its own instincts, misunderstands the world in an animistic sense, and therefore expects more dreadful punishments than ever occur in reality. However this may be, in all cases giving in to the instincts becomes connected for the child with the idea of danger. It is a danger which threatens from without, and the executors of it are, to the child's mind, its parents. The child is afraid that its parents may either punish it bodily (the so-called "castration anxiety"), or by a withdrawal of their affection. But later on there comes a time when the child begins to act as a "good child" even when the parents, who might punish it, are not present or will certainly not become aware of its behavior. Then fear has been turned into a feeling of guilt. The parents who might punish it are now, so to say, inside the child itself; they are always present and are to be differentiated from the real parents. Those "inner parents," who watch the child, who give commands and prohibitions, but also prizes and protection—they are the superego, and their "incorporation" is a result of a long instinctual development which we cannot discuss today.

Now I think you already understand why I am talking about this point at considerable length. It has much to do with "character analysis," in so far as the functions of the conscience are a very important component of the character of personality. Very characteristic for a personality are (a) what he considers good and what bad; (b) whether he takes the commands of his conscience seriously or not; (c) whether he obeys his conscience or tries to rebel against it, etc. On what does that depend? It depends, as all psychic structure does, on constitution and experience, and it is the experience part which we can investigate psychoanalytically. The structure of the superego, its strength, and the way in which the ego behaves toward its "id" depend in the first place on the actual behavior of the parents (for the superego, being the incorporation of the parents, is strict when the parents are strict). They depend in the second place on the instinctual structure of the child; and this in its turn depends on the child's mental constitution and all its previous experiences. The child who unconsciously hates his parents fears retaliation —his superego might act toward his ego in the same way as once his ego wished to act toward his parents. But for the most part the superego depends directly on the models which the child had before him in his environment and on the nature of his object relationship, the incorporations of which are represented in his superego. You know from the analysis of so-called criminals that in all probability the most severe deficiencies of the superego are to be observed in persons who in their childhood had no opportunity to develop lasting object relationships because they changed from one more or less loveless foster home to another. But it is not only the *content* of what is to be considered good and bad—what the father first teaches and the superego later demands—that is transmitted from one generation to the other through the superego structure; it is also the *idea* of good and evil itself and the way in which this idea is thought of in our society—it is the authority which asks obedience and promises protection if obedience is given—which are created through this change from fear into feelings of guilt.

We have spoken of the neurotic conflicts as conflicts between instincts on the one side and anxiety or guilt feelings on the other. In our structural terminology we should say that they are conflicts between the id on the one side and its ego, or an alliance between the ego and the superego, on the other. But sometimes there are also conflicts between the ego and the superego. Not all egos accept the demands of the superego without contradiction, and rebellions which were once attempted (or not attempted) against the parents may be continued against the superego. The extreme case of disunion between ego and superego is given in melancholia, where the whole weight of the personality is laid on an extreme pathological feeling of guilt which destroys the remainder of the personality. But you know that when the subject has a certain degree of such a feeling of guilt he may try to prove that it is not justified or to repress and to deny it. Many character anomalies turn out to be attempts of the ego to defend itself against a sense of guilt. There are personalities in whom the need to contradict the superego is so over-whelming that it overshadows all object relationships. They need "supplies of affection" from everybody in the same way as they needed them as little children, using the feeling of being loved as an argument against inferiority and feelings of guilt (and anxieties) into which they fall back when they feel that those supplies are denied. This continual passive asking to be loved— and in a very primitive way, asking to be loved by everybody, without evolving any real relationship to real objects, this being a regression into the ways in which the little child used to center regulation of its conflicts round its self-regard—this asking for love may either be a defense of the ego against the strong superego ("when I am loved, I cannot be as bad as that, after all"), or it may be a deficiency in the development of the superego, in the sense that the individual still is more governed by outer anxiety than by guilt feelings. Such a deficiency of supplies of affection blocks all real object relationships; and it also forms the basis for manifold secondary conflicts. The most characteristic of these is the conflict between the tendency to get by force the supplies which are denied and the tendency to repress every aggression, because the aggressed person might refuse all supplies.

I have repeatedly used the term "real object relationship," but we have not yet discussed what that means.

Love and hatred have a long history of development, and in every phase of this development disturbances may occur which are then reflected in the subject's character. The considerateness for the object which characterizes love is not present from the beginning. The infant's "love" consists only in taking and not in giving; he acknowledges the objects in so far as he needs them for his satisfaction, and when this satisfaction is attained they may disappear. The subject's first experiences in this respect, the way in which he got or did not get his satisfactions as a very small child, may be decisive for his later attitudes toward his objects. His general optimism or pessimism, his relationship to "getting," his capacity or incapacity for being patient, the dependence of his self-regard upon outer supplies, or its independence of them—all this may be determined by his earliest infantile experiences with objects. Later, in the so-called anal period, he is more obliged to take the objects and their demands into consideration. The training in cleanliness is the first occasion on which he has to give up primitive erotogenic pleasure for another person's sake, or rather, for the sake of getting the affection which he needs from his mother. Psychoanalytic characterology has especially studied the different ways in which those conflicts influence the later attitudes of the ego. Certainly here are the first social conflicts, whose specific nature has a formative force. But it would be an error to assume that it may be more or less a matter of chance that those social conflicts cover the anal phase. What we have learned is that it is precisely the anal instincts which, under the influence of these so-called social conflicts, change their aim or object, thus becoming incorporated into the ego. The "anal character traits" have developed, instead of anal-erotic instincts. It is not a "modern alchemy" that instincts may be turned into ego attitudes, as a critical author stated a short time ago. It is a clinical fact which can be observed again and again; and it is proved by the experience that an analysis of the conflicts which resulted in the development of defensive ego attitudes turns them back, after the interposition of overwhelming anxieties, into the original instincts once more.

The same is true for the relation between so-called "orality" and dependence. Their connection is not an accident but an essential one. Man is a mammal, and the human infant is born still more helpless than other mammals and requires feeding and care on the part of adults so that he shall not die. This undoubtedly provides a biological instinctual basis for the fact that every human being has a remote recollection that there were once powerful or, as it must seem to him, omnipotent beings on whose help, comfort, and protection he could depend in time of need. Later the ego learns to become independent and active and to use active means to master the world by itself. But the possibility of a "passive oral attitude" remains as a relic of infancy. Often enough the adult person gets into situations in which he is as helpless once again as he was as a child. Sometimes the forces of nature are responsible, more often social forces which have been created by people. Then he longs for just such omnipotent protection and comfort as was at his disposal as a child. He regresses, as we are used to saying and as we can prove by observing his instinctual behavior, to orality. There are many social institutions which make use of this biologically predetermined longing. To be sure, none of them promises the longed-for help without expecting some return. The conditions that they make vary greatly in different cultures. But all of them combine the promise of comfort and help with ethical conditions. The formula "if you obey me, I will protect you" is the one which all gods have in common with all earthly authorities. It is true that there are great differences between the idea of an almighty god or of a modern employer on the one side and the mother who feeds her child on the other: nevertheless it is the similarity between them, it is the instinctual bond between child and mother, which explains to us the psychological effectiveness of authority. It has been said that a man's character is formed by the social institutions in which he lives. The psychoanalytical instinct psychology does not contradict this statement in the least. On the contrary, it is psychoanalysis which makes it possible to understand how the social institutions work in detail in forming the characters of the individuals who live under their rule. The instincts are interposed between the institutions and the changes of the personalities. It is clear that the individual's character, which is the result of infantile instinctual conflicts, must depend upon the content and intensity of prohibitions and encouragements which the different instincts get in different social institutions. Actually, we see that various cultures produce various character formations.

But we must return from sociology to psychoanalytic practice. What are the basic consequences of what we have been discussing for psychoanalytic practice? It is clear that all mere talking about unconscious instincts or about reconstructions of the historical past of the patient cannot change anything, as long as the energies of those old conflicts, to liberate which is the aim of psychoanalysis, are bound in certain more or less pathological character attitudes. Where there are rigid attitudes instead of living conflicts, the latter must be remobilized. For that purpose it is necessary first to make the patient aware of the peculiarity of his behavior when he is not aware of it spontaneously. When the patient is aware of what he does, he has to become aware of the fact that he is forced to do so, that he cannot do otherwise; then he will understand that it is an anxiety which makes other behavior impossible, and that he needs the behavior in question for purposes of defense. He will learn to understand historically why these defenses were obliged to assume the form they have, and eventually what it is he is afraid of. If the mobilization succeeds he will experience anxiety; and later on, instead of the rigid and frozen attitude, there will appear once again the instinctual impulses in question, the old full emotions. I have shown elsewhere in detail that and how this procedure can be described by the formulas: we change character neuroses into symptom neuroses, and we change character resistances into living transference resistances, in order to handle them afterward as ordinary symptom neuroses and transference resistances are handled. The aim of this mobilization is the reduction of the ego attitudes to those historical situations in which they were originally formed. A special problem is the investigation of this historical situation and the so-called "defense transference"—the fact that the patient seems to "transfer" to his relation to the analyst not only his past instinctual demands but also the past situations in which he developed one particular form of defense. But the explanation of this fact is not very difficult. The character defenses in general have been developed precisely for the purpose of being applied again and again in every similar situation. The patients behave as if they were careful to make continuous application of a method which had previously proved useful against the danger, just as though they never could know when a similar danger might not reappear. What the patient is really striving for unconsciously is certainly the pleasure of instinctual satisfaction. But his past experiences (real or imaginary) force the ego to produce in every situation of temptation memories which once aroused anxiety, and against those memories the same defensive patterns have to be developed over again.

The next question is whether there are any analyses at all which are not "character analyses." And perhaps in a very strict sense there are no such analyses. A certain part of the energies which are bound in useless defensive conflicts and have to be put at the disposal of the individual once again, is always bound in certain defensive attitudes. But undoubtedly there is a difference of degree between real "character analyses" and "symptom analyses."

I should now like to attempt to illustrate by a few examples the historical genesis of character defenses and their treatment. But this is not an easy task. To demonstrate what is really meant, long case histories would be needed, for which the time is lacking. I must limit myself to relating the chief features of two cases which certainly do not offer any very special characteristics.

Similar features can be found in every analysis. And since the cases are rare in which the historical circumstances that necessitated certain attitudes are easily and microscopically understandable, you will excuse me if I use examples which I have once published in a similar connection. I hope that you have not read the paper in question.

The first patient I am going to describe could be called "a Don Juan of achievement." A successful and, in his own line, prominent man, he was in fact always dissatisfied with himself, always striving after higher achievements, with external success, but no sense of inward satisfaction. In a like manner, he was always trying to increase his quite adequate income and was unable to overcome his fear that it might be insufficient. He behaved in the same way in his love life: although women ran after him and he had one success after another, he always felt inwardly dissatisfied—which is understandable, since those relationships were completely lacking in tenderness and had none of the characteristics of a real object relationship. It is clear that the man was so dominated by an overwhelming narcissistic necessity that the libidinal aims of his instincts were completely overshadowed. The man was married to a woman considerably older than himself, who, in some ways, behaved toward him as a mother does to her child; she acted, that is, in many ways as a guardian to him, so that at home he, the big, successful man, was more like a little child. He found this dependence very oppressive, it is true, and was in the habit of revenging himself on his wife by attacks of rage, and by continual unfaithfulness, and by complete lack of consideration. Thus each of them made life a torment to the other. The first defensive function of his persistently unsatisfied wish to be a great man must therefore have been to deceive himself with regard to the fact that he was a little child in so many ways—one of which was his complete lack of consideration for the person who mothered him. This impression is strengthened by the knowledge that his wife was continually goading his ambition, just as his mother was in his childhood. The realization that there was something behind his continued dissatisfaction, which persisted despite all his external successes, and the truth of which he did not wish to admit, was gained in transference analysis. As in every other province, he was very ambitious in analysis and wanted to impress both me and himself by his quick success. At the outset, after he had read Freud, he was forthcoming with theories about his childhood; he grasped comparatively quickly, however, that this was not what mattered to me, and then began to observe himself and his behavior, and to behave like a "favorite pupil," continually stressing, however, the fact that the analysis progressed too slowly and that he was not satisfied with himself. On one occasion, at the last session before the holidays, he came late, because, just as he was starting for his analysis, he had a sudden attack of diarrhea, and this for the first time shook him very much. The bowels putting in their say made him experience the reality of the analysis in an entirely new way. He realized that his continual haste only served the purpose of drowning something else in him. The analysis explained this richly overdetermined diarrhea in the first place as an anxiety equivalent; it then brought this at first incomprehensible anxiety into relation with his fear of insufficient success, insufficient sexual objects, and insufficient earning. It was then discovered that the character formation of the patient had been complete in childhood. He had always been go-ahead, cheeky, outwardly successful; he had always been the first, even in being naughty, but had, nevertheless, always been dissatisfied with himself. In this behavior he had obeyed his mother, who had always been very ambitious for her son and had always urged him on to further deeds. When it appeared that, at bottom, his mother had despised his father, who was a tradesman, and had always said to the boy, "You must be better than your father," etc., it became clear that his behavior expressed a particular form of the return of the oedipus complex from repression; it was not yet intelligible, however, why it had taken this form—why it had this essentially narcissistic note. Various things soon became more obvious, however: his father had illegally sold certain goods, the sale of which was only permitted by special concession; the policeman, therefore, was a dreaded figure in the patient's childhood. In the eyes of the boy, this considerably reduced the power of the father; he determined not be frightened when he was big, but to make policemen afraid of him. (He remained faithful to this intention: as a motorist he loved to get policemen to intervene unjustifiably, and then afterward prove them to be in the wrong.) The circumstances in his home, moreover, were such that at times he had to stand behind the counter and serve when he was six years old. The customers liked the little boy and chose to buy from him; he felt this to be a triumph over his father, whom he already regarded as weak.

There were also two later experiences which particularly accentuated both the patient's continuous need to show his superiority in some such way and the impossibility of satisfying that need. The first experience was that when he was fourteen he was seduced by a maid, with whom he had regular sexual intercourse from that time on. This episode had been changed in memory to make it appear that it was he who had, at this age, seduced the grown-up girl. It needed analysis to convince him that it had happened the other way round, and that the whole of his later attitude to women was an attempt to alter this to him painful memory, in accordance with his wishes. This attempt, by the way, failed in a typical manner: he intended that the large number of women whom he persuaded to have intercourse with him should convince him of his active masculinity, which he unconsciously doubted; more detailed analysis, however, showed that he arranged things so that he seduced the women into showing their willingness, and that it was only when he saw this that he was not able to resist them. The second experience was that at seventeen he had an abscess on the lung for which he was operated on several times and which kept him in bed for months and convalescent for years—so that he had to be passively nursed like a little child.

The patient gradually became afraid of the transference in analysis, afraid that he might become "enslaved" to the analyst. His transference attitude was intended from the beginning to repudiate this anxiety. He attempted, even then, to disparage the analyst and to find "policemen" who were superior to him. What he expected with fear then turned out to have been true: the six-year-old salesman could not feel completely superior to his grown-up father in the role of tradesman. His father, who used to beat him a great deal, had been greatly feared by him in earlier years. His relation to him had completely overshadowed his relation with his mother, and, in consequence, his being needed by his father for business purposes had an additional libidinal value. The passive-narcissistic attitude was suggested to him in his early childhood by particular circumstances including, among others, illness, strict prohibition against masturbation, which put an end to his early phallic attempts, and the strictness of his father who beat him. It was, however, owing to the same set of circumstances that he feared this attitude. In this conflict, his mother's ambition, the disadvantageous comparison of his dreaded father with the policemen, and with his own successes as a salesman showed him a way out: by a continuous outward fight against his passive-narcissistic attitude, he was able to retain it at other points. The seduction by the maid and his illness after puberty then fixated these latter defensive attitudes in his character.

Another patient, a woman, was characterized by the haste with which she always undertook every more or less indifferent enterprise. She was physically, a well as mentally, always in a state of tension, always occupied with tomorrow, never living in the present. This continual activity of the ego remained on the surface to an amazing extent. Her associations spread in

every direction without ever getting any deeper. Her interests and occupa-
tions also bore the stamp of a superficiality which did not correspond to her
intelligence and talents. She avoided everything which had a "serious"
character. In describing her experiences she expressed a peculiar sense of
inferiority: "Nothing that happens to me can be serious or real." The
activity, restlessness, and continual worry about what would happen tomorrow served the purpose of forestalling any serious experience which might
happen, by means of her own, superficial, ego-determined, i.e., play-like
activity. This patient was passionately in love with a man. She could not
leave him, although serious conflicts were aroused in her as a consequence.
In all her anxiety and trouble, and, in particular, at the beginning of a
depression, she escaped—in the same way as a drug addict escapes by means
of his drug—with the help of real or imagined experiences with this man. It
soon became clear that it was not real love that drove her to him, but that he
satisfied narcissistic necessities whose fulfillment repelled anxiety or depression. However, it was not clear in what way he did this. Only gradually did
we realize that the chief quality of this man—and in this he was the diamet-
rical opposite of the patient's husband—was apparently that he was humorous, frivolous, and witty, and never called things by their right names. What
the patient really wanted from him was the reassurance: "I need not be afraid
of sexuality, it's only fun." In a first analysis the patient had from the very
beginning developed the resistance of not speaking, and no progress was
made. Only later did we understand that this had happened because the
analysis was "serious" and that its aim was to call things by their right
names, which the patient wished to avoid at all costs. The analysis with me,
on the contrary, appeared to make very rapid progress. It took us a long time
to understand that this progress was only apparent and was the result of a
particular resistance. I had, by chance, laughed at some remarks which the
patient had made during her first sessions. This enabled her to work "in
isolation." What she had with me was a "fun-analysis" (in the same way
that she enjoyed "fun-sexuality") without the analysis really attacking her
anxieties about her real instinctual life. When a child experiences something
that shakes it deeply, or when it is afraid of some occurrence, it "plays" this
occurrence afterwards. It forestalls in its fantasy what is expected, or repeats
the past occurrence, so changing its own passive role into an active one, in
order to practice mastering the dreaded tensions with the reduced quantities
which it measures out for itself. Our patient had apparently begun this
process but never ended it. Her anxiety was too great for her to make the step

from playing to reality. Just as another patient continually said to herself, out of fear of reality: "It is only an imaginary story and not true," so this one said: "It is only a game and not serious." The analysis showed that the "serious" sexuality had acquired its frightening character as the result of a sadistic component aroused by the birth of a younger brother at the end of the patient's fourth year. This had evoked unconscious anxiety that, if she gave in to her real impulses, she would tear the penis from men and the child from women. It is interesting to note that the escape into "playing" which was suggested to her by various circumstances in the external world was due, among other things, to a particular incident in the nursing of this younger brother. An elder sister had suggested to the patient that she should push over the perambulator and so get rid of the intruder. From that time on the patient was very much frightened of touching her little brother, particularly after she had once noticed how her mother and the nurse had laughed over the little boy as he was micturating. Her mother had persuaded her out of this aversion to touching him by saying: "Take him in your arms; I'm standing here; you're only playing at being his mother; you're not really his mother."

C. Current Views

8. A Psychoanalytic Classification of Character Pathology

Otto F. Kernberg

This paper is a proposal for a classification of character pathology which integrates recent developments in our understanding of severe forms of character pathology, especially the so-called "borderline conditions," with recent developments in psychoanalytic metapsychology. This classification attempts (1) to establish psychoanalytic criteria for differential diagnoses among different types and degrees of severity of character pathology; (2) to clarify the relationship between a descriptive characterological diagnosis and a metapsychological, especially structural, analysis; and (3) to arrange subgroups of character pathology according to their degree of severity. This system of classification should help in the diagnosis of character pathology by providing the clinician with more systematic information about the descriptive, structural, and genetic-dynamic characteristics of the different forms of character pathology. It should also help in the treatment of patients suffering from character pathology by singling out the predominant constellations of character defenses and other defenses peculiar to the categories of character pathology which I propose to describe. Last, but not least, this proposed classification should help in determining the prognosis for psychological treatment in these conditions by differentiating types of character pathology with varying degrees of indication for psychoanalytic treatment and for psychoanalytically oriented psychotherapy.

Freud (1908, 1931) and Abraham (1921–1925) described character pathology in psychoanalytic terms and suggested the first classifications of character pathology. These early classifications were based on their understanding of instinctual, especially libidinal, motivations. Fenichel (1945), after criticizing these and other attempts to develop a psychoanalytic typology of pathological character types, and after incorporating W. Reich's findings (1933), suggested a classification combining dynamic and structural explanations.

Reprinted from Otto Kernberg, *Object Relations Theory and Clinical Psychoanalysis* (New York: Jason Aronson, 1976), 139–60 by permission of Jason Aronson, Inc. Originally published in 1970.

From a dynamic viewpoint, Fenichel classified character traits into "sublimation" and "reactive" types, depending on whether the instinctual energy was discharged freely as part of the character trait or whether it was checked by some countercathectic measure forming part of that character trait. The sublimatory type of character trait, Fenichel stated, was mostly normal, and did not lend itself easily to further typing. In contrast, the reactive type of character traits reflected pathological developments of the personality. Fenichel suggested the subdivision of reactive character traits into attitudes of avoidance (phobic attitudes) and of opposition (reaction formation).

From the structural viewpoint, Fenichel defined character as "the ego's habitual modes of adjustment to the external world, the id, and the superego, and the characteristic types of combining these modes with one another." Accordingly, character disturbances were "limitations or pathological forms of treating the external world, internal drives, and demands of the superego, or disturbances of the ways in which these various tasks are combined."

Combining the dynamic and structural viewpoints, he proceeded to classify the reactive character traits into pathological behavior toward the id (including here among others the classical oral, anal, and phallic character traits); pathological behavior toward the superego (including here moral masochism, apparent lack of guilt feeling, criminality, and "acting-out" characters); and pathological behavior toward external objects (including pathological jealousy, social inhibitions, and pseudosexuality). Fenichel, however, appeared not to be fully satisfied by his proposed classification. He acknowledged that every person shows traits of both sublimatory and reactive types, and he suggested that the reactive characters may be "most satisfactorily subdivided by analogy to the neuroses, for the simple reason that mechanisms similar to the various forms of symptom formation are likewise operative in the formation of character traits." Following this statement, he described phobic and hysterical characters, compulsive characters, cyclic characters, and schizoid characters, as the characterological equivalents of the respective symptomatic neurosis (and psychosis).

Prelinger et al. (1964), in their comprehensive review of psychoanalytic concepts of character, comment that Fenichel's attempt to classify character types "is generally accepted in psychoanalytic theory today."

Because I believe that a re-examination of Fenichel's classification is in order due to the development of psychoanalytic understanding of the pathology and treatment of character disorders since the publication of Fenichel's classic work (Eissler, 1953; Erikson, 1956; Friedlander, 1947; Greenson, 1958; Johnson and Szurek, 1952; Rosenfeld, 1964; Stone, 1954), as well as the broadening of psychoanalytic understanding of borderline character pathology (Boyer and Giovacchini, 1967; Deutsch, 1942; Frosch, 1964, 1970; Knight, 1953; Zetzel, 1968), I shall attempt to incorporate recent findings regarding the degree of severity and the prognosis of character disorders into a psychoanalytic classification of character pathology. In so doing, I shall emphasize recent findings regarding the structural consequences to the ego and superego of pathological object relationships in these patients (Fairbairn, 1952; Giovacchini, 1963; Jacobson, 1964; Kernberg, 1966; Sutherland, 1963; Van der Waals, 1952), and I shall expand my earlier analyses of the structural disturbances in patients with borderline conditions (Kernberg, 1967, 1968).

My proposed classification will incorporate three major pathological developments: (1) pathology in the ego and superego structures; (2) pathology in the internalized object relationships; and (3) pathology in the development of libidinal and aggressive drive derivatives.

I shall describe three levels on the continuum from less severe to more severe character pathologies; for convenience, I have termed these as a "higher level," and "intermediate level," and a "lower level" of organization of character pathology. What follows is an outline of the assumptions underlying the proposed classification of character pathology.

THE ASSUMPTIONS UNDERLYING THE PROPOSED CLASSIFICATION

1. Regarding Instinctual Development

In contrast to earlier attempts at psychoanalytic classification of character pathology on the basis of the stages of libidinal development, the proposed classification assumes that, clinically, three main levels of instinctual fixation can be encountered: a "higher" level, at which genital primacy has been reached and predominates; an "intermediate" level, at which pregenital, especially oral regression and fixation points predominate; and a "lower" level, at which a pathological condensation of genital and pregenital instinctual strivings takes place with a predominance of pregenital aggression. This proposed classification incorporates the findings regarding instinctual developments in patients with borderline personality organization reported in an earlier paper (Kernberg, 1967).

2. Regarding Superego Development

The proposed classification assumes that a relatively well-integrated although excessively severe superego characterizes the "higher" level of organization of character pathology only, and that the "intermediate" and "lower" levels of organization of character pathology reflect the presence of varying degrees of lack of superego integration as well as of the predominance of sadistic superego forerunners over other superego components. Jacobson's comprehensive analysis of normal and pathological stages of superego development (1964) constitutes the basis for these propositions.

3. Regarding Defensive Operations of the Ego and, in Particular, the Nature of Pathological Character Traits

In concordance with the structural model elaborated on in an earlier paper (Kernberg, 1966), two overall levels of defensive organization of the ego are assumed: (1) a basic level at which primitive dissociation or "splitting" is the crucial mechanism for the defensive organization of the ego; and (2) a more advanced level at which repression becomes the central mechanism, replacing splitting. In the proposed classification, the "higher" level of organization of character pathology presents the advanced level of defensive organization, repression being the main defensive operation of the ego, together with related mechanisms such as intellectualization, rationalization, undoing, and higher levels of projection. The same is true for the "intermediate" level of organization of character pathology, except that, in addition, the patient shows some of the defense mechanisms which, in an even stronger, clearly predominant way, characterize the "lower" level. At that "lower" level, primitive dissociation or splitting predominates with a concomitant impairment of the synthetic function of the patient's ego, and the presence of the related mechanisms of denial, primitive forms of projection, and omnipotence. The proposed classification assumes a continuum of pathological character traits, ranging from the sublimatory type of character traits at the one extreme, through inhibitory or phobic character traits, reaction formation type of character traits, to instinctually "infiltrated" character traits at the other extreme. The implication is that the lower the level of defensive organization of the ego, the more there is a predominance of pathological character traits in which defense and direct impulse expression are linked, so that the primal impulse expression shows through the defense. The normal character shows a predominance of sublimatory character traits; the "higher" level of organization of character pathology presents a predominance of inhibitory and reactive character traits; in the "intermediate" level of organization of character pathology, character defenses combining reaction formation against instinct with yet a partial expression of the rejected instinctual impulses make their appearance; and at the "lower" level, instinctually infiltrated character defenses predominate.

4. Regarding the Vicissitudes of Internalized Object Relationships

No particular pathology of internalized object relationships is present at the "higher" level, at which ego identity and its related components, a stable self concept and a stable representational world, are well established; the same is true at the "intermediate" level with the exception of more conflictual object relations than at the "higher" level. At the "lower" level, severe pathology of the internalization of object relationships is present. Object relationships have a "partial" rather than "total" character, and "object constancy" has not been firmly established. Object constancy represents the child's capacity to retain his attachment to a loved person and to the internal representation of that person in spite of frustration and hostility in that relationship (Arlow et al., 1968). Object constancy also reflects the capacity for a total object relationship, that is, a relationship in which good and bad aspects of the object and of the self (and of their respective representations) can be tolerated and integrated. This capacity is missing in these patients, and the lack of integration of the self concept, as well as of the related object representations or representational world, is reflected in the syndrome of identity diffusion (Erikson, 1956; Kernberg, 1967).

What follows is an outline of the structural characteristics of the "higher," "intermediate," and "lower" levels of organization of character pathology, and the type of pathological character formation that belongs to each level. Bibliographic references will indicate sources describing these characterological types and their differential diagnosis.

HIGHER LEVEL OF ORGANIZATION OF CHARACTER PATHOLOGY

At the higher level, the patient has a relatively well-integrated, but severe and punitive superego. The forerunners of his superego are determined by too sadistic impulses, bringing about a harsh, perfectionistic superego. His ego, too, is well integrated; ego identity (Erikson, 1956) and its related components, a stable self concept (Jacobson, 1964), and a stable representational world (Sandler and Rosenblatt, 1962) being well established. Excessive defensive operations against unconscious conflicts center around repression. The character defenses are largely of an inhibitory or phobic nature, or they are reaction formations against repressed instinctual needs. There is very little or no instinctual infiltration into the defensive character traits. The patient's ego at this level is somewhat limited and constricted by its excessive use of neurotic defense mechanisms, but the patient's overall social adaptation is not seriously impaired. He has fairly deep, stable object relationships and is capable of experiencing guilt, mourning, and a wide variety of affective responses (Winnicott, 1955). His sexual and/or aggressive drive derivatives are partially inhibited, but these instinctual conflicts have reached the stage where the infantile genital phase and oedipal conflicts are clearly predominant and there is no pathological condensation of genital sexual strivings with pregenital, aggressively determined strivings in which the latter predominate.

Most hysterical characters (Abraham, 1920; Easser and Lesser, 1965; Shapiro, 1965), obsessive-compulsive characters (Fenichel, 1945), and depressive-masochistic characters (Laughlin, 1956) are organized at this level.

INTERMEDIATE LEVEL OF ORGANIZATION OF CHARACTER PATHOLOGY

At the intermediate level, the excessively punitive nature of the patient's superego is even stronger than that of the higher level disorders, but the superego is less integrated. His superego tolerates contradictory demands between sadistic, prohibitive superego nuclei on the one hand, and rather primitive (magical, overidealized) forms of the ego ideal on the other hand (Jacobson, 1964). These latter, primitive types of internal demands to be great, powerful, and physically attractive coexist with strict demands for moral perfection, and they can be observed in the patient's partially blurred superego-ego delimitations. Deficient superego integration can also be observed in the partial projections of superego nuclei (as expressed in the patient's decreased capacity for experiencing guilt and in paranoid trends), contradictions in the ego's value systems, and severe mood swings. These mood swings are caused by the primitive nature of the superego's regulation of the ego (Jacobson, 1964). The poor integration of the superego, which is reflected in contradictory unconscious demands on the ego, also explains the appearance of pathological character defenses combining reaction formations against instincts with a partial expression of instinctual impulses. At this level, the patient has fewer inhibitory character defenses than the person at the higher level, reaction formations are more prominent, and his character traits are infiltrated by instinctual strivings as seen in dissociated expressions of unacceptable sexual and/or aggressive needs, and a "structured impulsivity" in certain areas. Repression is still the main defensive operation of the ego, together with related defenses such as intellectualization, rationalization, and undoing. At the same time, the patient shows some dissociative trends, some defensive splitting of the ego in limited areas (that is, mutual dissociation of contradictory ego states) (Freud, 1938; Kernberg, 1966), and projection and denial. Pregenital, especially oral conflicts come to the fore, although the genital level of libidinal development has been reached. While pregenital, especially oral features predominate in the clinical picture, such features reflect to a major extent regression from oedipal conflicts; further, the aggressive components of pregenital conflicts are of a "toned down" quality, in contrast to the primitivization of aggression at the "lower level" of organization of character pathology.

Object relationships at this level are still stable in the sense of a capacity for lasting, deep involvements with others, and of a capacity to tolerate the markedly ambivalent and conflictual nature of such relationships.

Most "oral" types of character pathology (Abraham, 1921–1925) are organized at this level, especially what is now designated as the "passive-aggressive" (Brody and Lindbergh, 1967) personality type. Sadomasochistic personalities (Frank et al., 1952), some of the better functioning infantile (or "hysteroid") personalities (Easser and Lesser, 1965; Zetzel, 1968), and many narcissistic personalities (Kernberg, 1970; Rosenfeld, 1964) are at this intermediate level. Many patients with a stable, crystallized sexual deviation (Fenichel, 1945) and with the capacity to establish, within such a deviation, relatively stable object relationships are also at this level.

LOWER LEVEL OF ORGANIZATION OF CHARACTER PATHOLOGY

At the lower level, the patient's superego integration is minimal and his propensity for projection of primitive, sadistic superego nuclei is maximal. His capacity for experiencing concern and guilt is seriously impaired

(Winnicott, 1955), and his basis for self-criticism constantly fluctuates. The individual at this level commonly exhibits paranoid traits, stemming both from projection of superego nuclei and from the excessive use of rather primitive forms of projection, especially projective identification (Klein, 1946) as one major defensive mechanism of the ego. The delimitation between ego and superego is completely blurred: primitive, narcissistically determined forms of the ego ideal are practically indistinguishable from primitive forms of narcissistic ego strivings for power, wealth, and admiration (A. Reich, 1953). The synthetic function of the patient's ego is seriously impaired, and he uses primitive dissociation of splitting (Fairbairn, 1952; Jacobson, 1957; Kernberg, 1967) as the central defensive operation of the ego instead of repression. The mechanism of splitting is expressed as contradictory ego states alternating with each other, and this dissociation is reinforced by the patient's use of denial, projective identification, and unconscious fantasies of omnipotence (Klein, 1946). This omnipotence reflects a defensive identification of the patient's self concept with forerunners of his ego ideal, namely, idealized, condensed primitive self and object images. His pathological character defenses are predominantly of an "impulsive," instinctually infiltrated kind; contradictory, repetitive patterns of behavior are dissociated from each other, permitting direct release of drive derivatives as well as of reaction formations against these drives. Lacking an integrated ego and the capacity to tolerate guilt feelings, such patients have little need for secondary rationalizations of pathological character traits.

These patients' capacity for encompassing contradictory ("good" and "bad") self and object images is impaired, mainly because of the predominance of pregenital aggression as part of both ego and superego identifications. Excessive pregenital aggression also causes a pathological condensation of pregenital and genital conflicts with predominance of pregenital aggression (Kernberg, 1967) and is evidenced by sadistically infiltrated, polymorphous perverse infantile drive derivatives which infiltrate all the internalized and external object relationships of these patients. Thus, their oedipal strivings appear intimately condensed with pregenital sadistic and masochistic needs, and there may be direct expression of oedipal impulses such as in masturbatory fantasies involving the original parental objects.

Their inability to integrate libidinally determined and aggressively determined self and object images is reflected in their maintaining object relationships of either a need-gratifying or a threatening nature. They are unable to have empathy for objects in their totality; object relationships are of a part-object type, and object constancy has not been reached. Their lack of integration of self representations is reflected in the absence of an integrated self concept. Their inner world is peopled by caricatures of either the good or the horrible aspects of persons who have been important to them; and these exaggerated representations are not integrated to the extent that the person could feel that one of his inner objects had a "good side" and a "bad side." By the same token, his inner view of himself is a chaotic mixture of shameful, threatened, and exalted images. The absence of both an integrated world of total, internalized objects and of a stable self concept determine the presence of the syndrome of identity diffusion (Erikson, 1956). In fact, identity diffusion is an outstanding characteristic of this lower level of character pathology. The lack of integration of libidinal and aggressive strivings contributes to a general lack of neutralization of instinctual energy (Hartmann, 1950, 1955), and to a severe restriction of the conflict-free ego.

All these factors, in addition to the disintegrating effects of the predominant mechanisms of splitting and related defenses, and the lack of crucial ego organizers such as an integrated self concept and an integrated superego, contribute to severe ego weakness. Ego weakness is reflected especially in the patient's lack of anxiety tolerance, of impulse control, and of developed sublimatory channels as evidence by chronic failure in work or creative areas (Kernberg, 1967). Primary process thinking infiltrates cognitive functioning and, although not always evident on clinical contacts, it is especially manifest on projective psychological testing (Rapaport et al., 1945–1946).

Most infantile personalities (Easser and Lesser, 1965; Greenson, 1958; Kernberg, 1967; Zetzel, 1968) and many narcissistic personalities (Kernberg, 1970; Rosenfeld, 1964) are organized at this level of organization of character pathology. All patients with antisocial personality structure are at this level (Cleckley, 1964; Friedlander, 1947; Johnson and Szurek, 1952). The so-called "chaotic" impulse-ridden character disorders (Fenichel, 1945; W. Reich, 1933), the "as-if" (Deutsch, 1942) characters, the "inadequate personalities" (Brody and Lindbergh, 1967), and most "self-mutilators" (Kernberg, 1967) belong to this group. Patients with multiple sexual deviations, or a combination of sexual deviation with drug addiction or alcoholism, and with severe pathology of object relationships such as reflected in the strangeness or bizarreness of their sexual needs, are organized at this level (Frosch, 1964; Kernberg, 1967). The same is also true for the so-called "prepsychotic personality structures," that is, the hypomanic, schizoid, and paranoid personalities (Brody and Lindbergh, 1967; Shapiro, 1965).

The next "step down" along this continuum would carry us to the field of the psychoses. The lower level of organization of character pathology which I have been describing consists, in effect, of the group of patients who are generally included in the field of borderline disorders or "psychotic characters" (Frosch, 1964), or present "borderline personality organization" (Kernberg, 1967). The differential diagnosis between patients in the borderline field and the psychoses centers around the persistence of reality testing (Frosch, 1964; Weisman, 1958) in borderline patients, while reality testing is lost in the psychoses. This difference depends, in turn, on the differentiation between self and object representations (Jacobson, 1954, 1964) and its derived delimitation of ego boundaries: these are present in lower level of organization of character pathology, lost or absent in the psychoses.

The earlier-mentioned assumptions underlying the proposed classification outlined above are related to each other in a model of development of the psychic apparatus, a model centered on the development of internalized object relationships which has been spelled out in earlier papers (Kernberg, 1966, 1967, 1968, 1970). What follows is a brief summary of these propositions regarding the development of the psychic apparatus and the mutual relationships of the four kinds of assumptions enumerated before.

THE MUTUAL RELATIONSHIPS OF THE STATED ASSUMPTIONS: AN OBJECT-RELATIONS-CENTERED MODEL OF DEVELOPMENT

The internalization of object relationships represents a crucial organizing factor for both ego and superego development. Introjections, identifications, and ego identity formation represent a progressive sequence in the process of internalization of object relationships. The essential components of internalized object relationships are self images, object images, and specific affect states or dispositions linking each self image with a corresponding object image. Two essential tasks that the early ego has to accomplish in rapid succession are: (1) the differentiation of self images from object images; and (2) the integration of self and object images built up under the influence of libidinal drive derivatives and their related affects with their corresponding self and object images built up under the influence of aggressive drive derivatives and related affects.

The first task is accomplished in part under the influence of the development of the apparatuses of primary autonomy: perception and memory traces help to sort out the origin of stimuli and gradually differentiate self and object images. This first task fails to a major extent in the psychoses, in which a pathological fusion between self and object images determines a failure in the differentiation of ego boundaries and, therefore, in the differentiation of self from nonself. In the "lower" level of organization of character pathology, that is, the case of borderline personality organization, differentiation of self from object images has occurred to a sufficient degree to permit the establishment of integrated ego boundaries and a concomitant differentiation between self and others.

The second task, however, of integration of libidinally determined and aggressively determined self and object images fails to a great extent in borderline patients, mainly because of the pathological predominance of pregenital aggression. The resulting lack of synthesis of contradictory self and object images interferes with the integration of the self concept and with the establishment of "total" object relationships and object constancy. The need to preserve the good self and good object images, and good external objects in the presence of dangerous "all bad" self and object images leads to a defensive division of the ego, in which what was at first a simple defect in integration is then used actively for keeping "good" and "bad" self and object images apart. This is, in essence, the mechanism of splitting, an essential defensive operation of the borderline personality organization which is reinforced by subsidiary defensive operations (especially projective mechanisms) and thus determines an overall type of ego organization different from the more advanced type of ego organization that is normally reached in the "intermediate" and "higher" levels of organization of character and ego development and where repression and related mechanisms replace splitting and its subsidiary mechanisms.

The presence of "all good" and "all bad" self and object images interferes seriously with superego integration because under these circumstances, overidealized self and object images can create only fantastic ideals of power, greatness, and perfection, and not the more realistic demands and goals of an ego ideal constructed under the influence of more integrated, "toned down" ideal self and object images. Projection of "bad" self and object images determines, through reintrojection of distorted experiences of the frustrating and punishing aspects of the parents, a pathological predominance of sadistic superego forerunners, and a subsequent incapacity to integrate the idealized superego components with the sadistically threatening ones. All of this leads to a lack of superego integration and a concomitant tendency to reproject superego nuclei. Thus, dissociative or splitting processes in the ego are now reinforced by the lack of the normal integrative contribution of the superego, and contradictory internalized demands together with the insufficiency of the ego's repressive mechanisms contribute to the establishment of contradictory, instinctually infiltrated, pathological character traits. This development is maximally true at the "lower" level of organization of character pathology, and to some extent also is present at the "intermediate" level of organization of character pathology.

In contrast, when sufficient integration of "good" and "bad" internalized object relationships (involving self images, object images, ideal self images, ideal object images) takes place so as to permit an integrated self concept and a related integrated "representational world" to develop, a stable ego identity is achieved. At this point, a central ego core is protected from unacceptable drive derivatives by a stable repressive barrier, and the defensive character traits that develop have the characteristics of reaction formations or inhibitory traits. The development of this level of integration within the ego also creates the precondition for the integration of the sadistically determined superego forerunners with the ego ideal, and the subsequent capacity to internalize the realistic, demanding and prohibitive aspects of the parents. All of this fosters further superego integration and, eventually, depersonification and abstraction within the superego. The superego may now act as a higher level organizer of the ego, providing further pressures for a harmonious integration of any remaining contradictory trends within the ego. The "toning down" of such an integrated, more realistically determined superego permits a more flexible management of instinctual drive derivatives on the ego's part, with the appearance of sublimatory character traits. At the "higher" level of organization of character pathology the integration of the superego is still excessively under the influence of sadistic forerunners, to the extent that the superego, although well integrated, still remains excessively harsh and demanding. Repressive and sublimatory handling of pregenital drive derivatives, especially of pregenital aggression, is possible to a sufficient extent so that there is less infiltration of genital drive derivatives with pregenital, especially aggressive trends, and the oedipal-genital level of development clearly predominates. At this, the "higher" level of organization of character pathology, excessive severity of the superego centers around excessive prohibition and/or conflicts around infantile sexuality. Object constancy, a capacity for stable and deep object relationships, and a stable ego identity have all been reached at this level.

Normality represents a further, and final progression along this continuum, with a well-integrated and less severe and punitive superego, a realistically discriminating set of superego demands, ego ideal, and ego goals which permit an overall harmony in dealing with the external world as well as with the instinctual needs. The predominance of sublimatory character traits reflects such an optimum expression of instinctual needs, of adaptive and sublimatory integration of pregenital trends under the primacy of genitality, in the context of mature, adult object relationships. A firm repressive barrier against a residuum of unacceptable, infantile instinctual needs is complemented by a large sector of a conflict-free, flexibly functioning ego, and the capacity to suppress some realistically ungratifiable needs without excessive stress.

DIAGNOSTIC, PROGNOSTIC, AND THERAPEUTIC IMPLICATIONS

From a diagnostic point of view, the proposed classification of character pathology may help to differentiate types of character pathology which, at first, may present diagnostic difficulties in individual cases. Thus, for example, the differential diagnosis between hysterical and infantile character pathology is greatly helped by utilizing structural as well as descriptive considerations. The presenting pathological character traits may at first seem hysterical; however, a thorough examination of those traits in terms of what they reveal regarding the superego structure, the predominant defensive operations of the ego, and the kind of conflicts the patient is struggling with, may point to the fact that the predominant pathological character constellation is of an infantile rather than a hysterical type. Also, while certain types of character pathology typically coincide with a certain level of severity of character pathology, this may not be true in every case. Thus, for example, a patient with infantile personality may, on the basis of a structural analysis, appear to be functioning at the "intermediate" rather than the "lower" level of organization of character pathology, with consequences for the prognosis and treatment recommendations. One additional diagnostic advantage of the proposed classification of character pathology is the possibility, on the basis of the structural characteristics of the patient, to predict the kind of defensive operations that will predominate in the treatment, especially as transference resistances.

From the viewpoint of overall prognosis, the proposed classification reflects three levels of severity of characterological illness. The prognosis for psychoanalytic treatment of patients in the "higher" level of organization of character pathology is very good; these patients respond very well to psychoanalysis. The prognosis is less favorable at the "intermediate" level; these patients usually require lengthier psychoanalytic treatment, and the goals of analysis must at times be less ambitious. The prognosis for the "lower" level of organization of character pathology is always serious; at this level classical, nonmodified psychoanalytic treatment is usually contraindicated or a preparatory period of expressive psychotherapy is required (Eissler, 1953; Stone, 1954; Zetzel, 1968).

Some therapeutic implications of the proposed model have already been mentioned as part of the prognostic considerations. For patients at the "higher" level of organization of character pathology, psychoanalysis is the treatment of choice. These patients may seek treatment for symptoms of a rather recent, minor or situationally determined type, which may improve with brief psychotherapy. Ideally, however, they should be treated with psychoanalysis rather than one of the modified psychotherapeutic procedures because at this level the maximum improvement in personality functioning can be expected from analytic treatment. For patients functioning at the "intermediate" level of organization of character pathology, psychoanalysis is still the treatment of choice unless there is some special contraindication. These patients, however, will usually require lengthy psychoanalysis, and it may well be that in some selected cases a modified treatment is preferable either to start with or even as the only mode of treatment. For patients with the "lower" level of organization of character pathology, psychoanalysis is usually contraindicated. A special, modified psychoanalytic procedure with the introduction of parameters of technique (Eissler, 1953) is the treatment of choice at this level. (I have discussed this issue in detail in my 1968 paper.) A few patients at this level may still require or may be able to benefit from nonmodified, classical psychoanalysis. However, even in the case of these patients, the proposed classification may be useful, in that it highlights, in addition to the prognostic "warning," the typical defensive operations of these patients which are so predominant in their transference reactions, and the particular, severe pathology of their superego which may present extremely difficult treatment problems.

LIMITATIONS AND EXCEPTIONS

Several questions may be raised regarding the proposed classification of character pathology.

1. How Consistent Is the Relationship Between the Level of Organization of Character Pathology and the Actual, Overall Functioning of the Individual?

The actual functioning of the individual in adapting to his interpersonal environment and his intrapsychic needs depends largely on the level of his structural, intrapsychic organization. The higher the level of ego organization, the higher is the type of character defenses, and the more predominant the general manifestations of ego strength (impulse control, anxiety tolerance, sublimatory capacities).

Actual psychological functioning, however, also depends on the particular quality of the pathological character traits, and on the interpersonal environment within which such character traits express themselves. Thus, for example, a patient with a masochistic character structure and the higher level of character organization may appear much more disturbed in his interpersonal relationships than what his character organization would warrant, because his unconscious emphasis on self-defeat may bring about interpersonal situations of potentially disruptive or highly inappropriate nature for him. In contrast to this example, a patient with a narcissistic personality and a lower level character organization may function in a much better way than the ordinary patient with borderline personality organization, because of the protective and socially isolating nature of narcissistic character traits (Kernberg, 1970). In this case, the nonspecific manifestations of ego weakness (lack of anxiety tolerance, lack of impulse control, lack of sublimatory channels) may be absent, in spite of the presence of a typical defensive ego organization of the lower level character pathology and of severe superego pathology.

The actual functioning of the individual also depends on the degree of pathological superego pressures his ego is subjected to. Thus, for example, a patient with a depressive-masochistic personality structure and a particularly strict, sadistic but well-integrated superego may experience severe depressions of such a disorganizing nature that nonspecific manifestations of ego weakness make their appearance. Again, actual functioning may be much worse than what one would expect from the underlying level of organization of character pathology. Finally, the particular quality of a neurotic symptom also may influence the general functioning of the individual. Particular symptoms may have such a crippling effect on a person's life situation that his

overall functioning may be much more disturbed than his level of organization of character pathology would suggest.

A comparative study of a patient's actual functioning and of his underlying
level of organization of character pathology may be of great help in determining the analyzability of the patient. For example, in narcissistic personalities
with overt borderline functioning (such as indicated by nonspecific manifestations of ego weakness and clinical manifestations of primary process thinking) psychoanalysis is usually contraindicated. (In spite of their underlying
borderline structure, we expect a better surface functioning in narcissistic
personalities.) Other patients with nonspecific manifestations of ego weakness and with severe disturbances of their interpersonal life may, however,
have a good indication for psychoanalysis if, structurally, they belong to the
higher level of organization of character pathology, and their ego functioning
is disturbed because of massive pressures from a sadistic, though well-
integrated superego.

2. How Consistently Is a Descriptive Characterological Diagnosis Related to the Corresponding Level of Organization of Character Pathology?

While actual functioning does not reflect directly the underlying level of
organization of character pathology, the relationship between a descriptive
characterological diagnosis and the underlying level of character organization
is a much closer one. This close relationship is especially marked at the
higher level of organization of character pathology and at the lower level of
character organization. However, the relationship between the descriptive
characterological diagnosis and the underlying level of character organization
is less clear in the case of the intermediate level.

In general terms, the intermediate level of organization of character pathology is broader and more complex than either the higher or the lower one.
Subclassifications may be warranted at this intermediate level. I have observed at least two subgroups of ego organization within the intermediate
level of organization of character pathology. One type of ego organization is
represented by a "mixture" of defensive operations stemming from both
repression and splitting. This type of intermediate level character organization usually shows a combination of reactive character traits and instinctually
infiltrated ones. For example, there are some hysterical personalities with
infantile trends who present dissociative tendencies and episodic acting out

in which repressed sexual or aggressive impulses become conscious although dissociated from the usual self experience of the patient. The other subgroup of ego organization at the intermediate level is expressed by a layer of higher level ego organization centering around repression, underneath which is a layer of the lower form of ego organization centering around splitting. This form of structural organization is rather infrequent, but of great theoretical interest because it illustrates the mutual relationship of certain defensive operations of the ego and the nature of pathological character traits. Some patients with hysterical personality, generalized repression of some instinctual needs, and rather solid reaction formations experience occasional regressions or "breakdowns"; at such times, they may experience depersonalization, affect storms, strong paranoid trends, and present complex behavior patterns involving both defenses against and direct expression of rather primitive instinctual needs. What is so striking in these patients is that at the regressed level they still operate with complex ego patterns and defenses, and that reality testing is still preserved in the middle of serious malfunctioning. These cases present a failure of the repressive barrier and the activation of a more primitive ego structure when the higher level repressive structure fails.

3. How Stable Are the Three Levels of Organization of Character Pathology Outlined in this Paper?

Patients of the kind mentioned, who may abruptly shift in their level of structural organization as a consequence of a "double layer" of ego organization, represent one example of structural instability. In more general terms, there exists a minority of patients whose character organization is unstable. In these patients a higher level of organization of character pathology (and particularly of ego organization centering around repression) represents a defensive organization against a lower level of character and ego organization. The grouping of these patients into the intermediate level of organization of character pathology is not quite satisfactory.

In contrast to the cases, most other patients present a remarkable stability of their level of structural organization. Whatever changes in the level of organization of character pathology occur are slow, gradual developments within a psychoanalytic treatment or a psychoanalytically oriented psychotherapy. The transitory psychotic regressions that borderline patients present as an expression of a transference psychosis are not true structural changes, but rather a product of temporary loss of reality testing related to the pathological activation of projective and other primitive defensive operations. Such psychotic regressions are usually quite reversible (Frosch, 1970).

4. How Consistently Are the Structural Organization of the Ego and the Superego Related to Each Other?

In the section on "The Mutual Relationships of the Stated Assumptions: An Object-Relations-Centered Model of Development," I proposed that there exists, indeed, a close correspondence between the level of structural organization of ego and superego, and that the vicissitudes of internalized object relationships are a crucial organizing factor determining that correspondence. Thus, for example, a certain level of ego organization is a necessary prerequisite for the development of higher level superego structures on the one hand, and for the eventual integration and abstraction of the superego on the other. There are exceptions, however, reflecting irregularities in the development of some psychic structures, especially at the lower level of organization of character pathology. For example, there are patients with rather typical borderline organization of the ego who do have a better integration of superego functions than what one would usually expect at the borderline level. Such patients have a better capacity to tolerate guilt and concern for themselves and others and, while projection of superego pressures occurs, there is still a remnant of relatively integrated, abstracted superego functions which remains undisturbed. These patients have a better prognosis for treatment, and for some of them a nonmodified psychoanalysis may even be the treatment of choice.

SUMMARY

In this paper I propose a classification of character pathology in the attempt (1) to establish psychoanalytic criteria for differential diagnoses among different types and degrees of severity of character pathology; (2) to clarify the relationship between a descriptive characterological diagnosis and a metapsychological, especially structural, analysis; and (3) to arrange subgroups of character pathology according to their degree of severity.

This classification reflects a conviction as to the usefulness of a diagnostic study of patients involving structural and genetic-dynamic considerations in addition to purely descriptive ones. The developments in psychoanalytic technique and in modified, psychoanalytically oriented procedures have provided us with a broad armamentarium of psychotherapeutic tools. The development of diagnostic criteria derived from psychoanalytic theory could improve our capacity for optimal individualization of psychological treatment.

BIBLIOGRAPHY

Abraham, K. (1920), Manifestations of the female castration complex. *Selected Papers on Psycho-Analysis*. London: Hogarth Press, 1927, pp. 338–369.

————. (1921–1925), Psycho-analytical studies on character-formation. *Selected Papers on Psycho-Analysis*. London: Hogarth Press, 1927, pp. 370–417.

Arlow, J. A., Freud, A., Lampl-de Groot, J., & Beres, D. (1968), Panel discussion. *Int. J. Psycho-Anal.*, 49:506–512.

Boyer, L. B. & Giovacchini, P. L. (1967), *Psychoanalytic Treatment of Schizophrenic and Characterological Disorders*. New York: Science House, pp. 208–335.

Brody, E. B. & Lindbergh, S. S. (1967), Trait and pattern disturbances. In: *Comprehensive Textbook of Psychiatry*, eds. A. R. Freedman & H. I. Kaplan. Baltimore: Williams & Wilkins, pp. 937–950.

Cleckley, H. (1964), *The Mask of Sanity*, 4th ed. Saint Louis: Mosby, pp. 362–401.

Deutsch, H. (1942), Some forms of emotional disturbance and their relationship to schizophrenia. *Psychoanal. Quart.*, 11:301–321.

Easser, B. R. & Lesser, S. R. (1965), Hysterical personality: a re-evaluation. *Psychoanal. Quart.*, 34:390–405.

Eissler, K. R. (1953), The effect of the structure of the ego on psychoanalytic technique. *J. Amer. Psychoanal. Assoc.*, 1:104–143.

Erikson, E. H. (1956), The problem of ego identity. *J. Amer. Psychoanal. Assoc.*, 4:56–121.

Fairbairn, W. D. (1952), *An Object Relations Theory of Personality*. New York: Basic Books, 1954.

Fenichel, O. (1945), *The Psychoanalytic Theory of Neurosis*. New York: Norton, pp. 268–310, 324–386, 463–540.

Frank, J. D. et al. (1952), Two behavior patterns in therapeutic groups and their apparent motivation. *Hum. Relat.*, 5:289–317.

Freud, S. (1908), Character and anal erotism. *Standard Edition*, 9:167–175. London: Hogarth Press, 1959.

————.(1931), Libidinal types. *Standard Edition*, 21:215–220. London: Hogarth Press, 1961.

————.(1938), Splitting of the ego in the process of defence. *Standard Edition*, 23:273–278. London: Hogarth Press, 1964.

Friedlander, K. (1947), *The Psycho-Analytical Approach to Juvenile Delinquency*. New York: International Universities Press, pp. 183–187.

Frosch, J. (1964), The psychotic character: clinical psychiatric considerations. *Psychiat. Quart.*, 38:81–96.

————. (1970), Psychoanalytic considerations of the psychotic character. *J. Amer. Psychoanal. Assoc.*, 18:24–50.

Giovacchini, P. L. (1963), Integrative aspects of object relationships. *Psychoanal. Quart.*, 32:393–407.

Greenson, R. R. (1958), On screen defenses, screen hunger, and screen identity. *J. Amer. Psychoanal. Assoc.*, 6:242–262.

Hartmann, H. (1950), Comments on the psychoanalytic theory of the ego. In: *Essays on Ego Psychology*. New York: International Universities Press, 1964, pp. 113–141.

———. (1955), Notes on the theory of sublimation. In: *Essays on Ego Psychology*. New York: International Universities Press, 1964, pp. 215–240.

Jacobson, E. (1954), Contribution to the metapsychology of psychotic identifications. *J. Amer. Psychoanal. Assoc.*, 2:239–262.

———. (1957), Denial and repression. *J. Amer. Psychoanal. Assoc.*, 5:61–92.

———. (1964), *The Self and the Object World*. New York: International Universities Press.

Johnson, A. M. & Szurek, S. A. (1952), The genesis of antisocial acting out in children and adults. *Psychoanal. Quart.*, 21:323–343.

Kernberg, O. (1966), Structural derivatives of object relationships. *Int. J. Psycho-Anal.*, 47:236–253.

———. (1967), Borderline personality organization. *J. Amer. Psychonal. Assoc.*, 15:641–685.

———. (1968), The treatment of patients with borderline personality organization. *Int. J. Psycho-Anal.*, 49:600–619.

———. (1970), Factors in the psychoanalytic treatment of narcissistic personalities. *J. Amer. Psychoanal. Assoc.*, 18:51–85.

Klein, M. (1946), Notes on some schizoid mechanisms. In: *Developments in Psycho-Analysis*, ed. J. Riviere. London: Hogarth Press, 1952, pp. 292–320.

Knight, R. P. (1953), Borderline states. In: *Psychoanalytic Psychiatry and Psychology*, eds. R. P. Knight & C. R. Friedman. New York: International Universities Press, 1954, pp. 97–109.

Laughlin, H. P. (1956), *The Neuroses in Clinical Practice*. Philadelphia: Saunders, pp. 394–406.

Prelinger, E., Zimet, C. N., Schafer, R., & Levin, M. (1964), *An Ego-Psychological Approach to Character Assessment*. Glencoe: Free Press, pp. 11–36.

Rapaport, D., Gill, M. M., & Schafer, R. (1945–1946), *Diagnostic Psychological Testing*, 2 Vols. Chicago: Year Book Publishers, 1:16–28; 2:24–31, 329, 366.

Reich, A. (1953), Narcissistic object choice in women. *J. Amer. Psychoanal. Assoc.*, 1:22–44.

Reich, W. (1933), *Character Analysis*. New York: Noonday Press, 3d ed., 1949.

Rosenfeld, H. (1964), On the psychopathology of narcissism: a clinical approach. *Int. J. Psycho-Anal.*, 45:332–337.

Sandler, J. & Rosenblatt, B. (1962), The concept of the representational world. *The Psychoanalytic Study of the Child*, 17:128–145. New York: International Universities Press.

Shapiro, D. (1965), *Neurotic Styles*. New York: Basic Books.

Stone, L. (1954), The widening scope of indications for psychoanalysis. *J. Amer. Psychoanal. Assoc.*, 2:567–594.

Sutherland, J. D. (1963), Object-relations theory and the conceptual model of psychoanalysis. *Brit. J. Med. Psychol.*, 36:109–124.

Van der Waals, H. G. (1952), Discussion of the mutual influences in the development of ego and id. *The Psychoanalytic Study of the Child*, 7:66–68. New York: International Universities Press.

Weisman, A. D. (1958), Reality sense and reality testing, *Behav. Sci.*, 3:228–261.

Winnicott, D. W. (1955), The depressive position in normal emotional development. *Brit. J. Med. Psychol.*, 28:89–100.

Zetzel, E. R. (1968), The so-called good hysteric. *Int. J. Psycho-Anal.*, 49:256–260.

9. Character Analysis

Otto F. Kernberg

In line with earlier efforts to enrich an ego-psychology approach to psychoanalytic technique with object relations theory (see Kernberg, 1980, chap. 9), my aim here is to integrate my ideas regarding the structural characteristics of severe character pathologies with Fenichel's (1941) theory of technique. Fenichel's proposals for metapsychological criteria for interpretation both incorporated and critically revised Wilhelm Reich's (1933) technical recommendations for analyzing character resistances.

According to my understanding, unconscious intrapsychic conflicts are not simply conflicts between impulse and defense but are between two opposing units or sets of internalized object relations. Each of these units consists of a self and an object representation under the impact of a drive derivative (clinically, an affect disposition). Both impulse and defense find expression through an affectively imbued internalized object relation.

Pathological character traits carry out dominant, chronic defensive functions in the psychic equilibrium of patients with severe character pathology. All character defenses consist of a defensive constellation of self and object representations directed against an opposite and dreaded, repressed self and object constellation. For example, a man who is excessively submissive may be operating under the influence of a unit consisting of a self representation submitting happily to a powerful and protective parental (object) representation. But this set of representations is defending him against a repressed self representation rebelling angrily against a sadistic and castrating parental representation. These conflicting internalized object relations may, under optimal circumstances, become reactivated in the transference, in which case character defenses become transference resistances. Formulating the interpretation of these transference resistances in terms of their hypothesized internalized object relations may facilitate the reactivation of these component self and object representations in the transference, thus transforming the

Adapted from the *Journal of the American Psychoanalytic Association* 31: 247–71 by permission of International Universities Press, Inc. Copyright 1983 by American Psychoanalytic Association.

"hardened" character defense into an active intrapsychic and transferential conflict.

The severer the patient's character pathology, the more pathological character traits acquire specific transference functions and become both character resistances and specific transference resistances simultaneously (Fenichel, 1945, pp. 29, 537). The compromised formation between impulse and defense represented by these pathological character traits also leads to more or less disguised impulse gratification in the transference. The fact that in severe cases pathological character traits prematurely and consistently intrude in the transference situation means that the patient seems to enter prematurely a stage of severe distortion in his relation to the analyst, which resembles the ordinary transference neurosis but also differs from it. The typical transference neurosis in less severe cases takes some time to develop and is usually accompanied by a diminishing of the patient's neurotic manifestations outside the analytic sessions. The transference of the patient suffering from severe character pathology, however, seems to consist of the patient's playing out in the sessions a pattern that simultaneously persists in the rest of his life as well. In addition, the severity of the pathology is reflected in the degree to which pathological character traits are expressed in nonverbal behavior in the treatment situation rather than by means of free association.

To further complicate matters, the severer the character pathology, the more the patient's nonverbal behavior, examined over many weeks or months, also shows a paradoxical development. Chaotic shifts occur from moment to moment in each psychoanalytic session, making it very difficult to select the predominant material for interpretation. And yet, over a period of weeks, months, or even years, a strange stability in that apparent chaos can be detected. An unconscious, highly specific set of distortions emerges in the patient's relation to the analyst which reflects defensively activated, internalized object relations. These have to be resolved as part of the analysis of the transference in order to obtain significant structural intrapsychic change. Frequently, two contradictory sets of primitive object relations are activated alternately, functioning as defenses against each other; sometimes their mutual dissociation is the dominant resistance that must be worked through. Or else one specific primitive object relation acquires a long-term, subtle, but controlling influence over the patient's relationship with the analyst and expresses itself in a distortion of the psychoanalytic setting over time rather than in concrete developments that fluctuate session by session.

CLINICAL VIGNETTE

Mr. T. A professional in the field of social rehabilitation, an unmarried man in his mid-thirties, consulted because of difficulties in his relations with women and in his work with clients, a severely limited capacity for empathy, and a general sense of dissatisfaction expressed in experiences of boredom, irritability, and uncertainty over the meaning life held for him. He suffered from a narcissistic personality without overt borderline or antisocial features.

His initial attitude toward entering psychoanalysis and the method of free association was marked by strong ambivalence. On the one hand, he considered me one of the more desirable analysts in the relatively small local professional community where I worked; on the other hand, he thought that psychoanalysis was a rather old-fashioned and "passé" technique, and he regarded what he experienced as my rigid maintenance of a psychoanalytic stance as pompous and pedestrian. His own theoretical approach and background were almost diametrically opposed to psychodynamic views. In the early stages of his psychoanalysis, Mr. T was also extremely concerned about my interest in what he was saying; he suspected me of total indifference to him and interpreted any movement I made behind the couch as activity having no relation with him (such as balancing my checkbook). He became very angry when I failed to remember a name or an event he had mentioned in an earlier session.

Mr. T's free associations centered on his relation with his latest woman friend. At first he considered her very attractive and desirable, but he gradually discovered shortcomings in her that made him feel that she was getting much more from him than he was from her and led him to wish to terminate the relationship. In this context, his general suspiciousness of women, his fear that they were exploiting him, emerged as a major theme. This fear could be traced back to the relation with his mother, a locally prominent socialite who dominated his father and whom he had experienced as dominant, intrusive, dishonest, and manipulative. The patient described his father as a hardworking and effective businessman, withdrawn and chronically unavailable during Mr. T's childhood.

During the first two years of his psychoanalysis, the connection between his reactions to his girlfriend, his mother, and me became more and more evident. I was hypocritically pretending that I was interested in him when in reality I was using him for my own financial interest, or pretending to listen to him when I was engaged in my own activities. Similarly, his girl pretended to love him but was interested only in exploiting him socially and financially. Gradually it also became apparent that in his treatment of her he himself was dominant and exploitative, expecting her to guess his moods and respond to his needs without his paying attention to hers. Whenever I tactfully tried to make him aware of his contribution to their difficulties, Mr. T angrily accused me of trying to make him feel guilty and of acting the way his mother did toward him. He saw me as sly, intrusive, dominant, and guilt provoking, just like his mother.

In the transference, my enactment of the replica of his mother now seemed complete: Either I was silent, indifferent, and only pretending to be interested in him or I was actually interested in brainwashing him with my views by making him feel guilty and sadistically enjoying that control. Efforts to convey to him that he was attributing to me aspects of his own behavior toward women that he could not tolerate himself were futile. He broke up with his girlfriend and, several months later, established a new relationship with a woman which soon became a facsimile of the previous one.

Over the next year, the same issues seemed to repeat themselves endlessly in free association and in his relationship to me. I gradually reached the conclusion that the enactment of the relationship with his mother in the transference and with his girlfriends served powerful defensive as well as instinctual purposes. It was as if he managed to obtain some secret (at least partial) satisfaction of his unacknowledged needs for sadistic control from the women he saw. The women also served as receptacles for massive projection of his mother, thus providing rationalizations for his attacks on them.

In the third year of his psychoanalysis, I realized that Mr. T's relation to me in the transference had basically not changed since the beginning of treatment. Nor had his discovery of childhood experiences with his mother (which explained, apparently, his current relations to his girlfriends and to me) resulted in any change of his consciously held convictions about his present or past. I also noticed in his continuing suspicion and anger toward me an easy activation of fantasies of stopping the treatment. Although he never actually stopped, I did not have the feeling of certainty about his engagement in analysis that I had with other patients who might miss occasional sessions when acting out negative transference reactions but without shaking my conviction that they would return. With this man, I sensed both a fragility in our relation and a definite lack of deepening of it.

I also observed, over a period of months, that Mr. T listened to my interpretations eagerly enough, but he then either agreed with them, with the implication that he had earlier reached those very conclusions himself, disagreed with them immediately, or attempted to argue with me about them. Interpretations that he did not accept immediately he simply dismissed. At other times, he appeared very much interested in an interpretation and, in fact, attempted to use it in counseling his own clients, but he never gave any evidence of making use of it to deepen his understanding of himself in his hours with me. In short, his reactions to my interpretations reflected a chronic incapacity to depend upon me for further psychological exploration. Instead, he seemed intent on extracting interpretations from me and appropriating them for his own use. Abraham's (1919), Rosenfeld's (1964), and my own (1975) observations on narcissistic transference resistances clearly applied to this patient.

When I attempted to interpret these dynamics to him and to explore the functions of his attitude, it emerged that Mr. T was protecting himself against intense feelings of envy of me by utilizing for his own purposes whatever he saw as new and good coming from me. These envious feelings and the defenses against them reflected both preoedipal and oedipal conflicts. It gradually became evident to him that, although he could thus protect himself from feeling envious of me, he was precluding using my comments for his own self-exploration. This discovery led us back to his initial derogatory and critical attitude toward psychoanalysis as opposed to his affirmation of his own very different approach to clients.

Over a period of time, Mr. T began to understand that he was torn between his views of me as someone who might be instrumental in helping him to overcome his difficulties with women, someone he would therefore feel extremely envious of, which was intolerable, and someone he did not have to envy at all, which would reconfirm his conviction that nothing was to be expected from psychoanalysis. This analysis of his attitude toward my interpretations and, by implication, of his sharply contradictory and constantly oscillating attitude toward me intensified his sense of restlessness and loneliness in the sessions. He felt that even if what I was pointing out to him was accurate, my doing do implied a grandiose triumph over him and showing off on my part; as a result, he felt powerless, lost, and rejected by me.

In this context, in the fourth year of his psychoanalysis, the following rather protracted episode took place. Mr. T became increasingly alert to whatever he could experience as my shortcomings, both in and outside the sessions. Unbeknown to me, he developed a network of information about me that extended through various related groups in the small town where we both lived and culminated in his establishing contact with a group of disaffected members of the local psychiatric community who deeply resented the institution I was in and my role in it. Mr. T began to extract from one person who felt especially hostile to me information that the patient considered damaging to me, while feeding his contact information about my shortcomings as an analyst. When this information, amplified, came back to my patient through a third person, he became alarmed and "confessed" the whole process to me. That he had for weeks been withholding all these developments from me in itself illustrates the tenuousness of the therapeutic relationship, the limitations in the patient's free associations, and the distortion in the psychoanalytic setting.

My immediate emotional reaction to Mr. T's confession was intense. I felt hurt and angry, controlled by the patient, and helpless. It took several hours before I realized that Mr. T's relationship to his mother had now become activated with reversed roles, that he was now identifying himself with the aggressor, and that I, in the countertransference, was identifying with him as the victim of his mother's manipulations. I also became aware of the patient's intense fear that I might retaliate or abandon him and that this fear was clearly mixed with guilt feelings. After exploring his fantasies about my retaliating and rejecting him—he spontaneously remarked that that is what he would feel like doing in similar circumstances—I said that his description of his own behavior resembled his descriptions of his mother's treatment of him, an interpretation he could now accept. I also told him that his awareness that his curiosity about me contained aggressive elements made it less necessary for him to deny these feelings. Mr. T then said that he had found the exchange of information with the hostile group exciting. He had felt all along that he was transgressing our essential understanding about open communication, risking, as he saw it, the continuation of his relation with me but also experiencing a sense of freedom and power that was exciting, even intoxicating. In fact, he added, now that he was no longer afraid that I would throw him out, he could see something "good" in the entire experience.

Further exploration led to his awareness that his sense of satisfaction, power, and excitement came from his feeling that he could successfully control and manipulate me and I was really quite limited by my analytic attitude; he had never seen our relationship in this context before. This, in turn, led to further exploration of his now activated relationship to me in which he dared to identify with his mother, acknowledging a profound sense of power and satisfaction in expressing aggression that he had never dared to accept in himself, while I appeared in the role of himself, helplessly dominated by him as his own mother. This aggression included elements of orally determined envy and anal-sadistic impulses condensed with castrating impulses (which became dominant at later stages of the analysis).

For the first time, Mr. T was able to experience an identification with the image he had projected of his mother throughout all these years. At the same time, he achieved contact with the aggressive, revengeful components of his envy of me. Over the next few months it became possible to point out to him how his image of himself as helpless, empty, defeated, and lonely vis-á-vis exploitative women was a defense against the opposite self-image, in which he identified with his powerful mother and sadistically enjoyed himself in relating to women and to me as his (her) powerless slaves. The result was an integration of the previously dissociated and repressed sadistic self representation identifying with his mother and the empty, impotent self defensively set up against it. As a consequence, and in the context of the integration of these contradictory affects and self representations, Mr. T became more able to explore his relationship to me in depth and to deepen his understanding of his relationship to women and to his mother as well. Beyond that, a new image of me began to emerge in the transference. I became a tolerant and warm father toward whom the patient experienced dependent and sexual longings, marking, for the first time, a shift in the nature of the predominant transference paradigm and in his experience of the past.

Several technical aspects of this case might be highlighted. First, the early activation of transference resistances (Mr. T's anger and suspicion of my lack of interest in him) repeated aspects of his relations to women. I could therefore immediately integrate the analysis of character resistances with the main themes emerging through free association (his relation to his girlfriends). Next, the partial nature of his self representation, his related incapacity for deepening his emotional relationship to me as well as to his girlfriends, and the corresponding rigidly maintained version of his past gradually emerged as a self-perpetuating, global resistance to further advance in the treatment. Now my focus on the patient's attitude toward my interpretations permitted the interpretation of the most pervasive aspect of his narcissistic personality structure, namely, his identification with a sadistic maternal representation as a core constituent of his pathological grandiose self. The working through of that feature in the transference was necessary for any further move in the psychoanalytic process.

It should be stressed that the excited and sadistic behavior toward me, connected with a dissociated self representation, was available as a conscious experience in Mr. T's relations to various women, where it was expressed only in temper tantrums and protracted emotional storms that were "justified" by his massive projection of mother's image onto the women. Hence, this particular self representation was conscious yet dissociated from self experiences in which Mr. T felt lonely and inferior. He rationalized and protected himself against these feelings by primitive defensive operations, particularly projective identification. The expression of this grandiose and sadistic pattern in the transference and its integration, by means of interpretation, with contradictory self representations of the defeated, exploited child marked the successful completion of a systematic analysis of the corresponding character resistances that had first emerged in relation to my interpretations. In retrospect, the patient could understand that, in rejecting my interpretations as well as in coopting them, he had subtly enacted his mother's role and also his own role as a frustrated child.

This development also illustrates one interesting difference between the narcissistic grandiose self and the dissociated or repressed normal self representations against which the grandiose self is defending. The patient's dominant self-concept was of himself as a mistreated child entitled to compensation. This concept was hidden behind a self-righteous and well-rationalized exploitation of women and a derogatory dismissal of whatever might stir his envy. In contrast, the sadistic, angry, yet excited aspect of the self that emerged in the transference was also part of the normal, aggressively infiltrated self representation, paradoxically closer to authenticity and depth in relation to objects than the defensive surface self representation. At the deepest level, his concept of his sadistic mother included the projection onto her of his own rageful feelings from many sources.

From a still different viewpoint, the sense of stalemate I experienced throughout an important part of the third year of treatment could retrospectively be interpreted as the consequence of the mechanism of omnipotent control. The patient was successfully interfering with my interpretation of the dissociated aggressive aspects of his self, angrily accusing me of trying to make him feel guilty every time I attempted to interpret aggressive aspects of his behavior that he could not accept in himself. It was as if I had to function as a dominant mother or else remain impotently in the background. My hurt and angry reaction after his acting out of the negative transference aspects signaled, in addition to my own countertransference potential, the activation within me of his image of himself as the helpless, attacked, and hurt little boy faced with an overpowering mother. My emotional reaction could thus help me to further analyze an aspect of his experience of himself in relating to his mother, while pointing to his enacting the role of his mother in his relation to me. This formulation makes use of the concepts of concordant and complementary identification in the countertransference proposed by Racker (1957), which emphasized an object relations perspective in the analysis of countertransference.

STRATEGIES OF CHARACTER ANALYSIS

The severity of character pathology is not in itself sufficient to indicate whether interpretation of character resistances should be given early or later. In this regard, Fenichel's (1941, p. 67) proposal that character defenses be examined in accordance with what is predominant at any point in the analytic situation is a reasonable approach to the practical issue of when to interpret character resistances. He suggests first working with the patient's habitual and continuous character defenses in order to "release the personality from its rigidity" and working with other character resistances only when they have become transference resistances (p. 68). But one first has to know whether what one is confronting is character resistance and, if it is, whether it is economically predominant at the time.

Fenichel suggests working "at the point of the *most important* current instinctual conflicts. It is the point of the most important conflicts *at the moment*" (1941, p. 47). In my view the economic criterion for interpretation is determined by the point of highest affect disposition in the material. Insofar as drives (whether functioning as part of the defense or on the impulse side of the conflict) are manifest as affectively invested internalized object relations, the affectively predominant object relation in the analytic situation represents the economically dominant instinctual conflict as well. But affective dominance is not equivalent to consciousness or surface manifestations. As Fenichel put it: "For we must operate at that point where the affect is actually situated at the moment; it must be added that the patient does not know this point and we must first *seek out* the places where the affect is situated'' (1941, p. 45).

I propose that the evaluation of (1) the content of free associations, (2) the prevailing nature of the interactions in the patient/analyst relation—including the patient's nonverbal behavior during the sessions—and (3) the patient's overall relation to the psychoanalytic setting over a period of months or even years makes it possible to discern whether pathological character traits have invaded the transference, resulting in a condensation of transference and character resistances, and whether these character resistances have become affectively predominant, thus justifying the highest priority as the focus of psychoanalytic interpretations.

If free association is proceeding satisfactorily, if the resistances emerging in the context of exploring possible restrictions of free association can be interpreted—regardless of whether these are directly linked to the transference—and if the patient's awareness of his intrapsychic life as well as his emotional relationship to the analyst deepens over time, then the interpretation of nonverbal behavior in the sessions can wait until it can be incorporated naturally into the themes of the free associations and the transference.

Specific clinical situations are encountered in which nonverbal behavior strongly emerges in the sessions and in which the affect and object relations implied by the patient's nonverbal behavior and verbal communications are congruent or complementary. When a consonance exists between the nonverbal and verbal material, understanding the transference implications of both usually permits a deeper understanding of both. In other words, if both verbal and nonverbal material indicates the nature of the issues that predominate affectively in the content of the hour, the economic principle of interpretation in the sense of working at the point of the most important current instinctual conflict (Fenichel, 1941, p. 47) can be applied. Usually the material can also be understood simultaneously in terms of the dynamic principle—that is, in terms of a conflict between impulse and defense—and the decision can be made which aspect of the defense side of the conflict should be explored before the impulse aspect. Congruence between behavior and content and affective dominance in the hour usually means, by the same token, that the object relations "unit" involved is dominant in the transference as well. Clarification of the dynamic ordering of impulse and defense usually also has topographical aspects, permitting an interpretation from surface to depth, from consciousness to the unconscious. We usually find a consonance of verbal and nonverbal communications in patients with well-consolidated tripartite intrapsychic structure, whose conflicts also tend to be organized intersystemically. It is therefore possible to clarify which system—ego, superego, or id—the predominant defense organization corresponds to and which other system the impulse is stemming from. Thus the structural criteria of interpretation apply as well.

In other clinical situations, however, the conflicts reflected in the verbal content and the interactional material seem dissonant or incongruent. Strong affects in the verbal content and the development of acute or chronic affective interactions reflecting the patient's "frozen" character traits seem strangely unrelated to each other, thus raising the question of what material actually is predominant. Under these circumstances, applying the criteria proposed below usually permits one to arrive at a decision regarding which material should be dealt with first and how to approach it.

It is helpful to consider first whether the patient's free associations are proceeding satisfactorily or whether there is significant conscious suppression of material. Whatever facilitates understanding the motives for conscious suppression and the related transference implications takes precedence here. An understanding of the transference meaning of what is motivating the patient against full compliance with free association usually also provides an answer to what is affectively predominant in the session and whether it relates primarily to the verbal content or to aspects of the patient's nonverbal behavior.

Now, if free association seems to be proceeding satisfactorily, the question of what is predominant in the transference can be examined more easily and helps the analyst to decide whether verbal or attitudinal material predominates. I am suggesting that, with two simultaneous and parallel object-relations "units" revealed in the psychoanalytic situation (one in behavior, the other in the verbal content), the one with both transference dominance and affective dominance takes interpretive precedence. If, however, affective dominance and transference dominance diverge, I think affective dominance (the application of the economic principle) should have priority. I should stress that all defensive and impulsive, verbal and nonverbal, self- and object-related aspects of the material have affective components, so that "affective dominance" does not mean searching for some particular affect or a consciously dominant one, or one linked only with defense or impulse. It is the predominant affect in the total immediate situation that counts, not its access to consciousness. A hysterical temper tantrum, for example, may defend against another dominant affect in the immediate transference situation.

The approach I am suggesting differs from Wilhelm Reich's (1933) insistence that transference resistances anchored in character always be interpreted first. It also differs from Gill's (1980, 1982) insistence that transference always be given the highest priority for interpretation; there are times when affective investment is highest in extratransference issues or in the patient's exploration of aspects of his past. The fact that all analytic material has transference components does not mean that transference material automatically predominates. Sometimes a theme that has strongly dominated the transference for many hours—for example, a patient's chronic dissatisfaction about "not receiving anything from the analyst"—may suddenly shift into a displacement of that complaint onto a third person. Here, affective dominance and transference are still consonant, although the transference is—temporarily—displaced (which may actually facilitate its interpretation).

In addition, at times of rapid shifts in the transference itself, which complicates the task of detecting incongruity between verbal and nonverbal communication, waiting for a crystallization around one of the various affectively important issues present should eventually permit the analyst to decide what is affectively (and, therefore, economically) predominant. Here a "wait and see" attitude is preferable, in my view, to the exclusively topographical standpoint of focusing on what in the material is closest to consciousness. There is never just one "surface" to the material. There are many surface configurations, and the point at which to penetrate from surface to depth (the topographic criterion) depends on what is actually dominant in the total situation. Obviously, when the patient can be helped to acquire awareness of simultaneous, strongly unrelated emotional dispositions in the analytic situation, the exploration of his associations to this observation in itself illuminates the issues involved.

During periods of heightened resistance, the most important material may be relatively distant from consciousness (particularly in personality structures with strong repressive mechanisms). Although I agree that, once one has decided what material is most important, this material should be explored from its defensive side or aspects (which includes consideration of some conscious or preconscious configurations linked to it), access to consciousness does not in itself indicate thematic predominance.

I am here questioning a general tendency for the analyst always to proceed from the surface down, from conscious to unconscious material, disregarding what is economically predominant. However, I also question the tendency to arrive at premature genetic interpretations of the unconscious fantasies reflected in characterologically fixated object relations in the transference. Staying close to the surface manifestations of resistances is as problematic as searching for the "deepest level" of a certain conflict, "deep" usually meaning genetically early. I think the analyst should interpret in depth in the sense of focusing on the unconscious conflicts that predominate in any particular session, the unconscious aspects of the transference in the here-and-now. (But here-and-now must eventually be related to the there-and-then as well!)

Where important discrepancies exist between the verbal and nonverbal communication, when free association seems to be proceeding satisfactorily but without any real deepening of the material, and when, in addition, there are indications of stalemate in transference developments—or a loss of previously gained understanding of the current nature of the transference—I have found it helpful to give clear precedence to the analysis of the object relations aspects of the patient's attitudes over those derived from his verbal communications. The same "rule" applies to situations in which the patient either is repetitively acting out or seems to be developing strong potential for acting out. Giving precedence to nonverbal communication also applies to situations in which general emotional dispersal, an exacerbation of splitting mechanisms, results in affective fragmentation and becomes a major transference resistance, which occurs particularly in strongly schizoid personalities.

I would also give preference to the interpretation of behavior over that of dissonant verbal communications for patients with "living out" lifestyles, those whose free associations remain fixed at a surface level, or those who lack a thoughtful, cooperative attitude. In all these cases, Reich's recommendation that attitudes be interpreted before verbal content and that this be considered a special application of the principle of interpreting "surface" before "depth," "defense before content," still seems valid. Similarly, borderline character pathology, in which severe acting out colors the initial stage of the treatment, also requires rapid interpretation of the transference meanings of pathological character traits.

In other words, when free association "gets stuck" in the context of important activation of pathological behavior patterns in the analytic situation or in the patient's external life, analytic exploration of these behaviors and clarification of their relation to the transference are indicated. To put it still differently: From an economic viewpoint, discrepancies between verbal and nonverbal behavior require an interpretive approach to the total picture generated by these discrepancies. In practice, therefore, character resistances in the transference should be analyzed early on.

In other cases, severe distortions in relation to the psychoanalytic setting become apparent over a period of time. In the vignette presented earlier, after a period of progress in the third year of the analysis, a therapeutic stalemate highlighted the pathology of the patient's relation to interpretations and to the analyst in general (the subtle compromise solutions between envious idealization and devaluation). In still other cases, much like those described by Reich, the patient's free associations apparently flow, with abundant information about present and past and flexible shifts from affects to intellectual thoughts, from fantasy to reality, from the transference to the patient's external life, and so forth (thus imitating Ferenczi's 1919 and Glover's 1955 descriptions of optimal free association), but without any real deepening of the transference relationship or any manifestation of a particular nonverbal behavior in the sessions that would lend itself to exploring the transference.

In these cases, again it is the total relation to the analyst that is usually highly distorted, and it is this distortion that must be diagnosed, particularly as it affects the patient's relation to the analyst's interpretations. Here the interpretation of pathological character traits coincides with the interpretation of the patient's attitude toward the interpreting analyst. Under conditions of such stalemates, this subject matter has high priority. Otherwise, such patients typically acquire a superficial "learning" of the psychoanalyst's theories as a way of defensively resisting full awareness of their unconscious intrapsychic conflicts, with consequent limited therapeutic effects.

Under these circumstances, it is important to clarify the unconscious aspects of the patient/analyst interaction in the here-and-now as a crucial step to full understanding of the object relation that is being played out, without attempting prematurely to achieve genetic reconstructions. Here-and-now interventions should not be conceptualized as artificially cut off, dissociated from their there-and-then aspects. The issue of their relevance to the past should be kept in abeyance, however, until the unconscious aspects of the transference are fully explored. The patient often finds it easier to accept a transference interpretation if a tentative reference to the childhood origin of a certain attitude to the analyst is made; hence, genetic reconstructions should not be reserved for the final stages of analysis. But here I am stressing the need first to clarify the unknown in the present: a step erroneously bypassed in many patients with severe character pathology.

Spelling out a patient's unconscious fantasy on the basis of a specific object relation enacted by his chronic nonverbal behavior in the sessions corresponds to a psychoanalytic construction. But it is necessary to follow this construction with a genetic reconstruction only after the patient's associations gradually transform this fantasy into an antecedent object relation, with the appearance of new information regarding his past and a natural reordering of the new and old information in this area. Establishing the actual genetic sequence of such recovered material requires that the analyst actively order and reorder these genetic units of the patient's unconscious conflicts (Blum, 1980).

The analyst's exploration of his own emotional reactions to the patient under conditions of stalemate may be crucial to the diagnosis of both chronic countertransference distortions (which are more pervasive though less obtrusive than acute countertransference developments) and subtle but powerful transference acting out that might otherwise not have been diagnosed. In this regard the analysis of the analyst's total emotional reaction is a "second line" of approach when the first line of approach—direct transference exploration —proves insufficient (Heimann, 1960; Kernberg, 1975).

The analysis of an implicit and, for the patient, often completely unconscious "interchange" of role relations with the analyst highlights the advantages of studying the analyst's moment-to-moment affective responses to the patient. Such analyses also point the way to differentiating countertransference reactions in a strict sense (the analyst's unconscious conflicts activated in response to the patient's transference) from the analyst's global emotional response to the patient. We know that these two aspects of the analyst's reactions are complementary. For practical purposes, however, the distinction facilitates a more open exploration of the moment-to-moment shift in the analyst's affective responses to and fantasies about the patient's immediate attitudes and chronic attitudinal dispositions, thereby enriching the analyst's understanding of the verbal content of the patient's communication. Need I stress that the analyst's utilization of his own emotional reaction to the patient certainly does not mean sharing that reaction with the patient?

METAPSYCHOLOGICAL CONSIDERATIONS

I now return to consider Fenichel's economic, dynamic, and structural crite-ria for interpreting character resistances, combining these with the interpre-tation of internalized object relations represented in such character resis-tances. Regarding the economic criterion, I have stressed the need first to interpret the material that is affectively predominant, while simultaneously questioning whether closeness to consciousness is a significant criterion for determining such predominance of affects. This view underlies everything I have said regarding the difficulty in choosing economically predominant issues when information stemming from the patient's verbal and nonverbal communications is not congruent.

Regarding the dynamic criteria for interpretation, I reported earlier (1980, chap. 10) that, when transference regression is severe or in analyzable patients with borderline personality organization, the predominance of split-ting over repressive mechanisms permits the alternation in consciousness of the dynamically opposed components of intrapsychic conflict so that access to consciousness per se does not serve to indicate which is the defense and which the impulse aspect of the conflict. Defense and impulse can be rapidly interchanged in the alternating reversals of activated object relations that are typical of part-object relations, and conflictual impulses are conscious and mutually dissociated or split off rather than repressed. Here, consciousness and unconsciousness no longer coincide with what is at the surface and what is deep, what is defense and what is content. But while the topographic approach to interpretation (the ordering of the material from surface to depth) no longer holds for such borderline structures, the moment-to-moment deci-sion of which is the defensively activated ego state directed against which other "impulsive" ego state is very important. Hence, both the economic and the dynamic criteria of interpretation as spelled out by Fenichel are still fully relevant. This brings us to the structural aspects of interpretation of character resistances at various levels of severity of psychopathology.

The structural considerations regarding the interpretation of character resis-tances refer to the organization of the predominant internalized object relation activated in the transference in the context of a particular character trait or pattern. When we diagnose "units" of internalized object relations, we are diagnosing substructures of the tripartite structure. We are, in fact, applying a structural perspective where the overall tripartite structure may not yet (or may no longer) be operative. The patient's attitude, as mentioned before, reflects the enactment of a self representation relating affectively to an object representation or the enactment of an object representation (with which the patient appears to be identified at the moment) relating affectively to a self representation (now projected onto the analyst). One primary consideration here is the extent to which both self and object representations are rooted in broader aspects of the patient's ego or superego, reflecting broadly integrated concepts, values, and emotional dispositions of ego and superego or, to the contrary, the extent to which they are dissociated or split off from other self and object representations. Part-object relations are more disruptive, bizarre, fantastic than the total-object relations. The latter reflect more ordinary childhood experiences which, although repressed, become integrated with the child's ego and superego.

In the context of these elaborations of the structural aspects of pathological character traits in the transference, one important question arises. Does the object relation activated reflect intersystemic or intrasystemic conflicts? And in the case of intersystemic conflict, to which agency do the self representations and object representations correspond? Or, which object relation corresponds to the defense and which to the impulse side of the conflict, and in which agency is each embedded? In intrasystemic conflicts, split-off internalized object relations may at first appear mutually delimited yet intrinsically undifferentiated, intense yet vague, and always highly fantastic and unrealistic. They should be translated into an intelligible affective experience in the here-and-now, a fantasy enacted by them within which the defensive and impulsive aspects, in turn, have to be clarified in terms of which split-off object relation acquires a momentary defensive function against an opposing (impulsive) one. Attention to the interchange between patient and analyst of self and object representations—the alternation of complementary roles in the transference—should be integrated into the interpretation of these expressions of the conflict. That task often requires relatively rapid, imaginative tracking of what appear to be chaotic interactions. The analyst's systematically pointing out to the patient how he feels under the impact of a self representation and the particular object representation activated at different times may permit the analyzable patient with severe character pathology to achieve a degree of integration and empathy with himself and with his objects which will contribute to transforming part-object into total-object relations. In the clinical vignette presented earlier, Mr. T's gradually growing awareness of his identification with his sadistic-mother image as well as with his

mistreated and frustrated self-image led to his awareness and eventual tolerance and integration of contradictory tendencies in himself, of love and
hatred, and of his exploitive and devalued self experiences previously projected onto his girlfriends.

As regressive transferences emerge in the treatment, the patient's observing ego may be temporarily swept up by them. It is important for the analyst
to maintain a clear image of how a "normal" person would respond, under
the circumstances, to the analyst's interpretive comments. This theoretically
"normal" person is usually represented by the collaborative work of the
patient's observing ego with the analyst, but it may be almost totally missing,
temporarily in all patients, and chronically in patients with severe character
pathology. With severe cases, therefore, the analyst's evocation of a "normal" counterpart to the patient's actual regressive behavior becomes crucial.
This means that the analysts has to "split" himself. One part of him is
"experiencing"—accompanying the patient into regression and transforming his behavior into the construction of an enacted unconscious fantasy.
Another part of him is "distancing"—maintaining objectivity precisely at
times when objectivity is most challenged. The boundary function in the
analyst's mind between fantasy and reality requires his tolerance of primitive
fantasy and emotions and of internal discrepancies between the understanding
of what is going on and the level at which the patient can be approached. The
analyst must be able to maintain firm convictions together with flexibility.

In the long run, when character analysis is systematically pursued, a
paradoxical situation may emerge. Some patients find it much easier to talk
about their past than about the unconscious aspects of their current relationship to the analyst. The analyst himself may begin to wonder whether he is
neglecting the exploration of the past in his emphasis on the present. Other
patients may "jump" over the real past and link the conscious present with
what they assume are the deepest levels of past conflicts: they "easily"
connect current conflicts with, for example, "castration anxiety," but no
concrete and painful aspects of childhood emerge.

Careful working through of character resistances, maintaining constant
alertness to whether the patient is changing not only his current experience of
the psychoanalytic situation—thus indicating authentic shifts in transference
patterns—but also how he experiences his past—thus expressing the working through of transference patterns—may confirm the authenticity of psychoanalytic work, in contrast to a mechanistic translation of current difficulties into the patient's own rigidly maintained myths regarding his past.

REFERENCES

Abraham, K. (1919). A particular form of neurotic resistance against the psychoanalytic method. *Selected papers on Psycho-Analysis*. New York: Basic Books, 1953, pp. 303–311.
Blum, H. (1980). The value of reconstruction in adult psychoanalysis. *Int. J. Psychoanal.*, 61:39–54.
Fenichel, O. (1941). *Problems of Psychoanalytic Technique*. New York: Psychoanalytic Quarterly.
———. (1945). *The Psychoanalytic Theory of Neurosis*. New York: Norton.
Ferenczi, S. (1919). On the technique of psycho-analysis. In *Further Contributions to the Theory and Technique of Psycho-Analysis*. New York: Basic Books, 1952, pp. 177–189.
Gill, M. (1980). The analysis of transference: a critique of Fenichel's "Problems of Psychoanalytic Technique." *Int. J. Psychoanal. Psychother.*, 8:45–55.
———. (1982). *Analysis of Transference*, Vol. 1. New York: Int. Univ. Press.
Glover, E. (1955). *The Technique of Psycho-Analysis*. New York: Int. Univ. Press.
Heimann, P. (1960). Countertransference. *Brit. J. Med. Psychol.*, 33:9–15.
Kernberg, O. (1975). *Borderline Conditions and Pathological Narcissism*. New York: Aronson.
———. (1980). *Internal World and External Reality*. New York: Aronson.
Racker, H. (1957). The meaning and uses of countertransference. *Psychoanal. Q.*, 26:303–357.
Reich, W. (1933). *Character Analysis*. New York: Farrar, Straus & Giroux, 1972.
Rosenfeld, H. (1964). On the psychopathology of narcissism: a clinical approach. *Int. J. Psychoanal.*, 45:332–337.

10. The Treatment of Characterological Disorders

Peter L. Giovacchini

Opinions about the types of cases that can be psychoanalytically treated are constantly changing and the number is being enlarged. It is interesting to note that the contributors to this volume [see note below] have chosen to present clinical material that, if diagnostic categorizations were attempted, could be included under the rubric of character disorders, borderline syndromes, and even psychoses. These are all experienced psychoanalysts and some of them were raised in the classic tradition among the original pioneers of psychoanalysis. The fact that the clinical material presented for the discussion of psychoanalytic treatment comes from what we could broadly refer to as sick patients, regardless of diagnostic category, obviously indicates that many analysts believe that these cases need not be abandoned to other treatment modalities.

Since the clinical material I am going to discuss is familiar to most clinicians, perhaps diagnostic considerations are superfluous. Still, for the sake of clarity and precision, although *custom* may be the more precise term, I will briefly outline some nosologic distinctions.

I have in mind a group of patients who have what we might call character disorders. In contrast to the usual psychoneurotic patient, they do not present distinct symptoms; rather, they complain of general and vague dissatisfactions relating to who and what they are, where they fit in today's world, the purpose of their life, and the meaning of life in general. These are, of course, existential questions and they relate to the patients' identity. These patients may have symptoms, too—anxiety, depression, and paranoid preoccupations —but their primary concern is with difficulties in adapting to the world. Their maladjustment goes beyond social issues because they suffer substantially and feel truly miserable.

The question frequently arises as to how one distinguishes such patients from those diagnosed as borderline or psychotic. Once one understands the

Reprinted from P. L. Giovacchini, ed., *Tactics and Techniques in Psychoanalytic Therapy* (New York: Science House, 1972), 236–53 by permission.

character structure and the underlying psychodynamics of this group, the problem is more difficult rather than easier. This is not particularly unusual since there are often differences that manifest themselves on the surface but fade away as epiphenomena when looked at more deeply (microscopically). Still from a behavioral viewpoint, patients who suffer from characterological problems maintain an operational relationship to reality and, even though it may be constrictive, make an adaptation. They do not often become psychotic in the sense of suffering from florid delusions and hallucinations for protracted periods of time.

I am being purposely tentative because what I am calling character disorders can, at times, develop qualities that are phenomenologically indistinguishable from a psychosis. This happens most often during the course of therapy, but, as a rule, such episodes are transitory, and these patients seem to have considerable resiliency when compared with more traditional psychotic patients. It is equally difficult to distinguish the borderline patient. Unlike the character disorders, one usually thinks of this patient as one who can decompensate to a psychotic state rather readily. His ego state is never far from a schizoid disorganization and his adjustment is believed to be precarious. To repeat, these variations are imprecise and, in my opinion, not particularly useful except for statistical and classificatory purposes. When one wishes to study the therapeutic interaction—the main interest of the clinician—such diagnostic distinctions are of limited value.

Here, I would like to consider once more the question of specific therapeutic approaches that constitute variations of the psychoanalytic method but are not deviations or parameters. I plan to discuss initial strategy in detail. Some patients do not want the therapist to interject himself into their associations. They feel his interpretations or comments are intrusions. In some instances these patients are willing to answer questions about their histories or provide other factual information in the interest of clarity, but they become disturbed when the therapist makes a statement about what is going on inside their minds. Other patients who may be more difficult to treat behave in a completely different fashion, demanding that the therapist lead and manage them. Most patients can be placed somewhere between these two extremes, requiring specific therapeutic tactics. I will illustrate several types of psychopathology and various treatment maneuvers.

THE PATIENT AND THE NONINTRUSIVE THERAPIST

An example of a patient who resents any type of interpretative activity was a 35-year old businessman who believed that he was a chronic failure and felt markedly depressed and generally worthless. He reviled himself for his emotional lability and what he thought were totally unjustified bouts of anger. During the initial interviews he presented, without being asked, a well-organized, complete history. If I asked a question he would gladly answer it in relevant detail. Otherwise, I had the distinct impression that he would resent any comment that I might make about him. He could gratify my curiosity and give me information; however, he seemed to be irritated by even my most casual impressions.

I do not usually make interpretative comments early in the therapeutic relationship, although there are exceptions. This patient signaled to me in many subtle ways not to make any comments. At times I felt tantalized since he brought material that was so easily understood, yet he did not seem to see its significance. I very much wanted to say something, but I rarely gave in to this feeling; when I did, he would frown and otherwise indicate his annoyance. During the initial interviews he ignored my comments, sometimes with forbearance.

As he continued treatment on the couch, he sometimes credited me with having taught him something important about his relationship with some significant figure in his past (for example, his mother); he thought that this type of insight indicated progress and demonstrated my analytic skill. These were essentially nontransference interpretations but, rather curiously, I had not made them. These interpretations were the products of the patient's ruminations that he attributed to me and then praised me for having made.

His reactions were quite different, however, when I made my first *transference* interpretation. I pointed out that he needed to maintain a certain distance between the two of us, which he accomplished by drawing a curtain of intellectualism between us. My comment was not intended as criticism nor did he take it as such. As a matter of fact, I was intrigued by both the form and the content of his associations, and I was just as interested in the specific details of his defense as I was in the underlying anxiety that made him keep us psychically apart. His responses were especially interesting. At first, he was confused. Even though my statement consisted of a simple declarative sentence, he claimed he did not understand what I had said. He asked me to repeat it several times and, since I felt that his response was puzzling and full of anguish, I did. As he painfully and slowly grasped the meaning of my interpretation, he became increasingly sad.

Although the subsequent material more than abundantly indicated that the patient was, indeed, maintaining distance through intellectual control, he felt that he had been completely misunderstood. He resented the idea that I would have anything to say about his feelings and motivations; he felt that no one could know anything about them except himself. He believed that what I said could only be a projection of myself and not a true understanding of him. This, oddly enough, was the way he felt about every transference interpretation I made. Although this patient's reactions struck me as being particularly bizarre, I have since noted other cases who behave in a similar fashion, and sometimes in an even more circumspect fashion. For example, another patient, a professional man, told me during our very first session that he wanted me to remain silent. He did not want me to "intrude" into his thoughts; the time was his alone and I was not to introduce parts of my psyche into it.

Inevitably, the question arises as to how to handle such cases psychoanalytically when the chief therapeutic tool avowedly is the transference interpretation. Must our technique be modified when a patient apparently resents or "forbids" such interpretations? Several factors should be clarified. Although it may not be apparent, these two patients (as well as others I have subsequently seen) had a highly idealized attitude toward me. In some instances this idealization developed quickly during the beginning interviews. In others, they had already formed an idealized concept of me before the first interview. The first patient was referred to me by a former patient, one who praised me "to the heavens," apparently because of an unresolved positive transference. The second patient had read some of my writings and found himself very much drawn to them. Both patients had formed rather exalted pictures long before they actually saw me.

These patients seemed to present a paradox. On the one hand, the therapist is idealized but then whatever he wishes to impart is summarily rejected. In any discussions of therapeutic handling, one must first understand the psychopathology. In these cases, there is a specific type of relationship that has transference significance. Understanding the nature of this relationship should reveal a lot about these patients' specific characterological difficulties, and these insights might indicate the most reasonable therapeutic course.

To understand more, let us return to the clinical material. I found it prudent to take a wait-and-see attitude, and both the patients and I felt more comfortable after I decided to remain silent. The subsequent material emphasizes several themes. First, both patients indicated that I was intruding parts of myself into them. They perceived this as an assault and an attempt to rob them of their precarious autonomy; consequently, they had to keep me "at arms' length." Next, there was an antithetical factor in that they felt very close to me. They were referring to a symbiotic fusion where the boundaries between us did not exist. They saw the relationship as consisting of total unity between patient and therapist.

If I made an observation about our relationship, it indicated that a relationship between *two* people existed. If I commented about situations that were outside of the transference—that did not involve the two of us—it was not threatening. However, any transference interpretations upset the symbiotic unity that seemed to be so vital. Furthermore, the atmosphere of magical omnipotence seemed to be disturbed by a transference interpretation. To remain a deity one must stay concealed; gods do not reveal themselves if they are to preserve their omnipotence. If I said anything I ran the risk of being wrong and of exposing my frailty. My remarks about situations outside the transference did not particularly matter because they could be made within the context of symbiotic unity and so their validity didn't matter. Within the transference, however, my interpretations were intrinsically wrong.

When a patient laments that I do not understand him, from his viewpoint, he is correct. By intruding, I do not understand his need for symbiotic unity; therefore, his idealized view of me is shaken.

In a witty moment, Dr. Winnicott said that he makes interpretations for two reasons: one is to let the patient know that he is still alive and the other is to show the patient that he can be wrong. Perhaps in this pithy statement, Dr. Winnicott was summarizing the above points. To let the patient know he is alive points to the fact that the analyst exists, separate and apart from the patient, and the second reason indicates that he is not divinely infallible. These formulations remind me of an unusual situation that I hesitate to call clinical and yet may illustrate to an extreme degree the type of interactions described.

A colleague referred the husband of one of his patients to me for psychoanalysis. The wife gave her husband my name and he promised to call me. About two years later my colleague complimented me on the progress this man had made in his treatment. His patient would, from time to time, report about her husband's behavior which, at least descriptively, seemed to be much better integrated than before; certain phobic symptoms had disappeared. At times she would describe what happened during one of her husband's sessions, and the general movement seemed to be a gradual resolution of an idealized transference. In this case, there could be no question of my intrusion simply because the "patient" never called me and so I never even saw him! I was astonished at my colleague's remarks about a *proxy analysis* and an even more remarkable *proxy transference.*

I do not believe that these patients require a specific approach or basic alteration of the psychotherapeutic relationship. Once the analyst becomes aware of the transference and adaptive significance of the patients' reactions, they needn't hinder analysis. Even though the aim of analysis is to achieve further ego integration by acquiring insight, these patients can reach self-understanding in a setting where they do not feel intruded upon. Gradually, the analyst can augment the patient's self-observations, and eventually the patient will begin to view the analyst's interpretation as an extension of his own.

To reach such a state of mutual cooperation requires considerable patience and respect for the patient's autonomy. It can be an especially difficult analytic relationship because the analyst has to "suspend" his analytic operations and seemingly relegate his professional identity to the background. Once he recognizes, however, that his so-called lack of activity is, in itself, an active demonstration of his analytic forbearance—which may eventually help to clarify the patient's symbiotic needs—the analyst can relax and allow the analysis to continue unhampered by any intrusion.

OTHER CHARACTEROLOGICAL TYPES

In contrast to the inactivity demanded by the patients just described, there is another group that requires the analyst's intervention. These patients are in need of a panoramic prevision of the therapeutic course. Briefly, they need a unifying, cohesive experience during their first interview; without it, they seem to be unable to become engaged in treatment. The experience usually consists of interpretations of what will later be expanded into the main transference themes. Here I would like to discuss the manifestations of psychopathology that may help to determine our initial therapeutic approach.

Some patients do not want any intrusion; this is quite clear because of their reactions to our comments. Other patients may not resent interpretations and yet do not require an analytic demonstration "in miniature." Both types of patients will indicate, sometimes subtly and sometimes quite openly, that they want the analyst to participate in their psychopathological frames of reference; otherwise they will feel anxious.

A patient often seeks therapy not because he really wants to change; rather, he hopes to have his defenses reinforced in order to feel more comfortable with his psychopathologically determined adaptations. He doesn't want to give up his symptoms; he merely wants them to work better. However, when the therapist creates an analytic observational framework—a platform from which to view the psychic turmoil going on within the patient—instead of supporting the patient's defenses by educative or managerial activities, there is inevitably some tension. If the tension is very intense, analytic treatment may not be possible. The patient will indicate if he can tolerate the analyst's refusal to take sides with one or another aspect of his intrapsychic conflicts.

I believe that the occurrence of panoramic first dreams is a positive indication for analysis without intervention; it signifies a unity and cohesion of the personality. These patients may suffer from severe psychopathology, and there may be defective and primitive functioning (even considerable asynchrony among various ego systems), but there is a relative degree of integration reflected in their behavior and manner of relating. In retrospect, it seems that this group of patients tends to view both situations and feelings in a holistic fashion; they do not deal with certain matters in an isolated way. Even when they are markedly obsessional, they can still place their preoccupations in a larger context. This capacity is not necessarily a sign of psychic health because the larger context may be delusionally constructed.

For example, a young scientist was quite dissatisfied with the way he was being treated at work, especially by his immediate superior. He believed that this man was jealous of his creativity and was doing everything possible to hinder his advancement. There was an obvious paranoid element in this patient's feelings, and it resulted in a florid, paranoid psychosis later on. Although he spent considerable time marshaling evidence to support his view that he was being persecuted by the senior scientist, he did not restrict his associations mainly to this area. He was able to think about his work in relation to the other areas of his life. He hoped to achieve fame from his scientific discoveries, as well as money, prestige, and admiration; then he hoped he would be successful and popular with girls.

His paranoia was not confined to his mentor; he had a rather paranoid attitude about everything but his attitudes were not exclusively paranoid. Although he tended to be generally suspicious and mistrustful, he could also be friendly and cheerful. Sometimes he used his suspiciousness productively: since he didn't trust the motives or reliability of a colleague's reported data, he might repeat the colleague's experiment. He often obtained different results, which then permitted him to carry the formulations further. In retrospect this patient seemed to be able to coordinate the different facets of his life. Perhaps his chief adjustive (characterological) modality was paranoid, but it had many themes and variations. It even had a certain flexibility because it varied according to the situation and was determined by many factors.

This patient's early dreams were panoramic in the sense that they depicted the structure of his personality in a sweeping fashion and were predictive of the course of the transference. His first dream, which took place the night before his initial appointment, was long and involved. He was taking an ocean voyage with a very skillful and highly respected captain. However, somewhere during the voyage the patient found himself in the midst of a storm; he described the ship's precarious balance and indicated that it was in serious danger of sinking. The captain then became the villain because the danger being faced was his responsibility. The captain was not basically irresponsible or careless, but he knew he could save himself and did not particularly care about the patient's welfare. For the rest of the dream, the patient worked with the captain (the period of animosity having passed) and together they weathered the storm.

The dream was not quite this coherent. Some of its meaning was obvious from the patient's associations, and in presenting it here I undoubtedly used some of my secondary process. Nevertheless, there was a remarkable coherence between this dream and most of his others. *I did not feel it was necessary to do anything in particular except allow the transference to develop.* As the dream predicted, after an initial idealization, the patient became quite paranoid about me and had to be hospitalized briefly. However, he reintegrated and the analysis continued without any unusual complications.

Other patients may require a different initial approach. For example, one patient—an attractive, single woman in her thirties—was referred to me as a "classic" hysteric with phobic symptoms. She vividly described these symptoms; the main one was agoraphobia and there were numerous lesser phobias. She was afraid of riding in trains, automobiles, airplanes, or other form of public transportation. These fears, however, were overshadowed by

her fear of open spaces, which was equated with leaving home. As a consequence, she was virtually confined to home and continued to live with her
parents.

In view of her crippling symptoms, it seemed remarkable that she had
managed to come to my office. She, herself, complained about the great
effort and then said that she could control her anxiety somewhat if her father
were with her; he had driven her to the interview. This was the first time she
had sought therapy although her symptoms first appeared after she graduated
from high school. Because of her anxiety she did not go to college. The only
change in her life that seemed to be associated with entering treatment was
her father's illness. He had just recovered from a coronary, and it was fairly
obvious that the patient was very much afraid of losing him.

The patient, although soft-spoken and demure, seemed to create an air of
tension and urgency. At first, she appeared to be able to speak freely and to
impart considerable information; her attitude was pleasantly cooperative.
Nevertheless, I felt a vague sense of uneasiness and soon recognized that I
knew very little about her. The patient went into considerable detail about
her numerous phobias and gave an exact description of her house; however,
she imparted no feeling about her relationship with her patients, siblings, and
other significant persons. In fact, her descriptions of other people, which she
never gave spontaneously, were mechanistic and wooden; although initially I
believed I was learning something about her interpersonal relationships, later
I realized that this was not so.

It seemed that her life consisted of only her phobias and being at home.
She did not discuss the vocational, social, or sexual areas of life; I saw that
she seemed to be isolated in these respects, but I was reluctant to make any
inquiries. I may have been afraid of offending her or of upsetting a delicate
balance, although she presented a picture of sophisticated poise. She seemed
to have a delicate, porcelain veneer that appeared as if it could easily crack.

Although her symptoms were supposedly characteristic of a high-grade,
hysterical neurosis, I came to believe that I was dealing with a fragmented
person; I also saw her as a "difficult" patient. This feeling came to me
toward the end of the interview. The patient finally reached a point where
she had told me all she could and had nothing more to say. I would have
preferred to let her continue talking or to remain silent if she chose. However,
after she indicated that she had nothing more to say, I had the distinct
impression that if I remained silent I would lose her as a patient.

She looked at me with both an imperious expectancy and a pleading helplessness. Her narcissism was manifested by her straight, regal posture. She was immaculately groomed, with not one hair out of place. Still, the picture she presented was incongruous. When she turned her head, her profile impressed me, perhaps because of a hypnagogic distortion of mine, as that of a six-month-old infant. I thought I saw two distinctly separate ego states, indicating a serious fragmentation. She also convinced me that I would have to "do something" if I were sincerely interested in treating her.

This patient never had what could be considered a panoramic dream; they all dealt with circumscribed themes and had very little, if any, action in them. In the first dream she reported, she simply sat in her living room with a strange man; there was no movement or conversation. Later she had dreams in which she was imprisoned in a cave behind an iron grill. Further on in her treatment she dreamed of storms and holocausts, but she was always standing off at a considerable distance.

TECHNICAL CONSIDERATIONS

The phobic patient impressed upon me the need to do something definite, therapeutically speaking. It is sometimes difficult to ascertain why one feels such a need and what exactly is signaled by the patient, but the feeling is unmistakable. With some patients it is possible to sit back, relax, and adopt a wait-and-see attitude, but with others this cannot be done. These two types of patients cannot be distinguished by the severity of their psychopathology. It is clear that the first patient described had many obvious psychotic features, whereas the second one presented an almost classical picture of a hysterical neurosis with phobic symptoms.

From an ego-psychological viewpoint, there were distinct differences between these two patients in the degree and kind of psychic organization. In spite of the predominant primary-process thinking in the first patient, his ego was fundamentally unified. On the other hand, the second patient was markedly fragmented. Her ego used the defense mechanism of splitting to keep various facets of her life separate from each other. The outside world was no longer part of her experience since she confined herself to her parental home, where her father, in particular, represented a lifeline.

As treatment later indicated she had split off parts of herself—unacceptable, destructive fragments—and then phobically isolated herself from them. The paranoid scientist also projected parts of himself but he did not separate himself completely from them. He interacted with others actively, which required the maintenance of inner unity. The so-called hysterical patient withdrew from and, to some extent, even denied the outside world, which she equated with the unacceptable within her. Thus, she lived a highly constricted life with only part of her total ego. She sought treatment because the equilibrium of even that part was being threatened by her father's illness and possible death, and if she split off a painful part, this time she would have nothing left, so to speak, for herself.

One is reminded of a situation in organic medicine where a patient may not be able to function efficiently because he is missing a part of himself, perhaps a limb; the problem for that patient is rehabilitation. My phobic patient was missing parts of herself but, unlike a missing limb, they were potentially recoverable.

My patient wanted treatment so that she could continue to live with her constrictions. As her first dream indicated, she wanted to have me simply replace her father without establishing a relationship; the dream was set in her living room, and she and the stranger did not communicate.

These constructions are all retrospective; actually I understood very little during the first crucial interview except: (1) I could not wait for understanding to come, and (2) I was dealing with an ego with many split-off components.

In contrast to the first dream (which was reported at a later session), she felt uneasy with and did not seem to tolerate silence. I definitely felt she wanted me to talk *to her,* which is quite different from communicating with one another. I could feel an immense dependency when she expressed needs that are so primitive (and belong to preverbal developmental stages) that they cannot be articulated. Still she wanted something verbal from me; in this instance words would have concrete, magical powers. Her fragmentation seemed obvious in spite of the fact that such structural characteristics were part of a neurosis that is supposed to represent the highest order of psychosexual integration. Many psychoanalysts have noted the close proximity of a surface hysterical picture and an underlying, often malignant, schizophrenia.

As mentioned above, I did not know how to meet her expectations for silent, magical support. I wondered if such a part-ego could tolerate both a regression inherently stimulated by the psychoanalytic setting and an analyst who would not actively try to provide such elemental support. I knew that this patient would attribute (in fact she had already done so) omnipotent qualities to me, but how would she respond if I maintained an analytic stance and did not try to respond within her frame of reference?

From my theoretical understanding, although minimal, I surmised how a fragmented ego might respond to the psychoanalytic approach. This patient seemed to be able to generate considerable and disruptive anxiety if her needs for magical subsistence were not met. I soon realized that if I could give her what she wanted, she would probably have a fixation, perhaps a delusional one. However, the idea of giving her what she wanted was simply an academic conjecture for me because I would not have known where to begin if I had decided to respond to her at the level she herself presented.

I felt that it was not feasible just not to respond at all except with analytic expectancy. A fragmented ego, per se, does not exclude an analytic approach, but the analytic patient has to learn to see the outside world and his reactions in terms of what is going on within himself. In other words, there has to be some cohesion among the parts of the self and a recognition of the external world toward which he is responding. My phobic patient did not seem to be able to discriminate between different parts of herself and the qualitative and quantitative aspects of her environment. She did not understand how situations are related to one another and how one event determines another; it could be said that she had little concept of dynamic interrelationships.

Psychoanalysis as a procedure seemed to be incomprehensible to her. I now believe that this fairly common phenomenon among patients suffering from characterological problems is the product of the patients' fragmented view; they have no appreciation of deterministically related interactions. Psychoanalytic treatment requires an observational frame of reference where connections between parts of the self and feelings and behavior toward external objects are made. The analytic process has, in a sense, a unity of its own. My patient and many others have no feelings about analysis because they have none of the unity that is inherent in the analytic process. However, it is precisely this type of patient who needs the unity that analysis offers. Although they can only fragment (and this may prevent them from tolerating an analytic approach), they are in dire need of a unifying experience.

I became aware of an impasse in my thinking and had a strong desire to try analysis even though it might be beyond the patient's capacities. I also realized that I wanted to impress her with my wisdom in knowing what was best for her—in this case, analysis. Without being completely aware of what I was doing, I asked the patient why she put herself entirely in my care on such short acquaintance. The patient was not at all astonished to have me speculate about her trust in me; she simply wondered why I felt her trust was naïve and why I questioned her at all. To her it was perfectly natural to see me as a father substitute and she was incapable of questioning her own motivations or the defensive and adaptive functions of such an interaction.

After she replied, there was a period of silence. This time the silence didn't seem to bother her. On the other hand, I felt a need to collect my thoughts, and as I struggled with them, I became uncomfortable. Later that day, I recognized that the patient was displaying total dependence upon me and was making me responsible for her life; I felt uneasy because of the magnitude of that responsibility.

During later sessions I also felt inhibited about making interpretative comments if I had something to say. My reluctance to look for intrapsychic sources of behavior and attitudes became quite intense. I finally concluded that I was responding to her fragmentation and that if I continued doing so, analysis, at least with me, would not be possible. Consequently, I told her that she had an inhibiting effect upon me, which I believed she purposely, although unconsciously, created in order to keep me under control. At the same time I implied that she had to render me powerless because she was afraid I would attack her.

Again, she did not seem to be upset by my observations but was able to relax and speak freely. For the next ten minutes, she was warm and friendly and made many positive statements about me and my office. I had the distinct impression that she was in a state of starry-eyed idealization; I found this oppressive rather than narcissistically enhancing. Although I felt controlled by her idealization, I decided to wait and see what would happen.

The patient began to have periods of silence, and it became obvious that she was visibly struggling with certain feelings or thoughts. I said that maybe she had feelings about me that were difficult to express. I also indicated that I would respect her decision if she chose not to express them. Her affect changed immediately and she became increasingly angry. She confessed that she felt I had suddenly become unsympathetic and was not the least bit interested in either helping or understanding her; she believed that I actively disliked her and would do her harm if I could. Just then I felt much more relaxed and believed that analytic contact had finally been made, if the patient did not, in the meantime, walk out on me. I felt impelled to make an interpretation that would "pull together," that is, unify her fragmented behavior. Therefore, I told her that her reactions were understandable in view of her intense need to see me as a god-like protector, a need that would be disappointed as she became more aware of my limitations. To some extent, she perceived my ineptness as dangerous.

At this time the patient relaxed and seemed pleased; we had reached the end of the session and there was no doubt about further interviews. We both assumed that therapy had begun. In fact, I felt that she was a long-standing patient and that all we needed to do was to set up a schedule. I emphasize this point because initially she had asked many questions and raised objections about treatment hours and how to get to and from my office. She said nothing more about such difficulties and was quite flexible about fitting into my schedule.

The next session seemed to be a continuation of the material she had presented before she became angry; her associations repeatedly referred to her need to both idealize and control me. Although no treatment proceeds with predictable regularity, this woman's treatment went through various phases. For a long time she was extremely dependent and attributed omnipotent powers to me. There was often marked evidence of a symbiotic fusion. After this she displayed increasing anger which finally reached paranoid proportions. She became delusional about me and developed somatic delusions. She believed that a small freckle on her left forearm was a cancerous mole and sought verification from me and other physicians. Her paranoia increased tremendously and she bitterly reviled me. Strangely enough, however, these attacks were usually confined to my office. She talked of quitting treatment but never too seriously. She went only so far as to demand a consultation. In spite of my lack of understanding and competence she asked me to make the referral.

At first, the patient idealized the consultant but, during the course of the consultation, she developed a paranoid distrust. She finally considered him an ally of mine and, therefore, worthless. The consultant's description of their one-hour interview was an exact replica of the three years she had been in treatment with me. (He had had no previous information about my patient.) It was also remarkably similar to what I had experienced with her during our initial interview.

Although she was angry, she was impressed when I spoke of the similarity of her reactions toward me and the consultant and the similar movement in the two first interviews. Recalling our first interview made it easier for her to see that there was a preordained quality to her reactions. From this point on, there was nothing unusual in her treatment. She experienced regressive fluctuations but was consistently able to recognize them, often with considerable affect, as transference manifestations.

GENERAL COMMENTS

Patients who suffer from characterological problems bring into focus both diagnostic factors and technical considerations. My phobic patient illustrates the fact that symptoms alone do not provide an adequate understanding of the more subtle aspects of psychopathology. It is preferable to rely on the patient's reactions toward the therapist as they occur in the here-and-now of the consultation room. My patient presented an interesting sequence of reactions during our first interview that were identical with the later unfolding of the transference. The young scientist, however, reacted in a more conventional fashion. Each patient's reactions and the resultant technical approaches were attributed to certain structural qualities best described in terms of their egos. Holistic unity, as compared with ego fragmentation, led to a different course of therapeutic events.

It can be asked whether all patients with fragmented egos will react in the same fashion as the woman described here; one can also examine the criteria for treatability. I can recall other patients whose egos were probably fragmented who reacted differently from this woman. In fact, it has been reported that these patients cannot tolerate an analytic relationship and that they require a modified therapeutic technique in order to derive any support from the relationship.

Patients' reactions are determined by many factors. My phobic patient might have responded quite differently if I had actively probed or tried to be reassuring. *Her reactions seemed to be a response to my nonintrusive approach.* I have also treated other patients with fragmented egos. *Maintaining an analytic attitude (which simply means relating the patient's attitudes and behavior to his feelings toward the analyst and analytic setting) seems to be the instrumental factor that produces a sequence of reactions that indicate the development of the transference. I have repeatedly noted such reactions whenever I was able to respond as I did with the patient discussed here.*

The criteria for treatability cannot be dealt with on an absolute basis. The qualities that make a patient treatable or nontreatable do not reside wholly within the patient. Rather, it is important to look at the reactions and counter-reactions; the relationship itself between the patient and therapist may determine whether the patient is treatable. This perspective emphasizes the interpersonal factor. A patient may be nontreatable by one therapist but treatable by another. The responsibility for success or failure, from this viewpoint, resides in their interaction. This does not mean that technical issues and the structure of the patient's personality are not important. Nor does it mean that therapeutic failure is always due to some idiosyncratic countertransference element. Because of specific defenses or ego defects certain patients cannot respond to any approach that is designed to foster self-observation and introspection.

On the other hand, many patients who seem to be analytically inaccessible may respond very well to analysis. Therapists, of course, may abandon the analytic approach for a variety of reasons. *Some patients (and I believe those with fragmented egos can be included in this category) are especially skillful in stimulating the therapist's ambivalence about analysis.*

If a patient's ego is fragmented, the therapist tends to be protective toward him. The therapist senses his helplessness and his relative lack of adaptive techniques to cope with the exigencies of the external world. The patient may create further frustration by not being able to articulate his needs; if he can, the therapist may still not understand what he is seeking. Consequently, the therapist's wish to be protective and helpful while not knowing how, creates an impasse that is of greater urgency than conducting analysis. The therapist may be impressed with the patient's needfulness and, for some reason, believe that it is inconsistent with an analytic approach. Consequently, there is a tendency to want to offer the patient a constructive experience but not an analytic one; it may be experienced intensely as an urge to "do something," which dominates the entire treatment setting.

The primitive fixations of these fragmented patients involve preverbal ego states. The urge to "do something" for them cannot lead to constructive gratification in the sense that it will produce higher states of psychic integration. At best, the patient may achieve a defensive stabilization which may be reflected in greater comfort. However, this is usually a precarious and temporary adjustment.

I have found that once I become aware of my inability to respond to needs that neither the patient nor I understand, the easiest path to follow is that of analysis. I find it is an effective way out of a dilemma since the analytic viewpoint does not require me to become involved at the level of content. Instead, I can view the patient's overt and covert demands in terms of intrapsychic forces and their relationship to the defective functioning of various ego systems. The patient's material is not seen as a problem per se but his productions are viewed in a broader perspective. Using analysis the therapist is not faced with an impossible request; rather, he tries to understand what is happening in terms of psychic determinism. Engaging once again in a familiar frame of reference makes the analyst more comfortable, his comfort is transmitted to the patient; this, in itself, may be instrumental in making the patient analytically accessible.

PART IV

TYPES OF CHARACTER PATHOLOGY AND TREATMENT TECHNIQUES

11. Transference Resistance in Hysterical Character Neurosis—Technical Considerations

B. Ruth Easser and Stanley R. Lesser

Hysteria was considered for many years the diagnostic entity most amenable to the psychoanlytic method. In the more recent past, clinical experience has questioned this postulate. Therapeutic failures have led to a reassessment of the prognosis;[7] a questioning of the original dynamic and developmental etiology of the disorder;[8] also to the promulgation of modified therapeutic techniques and therapeutic emphasis.[12] Thus Knapp, et al., suggest that prognostic evaluation is extremely capricious. Marmor[8] places the primary conflict in the oral rather than the oedipal phase of development. Winter[12] advises that technically the analysis should be based upon the oral relationships with the mother and the triangular relationships of the oedipal conflict be de-emphasized, i.e., the father left out.

We believe that there are two prime reasons why the clinical analytic method has, in many instances, failed to effect a resolution of the underlying conflicts which produce both hysterical character traits and hysterical symptomatology. The first is diagnostic misevaluation, lack of differentiation of the hysteric from other groups displaying similar overt traits and symptoms. We have attempted in a previous paper, "Hysterical Character: A Re-Evaluation,"[2] to discriminate the hysterical character neurosis from other diagnostic categories which we have lumped together under the rubric "Hysteroid." Two, even when a correct diagnosis has been established, we feel that inadequate attention has been given to the ego attitudes and relational modes of the hysteric personality. These attitudes and modes, if unattended, preclude the development of a transference neurosis which would enable the resolution of the underlying conflicts.

The question of the nature of the transference in the hysteric is, we believe, a key issue. The zest with which the hysteric approaches the therapeutic task and so readily seems to absorb insights frequently obscures a relationship in

Reprinted from G. Goldman and D. Shapiro, eds., *Developments in Psychoanalysis at Columbia University* (New York: Hafner, 1966), 69–80 by permission of Columbia University Psychoanalytic Center.

which the patient has indeed been an onlooker observing and reacting to the analyst at work rather than working through his own problems. There may be some change in the behavior but the basic inhibitions, the quality of object relations and the emotional way of life remain unmodified.

Wilhelm Reich[9] stressed that character traits, "character armor," must first be analyzed since he visualized that its function was to defend the patient against the stimuli of the outer world and against repressed inner impulses. Nevertheless, he followed Freud's original dictum in stating "apprehensiveness and coquetry defend against genital sexuality and that one should interpret more or less directly the genital sexual nature of the defense . . . the fact that this sexual behavior also expresses other, secondary strivings, such as primitive narcissism, or the wish to dominate or to make an impression is not important in this context." We would agree with Reich as to the core sexual problem. We also agree with the need to loosen the "character armor" before the patient can allow himself to enter a therapeutic alliance. We would most emphatically disagree that the so-called "secondary strivings are not important to this context." Rather we feel that the analysis of these "secondary strivings" e.g., "the need to impress" are resistances which, if not resolved, will color, impede and frustrate the entire course of the analysis.

Edward Glover,[6] in his concept of "transference resistance," describes an aspect of transference in which childhood reactivity bedevils the analyst as infantile memories are approached, particularly those about the oedipal situation and leads to stagnation or exacerbation of the symptoms. He regards this transference resistance as a regressive phenomenon concomitant with the development of a transference neurosis. This would imply that these character resistances are necessarily secondary to the formation of a transference neurosis. Our observations lead us to emphasize that the character resistances confronting the analyst are an integral part of the life style of the hysterical patient both before he encounters the analyst as well as immediately present in the opening phases of the analysis. In this, our concept would be much closer to the concept of resistances to the transference. In other words, we suggest that the therapeutic behavior in analysis is usually a mere repetition of the patient's behavior in numerous contemporary and past interpersonal transactions rather than the manifestations of a transference neurosis.

In this paper we wish to highlight certain common ego maneuvers and ego attitudes that are utilized in resistance to the transference and must be differentiated from transference phenomena:

1. The ease of emotional lability;
2. The maintenance of the child self-image;
3. The derivatives of the unconscious construction of a fantasied role;
4. The ability to evoke a response in the analyst that establishes and maintains the gratifications from secondary gains.

The hysterical character depicts what may be characterized as "the emotional way of life." The understanding of the emotional way, in analysis, is a prime requisite for successful treatment. Manifest emotionality or, more properly, emotional reactivity is the outward manifestation of the self as an involved emotional participant. Obversely, the interreactivity with the object (in this case the analyst) seems to the patient essential for his immediate security, the perpetuation of the character mode and the defensive guarding against specific unconscious conflicts. The latter concept of emotionality as a defense is similar to Valenstein's[11] proposal of the term "affectualization" as a defense mechanism. ". . . affect, and its intensification and excessiveness, with unconscious use or exploitation for defensive purposes to avoid the cognitive appreciation of emotionally charged issues and the rational recognition of explanatory connections, i.e. affectualization." The ubiquitous proneness to this behavior in every relational and adaptational aspect provides a most effective character armor. Dreams, associations, symbolizations, infantile memories, transference reactivity, current events are all pervaded. Interpretations presented without a constant alertness to this proclivity will only become new grist for this already well-established emotional mill. Since affect-laden ideation is in most instances a principal road to effective interpretation, it is easy for the analyst to view these highly emotional associations as meaningful. However, the hysteric has the tendency to relish the emotive role of a dreamer, free associater, a creator of symbols or an abreactor, or counterwise: a resister, antagonist, provocateur, or for that matter, any role that seems necessary or appealing. The analysis may seem to be going well or badly but in fact is not going at all.

The hysteric views (consciously and unconsciously in varying degrees) this emotionality as a jewel to be exhibited, fondled and cherished. Any attempt to move beyond it or to remove it is viewed as an attack and is defended against with the total personality, i.e., with a new surge of affectivity. The tenacity with which this character trait is guarded is not surprising when one considers its multi-determination and the multiple psychic functions served. Analogously to a neurotic symptom it provides a source of pleasure (even when seemingly painful), a source of pride (even when consciously disparaged and deplored), and a preservation of the self-image as an affectively involved being, which becomes a useful commodity in evoking the interest and involvement of others (even when viewed by others as an irritant). Most importantly, for analytic consideration, it provides a secondary defensive barrier against the experience of the more painful and feared core affects; the illumination of unresolved infantile conflicts and the true awareness of their role in present and past relationships. Siegman[10] in is paper, "Emotionality—A Hysterical Character Defense," both emphasizes the defensive use of the histrionic emotionality and also suggests a developmental line through which the hysteric may avoid responsibility for his dyscontrol and the internal pangs of conscience:

Patients are sometimes surprised to find that not everyone experiences similar emotions and that the particular stimulus does not really warrant all the emotionality. At the same time, the patient may be able to distinguish these "hysterical" emotions from other affects and may also become aware of a certain attractiveness and pleasure in the experiencing of these feelings. . . . the hysterical affectivity is utilized by the ego as a fixed mode of adjustment to the demands of the superego, id, and reality. Hysterical emotionality is a dramatic and exhibitionistic demonstration to the superego that the ego is "well-behaved," "proper," and experiences the correct emotions, in order to avoid the displeasure of guilt or loss of love. Similar demonstrations are offered to superego surrogates, parents, the public, or fate. . . . The hysterical defense seems to be directed toward, and to have its genesis in, the oedipal period. Hysterical behavior is strongly reminiscent of the child's dramatic and exhibitionistic efforts to win the parent's love and approval and avoid rejection and punishment by showing the expected behavior and emotions after having done something bad.

A reciprocal relationship exists between the emotional lability and the defensive uses of a child self-image. "If I am a child how could I indulge in adult sexual activity, and moreover, if I find myself there I cannot know what I do; how to do it; why I do it; or to be responsible for my actions." The emotionality lends a childish cast to the patient and the patient utilizes this childish self-image in several interlocking defensive maneuvers. Many of these defensive maneuvers are utilized to sustain inhibitions and to avoid the acceptance of adult responsibilities. An emotional storm ensues whenever there is an internal impulse toward or an external demand for the adult role, e.g., a housewife panics because after preparing for a dinner party, she forgot to light the oven; a young man flies into a rage at his girl friend while she is engaged in a provocative strip because he suddenly recalled that she had been critical of the restaurant he had chosen for dinner. The childish emotionality and juvenile coquetry provokes others into an adoptive role. The hysteric then renews his pride by seeing himself as more sensitive, more empathic, more responsive than the parentified object. Rather than hide the anticipated non-fulfillment of duties the hysteric dramatizes and exhibits his incompetence. The emotional dyscontrol itself is proffered to himself and to the external world as a "logical" rationalization for his inability to engage in unemotional thinking and behavior and hence he is incapable of adult tasks or role fulfillment. Furthermore, a role reversal takes place in which the hysteric induces others to seemingly force him into an area of his own desire, e.g., the competitive or genital-sexual.

The patient is at once using his emotional lability to deny that he sees or knows what lies in these inhibited adult areas; that he himself has desires to enter these areas; that he is capable even if he did wish to break through these inhibitions; that the emotionality itself gives him substitutive satisfaction and even pride. Furthermore, he is able to induce parental attitudes in those with whom he is close. These parental responses are first converted by the patient into demands for maturity, responsibility and adult action. At this point he attacks the surrogate parent for making unrealistic and unattainable demands. The analytic situation presents a tailor-made forum for a repetition of these dynamics. Unless the analyst can go behind these resistances he runs the danger of falling into the Scylla of being viewed as an indulgent parent or the Charybdis of being viewed as a taskmaster in his activity should be agree or confirm what the patient has already underlined as his "irresponsibility."

The key to the solution of this resistance lies in the understanding of the specific utilization of these ego maneuvers by the hysteric. Repression and inhibition are the core defenses. These cannot be attacked frontally without arousing the aforementioned secondary defensive cycle. The externalized defensive cycle depends upon the use of the mechanisms of denial, projection, and reversal of roles. Insight into the use of these projections and distortions in his current life experience, both within and without the analytic situation, is the first order of business.

A school teacher raged at her principal for demanding that she correct her chronic lateness. She rationalized her lateness as a life-long characteristic. Why couldn't she be accepted as she was and secondly why should this be demanded of her when it was well known that she was a superior teacher.

On further exploration clarification ensued. She had provoked her principal to phone and awaken her each morning.

Interpretation and formulation allowed the patient to accept her own role in inducing the principal to replicate the childhood situation and to shift the responsibility for promptness from herself to the principal. In treatment the external situation is presented as a defense and a confirmation of her own incompetence. She is still a child, accepted as a child and thus incapable of assuming responsibility for her own behavior, desires or feelings. It is at this point that a challenge to this self-image is possible and often mandatory. This working through process is repeated in various behavioral areas each time a seeming demand for more mature functioning is perceived. A gradual recognition of the defensive use of the infantile self-image becomes possible, which in turn, increases awareness of greater competence and permits confrontation of the areas of inhibition.

Exaggerations, pseudo-ignorance and perceptual distortion are well-known attributes in the hysterical presentation. This presentation, while often at first appearing ubiquitous and randomized, soon, when closely observed, is the manifest form of underlying fantasies. These fantasies when grouped, epitomize a preconscious and/or unconscious role in which the patient has cloaked himself. These roles, which determine many aspects of the distorted ego function, are centered around such images as that of "the prince," "the femme fatale," "the hero," "the martyr." Dramatizations and distortions protect the patient from reality confrontation, conscious awareness which might expose his role playing and limit the ease with which he turns the world to his psychic purpose. His illusions determine many attitudes (often unconscious) that are derivatives of this central role. In turn, as with the child self-image, they compensate for and protect against insight into the primary conflicts and inhibitions.

A young matron emphasized her personal dedication to humanitarian and philanthropic causes. She entered an analytic session distraught and grieved at having encountered what she described as a wretched, deprived group of people marching up the street before the analyst's building. She was particularly moved by her "empathy" for these people who were being superciliously watched in this wealthy neighborhood.

When this unhappy scene was further explored there unfolded a description of a group of festive marchers on their way to the annual political picnic. Upon seeking the motivation for such obvious distortion, it became apparent that this patient had retained the fantasy that she herself was of true aristocratic character and feeling, relegating the analyst and his co-tenants to the category of upstarts. She could afford to practice *lese majeste*. Interpretation led to the production of new material, the essence of which was that this lady had been pursuing a covert mode of life through purchases indicative of high aesthetic taste, such as elegant furnishings and gourmet foods in accord with her fantasied, aristocratic, high-born self-image and in marked contrast to the sympathetic, suffering worker of humanitarian endeavors. Furthermore, it shed new light on her sexual refusal of her "peasant" husband. By presenting to the world and particularly to her husband, confusion, incompetency, inability to keep house, to maintain household budget, she successfully diverted her husband and others from any knowledge of this secret, highly invested and carefully maintained, aristocratic self-image. Better to be an exasperating little girl than to be challenged and perhaps ridiculed for these strivings.

As long as such a fantasy remains unrevealed and unexplored, interpretations actually fortify the fantasy and maintain the analyst as inferior and impotent. Exploration of behavioral and perceptive modes and confrontations of distortions and non-perceptions are a *sine qua non* enabling the therapist and the patient to ferret out and expose underlying attitudes and their correlated fantasies. These fantasies and attitudes are invested with guilt and shame in contrast to the child self-image which is often quite ego syntonic. They are moreover, heavily narcissistically invested for they are derivatives and residual bastions of strong excitatory infantile experiences. They are a mode through which the oedipal situation is perpetuated and unresolved. If these character attitudes are not worked through, they permit parallel attitudes to prevail in the "transference" which effectively blocks the analysis. Furthermore, these character attitudes often carry within themselves exaggerated and labile emotionality. Once these fantasies are confronted, one begins to observe rages, sorrows, injured feelings, etc., which become more meaningful to the patient and to the therapist.

As these fantasies are derivatives of childhood experiences and conflicts they serve as a bridge to forgotten and distorted childhood memories. The aristocratic fantasies of the aforementioned young matron led to a recall of a formerly repressed memory of her father fostering and cultivating this aristocratic pose through his own elegance and the stimulation of this elegance in her. This allowed for the undoing of a tenaciously held image of her father as unfeeling, uncouth, and obstructing her femininity. In turn, this revived a flood of bodily excitations emanating from the recollections of her relationship with her father.

One must anticipate that at each point of exposition, the analyst is confronted by a new round of hyper-emotionality, hyperincompetence and irresponsibility and, not infrequently, symptom formation. This display is usually accompanied by the oral demands expected of an angry child, a whining child, a suffering child and a frightened child.

Of course, transference behavior by the patient finds a potential echo in the countertransference attitudes of the analyst. There is no patient like the hysteric to prove Franz Alexander's[1] dictum, "Since the phenomenon of countertransference has been recognized, we know that a completely objective attitude of the analyst exists only in theory no matter how painstakingly he may try to live up to this requirement." The evocation of emotionality in others is, as has been mentioned above, prime psychic stock and trade of the hysteric. The analyst finds his day enlivened by this patient's hour. He is courted and flattered. He is made a cherished spectator to an ever unfolding psychic drama. He is invited to become a principal player within the drama, the key to its resolution. Almost no analyst is beyond these temptations. Secondly, the analyst's expectations of his curative powers are mobilized by the apparent simplicity of the defenses, the clarity of the meaning of the behavior, the lucidity of the symbols, the openness of the underlying conflict and the obviousness of the sources of gratification, both conscious and unconscious. Furthermore this therapeutic zeal is abetted by the inference of suggestibility as the patient reiterates the ease with which he is supposedly influenced and led by others.

Even as the analytic drama is being enacted one notes that large and significant areas are avoided, cloaked in vagaries and/or presented but never pursued. A mother may not be mentioned; sexual behavior cannot be discerned. One patient would not use the word "woman," always substituting lady or girl. Amnestic material is presented with large sectors forgotten. Situations both past and present are given preliminary exposition but their resolution remains buried. The dreams have similar vagueness, incompleteness and lack of resolution. It is in attempting to probe the clearly distorted, displaced and repressed that the true intransigence of the defensive structure becomes apparent. It is at these points of resistant roadblocks that the analyst may find himself prone to, or in fact, replicating the emotional attitudes of the parents or later parental surrogates, in fact responding as would the patient's friends, mate, employer or relatives. He may protect his patient from shame and anguish; he may exhort; he may reassure; he may threaten. In each he is conspiring in the maintenance of the patient's neurotic defense.

This by-play, i.e., the actualization within the transference, is in fact a repetition of the secondary gains which have enabled the patient to maintain his conflicts and inhibitions. Whenever the manifest content of the dreams contains the same elements of seductiveness and flattery it is strongly indicative of an intact defensive structure. The secondary gains achieved by the hysterical character neurotic are almost exactly analogous to the classical description by Freud of the secondary gains achieved through a conversion symptom.[3-5] However little attention has been paid to the analyst's indulgence in his own secondary gain as enhancing and endangering the resolution of the neurosis. In fact, the major mechanism through which the hysteric achieves his secondary gain is the evocation in others of emotional interest, responsiveness and pleasure. The analyst's emotional response reassures the patient that he is, as he was in childhood, continuously cherished without the necessity of intrusive physical sexuality nor of the harsh reality that might shake those illusions and fantasies that have been substituted for genital sexuality. If this undersirable transference situation should eventuate, the patient has a repetitive experience rather than a corrective emotional experience; he sustains those inhibitions and repressions that allow him the relational experiences which have been his stock and trade from childhood until his entrance into analysis, and permit him a continued self-imposed blindness to the motivations underlying his behavior.

Although this paper is primarily devoted to the mechanisms of the secondary gains, facades and hyperbolized emotional reactivity of the hysteric, nevertheless, to avoid a therapeutic and theoretic skew, it is essential to stress the psychic pain endured by these patients and to touch upon some of its sources. The therapeutic danger of accepting secondary gain as primary gain is matched by the danger that the therapist's disillusionment and frustration may lead him to ignore and deny the quality of his patient's pain. Hysterics hyperbolize their responses to external events. This externalization defends against the arousal of anxiety-laden body sensuality. This body sensuality is of course much more closely related to inner impulses. These inner impulses are unconsciously assumed to be perenially in danger of arousal and once aroused are feared to be uncontrollable and overwhelming. These diffuse and specific somatic excitements and pleasures are poorly discriminated from sexual impulses and the sexual arousal of the body. These interconnections are not surprising when one considers the developmental pathogenesis of this disorder. Repression and displacement occurred in childhood in response to the genital sensations that were evoked in relation to parental figures. Pleasure derived from the genitals and other parts of the body hazily discriminated during childhood have, for the hysteric's ego, remained but little further discriminated. Two sources of sensuality have remained less re-pressed and inhibited: (1) The evoking in others of sensuality and even more its concomitant emotionality. The patient's sensation then is limited mainly to the reflexion of this arousal in others;[13] (2) The expression of emotionality dissociated from sensuality is permitted and is, in fact, hypertrophied.

Certain milestones mark the penetration of the emotional character facade of the hysteric. It is at these points that a therapeutic alliance and a working transference are established. One sign of the development is the dampening and deepening of the florid emotionality. The emotions are more enduring and tend to be focused on the analyst and a few close affective objects. The patient's assumption of responsibility for his own emotionality lends greater self-consciousness to his behavior and emotional display. Guilty apprehen-siveness begins to become manifest through the increased concern and feared anticipation of retaliation and threatened withdrawal by the therapist. As the patient becomes more conscious of the relation between his own emotionality and the response of others his emotionality becomes more tentative and better controlled. This increased consciousness of the significance of his role leads to increased self-awareness and awareness of bodily feelings and sensations. Transient conversion symptoms and psycho-physiological responses often occur (e.g., urinary frequency).

Bodily feelings, beginning genital sensations instigate body exploration and arouse masturbatory temptations. The gratification of these impulses within a strong affective tie arouses the original fears and guilts. These tend to manifest themselves in feelings of loneliness and the expectation of with-drawal by the analyst. One patient rather succinctly stated, "Orgasm is my graduation and I am not ready to be graduated." This separation anxiety, with its depressive hue, marks the onset of the second stage in the analysis of the hysteric. Paradoxically, in the face of mounting guilt and anxiety, there is a growing sense of pride and gratification. This pride and gratification is the resultant of decreasing inhibitory barriers both internal and external. These positive affects permit further analytic work and increase the scope of interests, accomplishments and pleasures both within and outside of the analysis.

CONCLUSION

Particulate ego reactivity and ego maneuvers characterize the defensive or-ganization of the hysterical character neurosis. These same characteristics serve as a resistance to the development of an effective analytic transference. This defensive purpose is often difficult to discern and, if discerned, to modify. The hysteric's use of emotionality as a defense often results in important secondary gain for the patient. This secondary gain is the evocation in others of affective counterreactivity. As in all interpersonally useful secondary gains it is difficult in itself for the patient to forswear in the expectation of lessened future suffering.

In the hysteric a special analytic difficulty in this regard is operant. The analyst himself is potentially susceptible to this form of stimulus and evocation of emotional response. It is this very mutuality of gratification that tends to permit the acceptance of quasi-transference in the same way that the defensive emotionality is misread as basic emotional response. Furthermore, the quasi-transference does not permit the analysis of the defensive use of the self presented as a child, rather, it reinforces and sustains it. As long as the child role is indulged, interpretations are rendered impotent and neither the underlying fantasied role, nor its attitudinal derivatives can be explicated. The authors deem it necessary for this fantasy complex to be brought into conscious awareness before the infantile memories and emotional experiences long since repressed can be recovered. Once this phase of the analytic task has been accomplished, a transference neurosis evolves and the second phase of the analytic process can proceed.

REFERENCES

1. Alexander, F. *The Scope of Psychoanalysis.* New York: Basic Books, 1961, p. 264.
2. Easser, B. R., and Lesser, S. R. Hysterical personality: a re-evaluation. *Psychoanal. Quart.* 34:390–405, 1965.
3. Freud, S. A case of hysteria. *Standard Edition,* Vol. 7. London: The Hogarth Press, 1953.
4. Freud, S. *A General Introduction to Psychoanalysis.* Lecture 24. New York: Liveright Publishing Corp., 1935.
5. Freud, S. Inhibitions, symptoms and anxiety. *Standard Edition,* Vol. 20. London: The Hogarth Press, 1959.
6. Glover, E. *The Technique of Psychoanalysis.* New York: Int. Univ. Press, 1958, p. 68.
7. Knapp, P., Levin, S., McCarter, R., et al. Suitability for psychoanalysis: a review of one hundred supervised analytic cases. *Psychoanal. Quart.* 24:459–77, 1960.
8. Marmor, J. Orality in the hysterical personality. *J. Amer. Psychoanal. Assoc.* 1:656–71, 1954.
9. Reich, W. *Character Analysis.* New York: Orgone Institute Press, 1949, pp. 189–192.
10. Siegman, A. Emotionality—a hysterical character defense. *Psychoanal. Quart.* 23: 339–54, 1954.

11. Valenstein, A. The psycho-analytic situation. *Int. J. of Psychoanal.* 43:315–324, 1962.
12. Winter, H. Pre-oedipal factors in genesis of hysterical character neurosis. *Int. J. of Psychoanal.* 45:338–42, 1964.
13. Wisdom, J. A methodological approach to the problem of hysteria. *Int. J. Psychoanal.* 42:224–37, 1961.

12. Obsessional Characters and Obsessional Neuroses

Humberto Nagera

The obsessional character is one of many possible outcomes in normal personality development and, where it remains within limits, a useful and desirable form of personality organization.

On the other hand, obsessional character formation can overstep these limits and come closer to the so-called character disturbances, character disorders or character neuroses of the obsessional type. Nunberg in his *Principles of Psycho-Analysis* (1955) defines individuals with a character neurosis as those "who are free of neurotic symptoms but who behave pathologically." Reich (1928) in distinguishing between character neuroses and symptom neuroses remarks that the subject only feels ill when the trait that has been built into the character becomes magnified. He says: "It is only when the characterological shyness rises to the pitch of pathological blushing or the obsessive orderlings to a compulsive ceremonial—that is, when the neurotic character undergoes exacerbation to the point of the development of symptoms—that its subject feels ill."

In the obsessional character disorder the limits compatible with normal ego functioning and normal object relationships have been transgressed, and the character traits belonging to the normal obsessional character are exaggerated to the point of becoming its caricature. Although the individual himself may experience no neurotic suffering or anxiety, other people will notice that there is something wrong with him and find him difficult to deal with. Such characters are hard taskmasters for others, while their own ego performance is usually affected to some degree. Also, their increased orderliness and meticulousness is disturbing to their environment, while they themselves take it as a matter of course.

Nevertheless, neither the obsessional character nor the obsessional character disorder should be confused with the obsessional neurosis proper, since the latter state implies a great deal of anxiety and suffering largely absent in

Reprinted from Humberto Nagera, *Obsessional Neuroses: Developmental Pathology* (New York: Jason Aronson, 1976), 139–42 by permission of Jason Aronson, Inc.

the former. It is characteristic of the obsessional neurosis that it represents an actively ongoing conflict, in Freud's terms "an interminable struggle" between internal forces, while obsessional character formation represents a more or less successful attempt at solution of specific developmental conflicts which are brought to a halt by it.

Nunberg (1955) has pointed out that "character traits or habits are much better assimilated than symptoms, and form an integral part of the ego. The assimilation is frequently so complete that the distance between character and ego disappears. Then the character seems to be identical with the ego, which is never true of symptom and ego" (p. 318).

I have noted elsewhere (Nagera, 1966) the frequency with which certain neurotic conflicts or even neuroses proper are solved in childhood and adolescence by incorporating into the character structure certain traits and attitudes that avoid the ongoing conflicts. At the expense of accepting some limitations, inhibitions, and alterations in the ego organization, acute anxiety, neurotic conflicts, etc., are brought to a halt and a new solution is introduced that may be more or less permanent in nature. Nunberg (1955) has pointed out too that "the conflict between hetero- and homosexuality may be brought to an end either through neurotic symptoms or by character changes," as happens also with conflicts between erotic and destructive instincts (p. 319).

How far such a solution is permanent depends on numerous factors, among them its relative success. Sometimes the transformation of neurotic conflicts into character structures is only partial and perhaps therefore easily reversible. Many patients are known to oscillate between openly anxious and florid states of obsessional disturbance and more controlled ones without manifest anxiety, where it seems as if temporarily some of the well-known obsessional character traits had hardened up and replaced the more disturbing obsessions and compulsions.

Nunberg has made it clear that the "anal character traits" can be a continuation or repetition of instinctual drive gratification in an aim-inhibited or sublimated form (a child who retains feces may become an overpossessive and avaricious adult). Or these traits may be the result of reaction formations of the ego, with the anal instinct turned into its opposite (p. 305). A combination of both types in the same patient is not unusual.

What leads from these neurotic conflicts, or developmental conflicts, to character developments of an obsessional type seems to remain a two-way process. We have all observed well-established obsessional characters who have backtracked from the obsessional character to an obsessional neurosis at different speeds. Here the obsessional character organization has crumbled because of renewed pressure on the economy of the personality structure, due sometimes to unexpected and traumatic experiences and life situations, excessive frustrations, etc. In some cases this occurs at the time of "change of life." Many others have pointed out this relationship between character and neurosis. Nunberg, to quote but one example, says, "There exists some kind of relationship between character and neurosis, particularly when we learn that a character trait may degenerate into a neurotic symptom. Normal and useful curiosity, for example, may deteriorate into obsessional questioning" (p. 315).

In the limited number of observations I have made of this reversal from an obsessional character to a florid obsessional neurosis, or to neurotic conflicts on the way to the development of a possible obsessional neurosis, it invariably happened that the "normal" obsessional character transformed itself in the first instance into a less normal one, i.e., into something more akin to a character disturbance of an obsessional type, and remained static as such for some time. Such a development points to the economic strengthening of the forces involved in the solution represented by the obsessional character. In this, all personality traits, reaction-formations, etc., become exaggerated, the individual becomes more obsessed with doubts and uncertainty, orderliness becomes excessive, and ego functioning can be brought to a complete halt. The degree of the changes that take place varies from one patient to another; it may happen that the process will develop no further but can be contained at this intermediary stage. A return to the more normal obsessional character _organization_ is sometimes possible as soon as the reasons responsible for the increase in the drive and defense activity disappear.

In other cases the above stage is just a station in the transit to the further development of a neurotic type of conflict or an obsessional neurosis proper. It is the neurotic suffering and anxiety suddenly present that mark the change from the character solution to the neurotic solution of the conflicts.

REFERENCES

Nagera, H. 1966. _Early Childhood Disturbances, the Infantile Neurosis and the Adulthood Disturbances. Problems of a Developmental Psychoanalytic Psychology._ Monograph no. 2 of _Psychoanalytic Study of the Child._ New York: International Universities Press.
Nunberg, H. 1955. _Principles of Psycho-Analysis._ New York: International Universities Press.
Reich, W. 1928. On character analysis. In _The Psychoanalytic Reader._ London: Hogarth Press and London Institute of Psycho-Analysis, 1950.

13. Comparing Obsessional and Hysterical Personalities

Humberto Nagera

The point is frequently made that the obsessional rearrangement of the structure of the personality leads to a "better," "stronger," "more desirable" personality organization than that made by the hysteric.

This conclusion is partly due to the correct assumption that the development of an obsessional neurosis requires an ego organization of good quality, and partly to the well-known statement by Freud that a "precocious" ego development is among the *predispositions* to the development of an obsessional neurosis.

As mentioned before, certain obsessional character traits are in many ways assets to the personality when present in specific quantities, combinations, and proportions. On the other hand, it is only too well known that other obsessional characters offer combinations of traits of a less desirable nature, which in some cases lead to severe limitations even where a good potential of ego performance exists. What is true of the obsessional character is true in a similar way for neurotic disturbances. According to Ernest Jones (1918) both valuable and disadvantageous qualities derive from "the interrelations of the different anal-erotic components with one another and with other constituents of the whole character." He thinks that among the valuable "may be reckoned especially the individualism, the determination and persistence, the love of order and power of organization, the competency, reliability and thoroughness, the generosity, the bent towards art and good taste, the capacity for unusual tenderness, and the general ability to deal with concrete objects of the material world." Among the disadvantageous "belong the incapacity for happiness, the irritability and bad temper, the hypochondria, the miserliness, meanness and pettiness, the slow-mindedness and proness to bore, the bent for dictating and tyrannising, and the obstinacy. . . ."

The obsessional neurosis is more severe, more ego-encompassing and

Reprinted from Humberto Nagera, *Obsessional Neuroses: Developmental Pathology* (New York: Jason Avonson, 1976), 193–96 by permission of Jason Aronson, Inc.

crippling than the hysterical neurosis. The prognosis of the former is always more serious than that of the latter for the same reasons. From the point of view of drive organization the obsessional neurosis always implies an important fixation point at the anal-sadistic stage to which an important regressive move has taken place in later development. Here again the hysteric patient's fixation point is at a higher level (the phallic-oedipal) and in this sense compares favorably with the obsessionals.

Nevertheless, and in spite of all that has been said above, clinical observation and experience still points to the special quality of the ego of the obsessional neurotic.

I think that a reconciliation of these apparent contradictions is reached if we state that a minimum "quality" of ego development is required to "produce" an obsessional neurosis, a minimum which is relatively high compared with other forms of psychopathology including hysterias. This requirement refers even to the most poorly organized forms of obsessional neuroses, let alone the more highly organized ones.

Considering now the hysterical developments from the ego side, there is no doubt that they can start with a lower "quality" than that required for the ego of an obsessional neurosis, provided that their drive organization has proceeded to the appropriate point in its development. But though clinical experience shows that some hysterical disorders occur in otherwise very primitive and poor ego organization, it must be remembered that these are only cases that occur at the lower end and that many other forms of hysterical personality are of the highest order. In short, at the higher end of the scale, hysterics can be as good as, perhaps at times better than, obsessionals from the point of view of the high quality of their ego organization.

It is for the above reason that I think it is a fallacy to assume that the obsessional outcome always implies a better ego or a better personality than the hysterical one.

If we were artificially to express ego quality in grades (grade 1, poor ego development; grade 2, medium ego development; grade 3, good ego development; and grade 4, excellent ego development), then a diagram (Figure 1) would show at one glance that the minimum ego quality required for an obsessional neurosis is grade 3 (good) while the hysterical patient can go down the scale as far as grade 1 (poor).

On the other hand, an obsessional patient with ego development of grade 3 (good) will have a less rich personality, capacity, etc., than the hysterical of the highest order, though it should be clear from the schema that obsessionals can also reach grade 4.

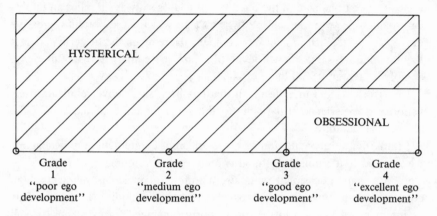

| Grade 1 "poor ego development" | Grade 2 "medium ego development" | Grade 3 "good ego development" | Grade 4 "excellent ego development" |

FIGURE 1. EGO QUALITY

A similar argument as to the necessary "quality" of ego required applies to other forms of psychopathology. Homosexuals, for example, can like hysterics show a much wider range of variation than can obsessionals as far as the quality of ego organization is concerned; some homosexuals are highly developed while others show a poor ego organization.

I believe that a closer and more detailed study of the ego organization is necessary, as Hartmann (1950) and others have pointed out, to specify what degree of development of what ego functions has been reached, as well as their interaction with the drives and with one another, etc. It is here that many clues are to be found as to the possible outcomes of the developmental and neurotic conflicts of the child. Although *a priori* it looks as if variations are possible ad infinitum, I am inclined to think that certain general and common groupings, combinations and patterns will be discernable.

REFERENCES

Hartmann, H. 1950. Psychoanalysis and developmental psychology. In *Essays on Ego Psychology*. London: Hogarth Press and The London Institute of Psycho-Analysis, 1964.

Jones, E. 1918. Anal-erotic character traits. In *Papers on Psychoanalysis*. London: Balliere, Tindall and Cox, 1948.

14. An Object-Relations Perspective on Masochism

Theo L. Dorpat

This chapter presents clinical data to illustrate and discuss an object-relations perspective for understanding masochism. Object-relations theories are probably the most critical and essential aspect of psychoanalytic clinical theory (G. Klein 1976). Klein distinguishes between clinical theory, which is derived from psychoanalytic data, and metapsychological theory, which expresses Freud's philosophy of science. In contrast to metapsychological theories, object-relations theories are testable by clinical psychoanalytic methods.

CLINICAL MATERIAL

Mr. A., a 39-year-old C.P.A., worked for a large corporation when he began analysis. He was married, but separated from his wife and three children. He had low self-esteem, frequently felt depressed, and experienced a long-standing dissatisfaction with his job and marriage. He complained that his wife did not respond to him either emotionally or sexually and that he had not had sexual relations with her for several years. He alluded to having engaged in abnormal sexual acts with prostitutes, but was unable to divulge the details of these practices until he had been in analysis for over a year.

Mr. A. had grown up in a large Texas city, the second son of an Armenian family. Both sets of grandparents had emigrated to the United States early in this century. He described his father as an easy-going, intelligent owner of a small business firm, and his mother as a hot-tempered woman who, although rarely affectionate, was fiercely loyal to and protective of her family. When Mr. A. was 13, his father died of a heart attack.

In the first weeks of analysis, the patient would discuss some problem and then ask, "What should I do?" or "Don't you have some advice for me?" It

Reprinted from P. L. Giovacchini and L. B. Boyer, eds. *Technical Factors in the Treatment of Severely Disturbed Patients* (New York: Jason Aronson, 1982), 490–513 by permission of Jason Aronson, Inc.

became abundantly clear that he wanted me to give him directives on how he should lead his life and behave. Initially, I used the customary methods of silence or turning the question back to the patient to deal with his questions and demands. When his questions intensified, I explained the analytic contract and frame to him, telling him why I thought it would not be helpful to him or the analysis for me to provide answers. My efforts were fruitless and he became more demanding of marital advice. Finally, I told him, "You feel so anxious and uncertain about your relationship with your wife that you are trying to control and pressure me into giving you an answer about what you should do." He then relaxed and talked about how troubled his conscience was about his marriage. However, this interaction did not resolve his need to control the analyst and seek magical answers to his problems.

The patient's relative lack of psychological separateness from others characterized many of his important interpersonal relations. In the thirteenth month of analysis, Mr. A. became disturbed over the learning difficulties his 10-year-old daughter was experiencing in her language class. She spoke and wrote in fragmented, incomplete sentences. After her teacher pointed out this problem to her parents, they noticed that the other two children and the mother also talked in this fragmentary manner. They would typically wait for each other, and especially the father, to finish the sentences they had begun. For example, the wife would start to say something and hesitate. Her hesitation served as a cue for Mr. A. to finish her sentences. In this way, all of the family members shared in maintaining pathological symbiotic (or self-object) relationships in which they thought and spoke for each other. The same interaction was transferred to the analytic situation, where, for the first three years of analysis, the patient persistently wished, and even demanded, that I think and speak for him.

Childhood Trauma

One of the major causes of Mr. A.'s chronic depression was an unresolved and pathological mourning reaction to the death of his father. As his attachment to me became more stable and important, long-repressed memories of his father and his death came to the fore. Mr. A. had not completed the "work" of mourning; he had not grieved for his father and had been unable to accept the reality of his death fully.

Even on the day of his father's death, he had been unable to cry over the loss. Limited space does not allow full documentation of the hypothesis that the death of his father and his pathological mourning response to the loss severely blocked the patient's psychosexual development. For studies on how denial of death and pathological mourning reaction retard psychosexual development, see Altschul (1968), Dorpat (1972), and Wolfenstein (1966, 1969).

The mobilization and reactivation of the mourning process for the death of his father had two positive consequences, both involving progressive steps in his development. Whereas formerly he had repressed memories of his father, he was now able to remember his father as a warm, affectionate man. Memories of sitting in his father's lap and talking and playing with him came back. He identified with this loving aspect of his father and became much closer to and more affectionate with his own children. To some extent, identification with this loving imago supplanted his defensive identification with the hostile, controlling aspects of his mother.

While working through his mourning, the patient unconsciously and pathologically identified with his father's illness and mode of death. Early in the analysis, he talked seriously about his fears that he would not live beyond 52, his father's age when he died. One day Mr. A. came to an analytic hour breathless and tired from playing racquetball. He feared that he would have a heart attack, as his father had. "Living means more to me now," he said. "Before, I didn't think I would live a longer life." The above vignette and other clinical evidence indicated some working through of his pathological identification with his father's age at death. Such pathological identifications with the illness or death of a lost loved one are frequently found in unresolved mourning reactions (Anderson 1949, Krupp 1965).

The revival and gradual working through of grief for his father had another constructive outcome. He began to identify consciously with his father as a trader and businessman. For over fifteen years, Mr. A. had carried out a double work life. By day he worked as an accountant; at night, he quietly and secretly did what he really enjoyed—investing. In the second year of analysis, he confided that he had accumulated a small fortune through investing, mainly in real estate. He had never liked being an accountant, and he especially disliked filling out tax forms and taking orders from his superiors. In the twenty-first month of analysis, he resigned his position in the corporation and opened a private office as an investor and real estate developer.

His move to a business career also marked another forward step in his emancipation from his mother. She had wanted him to be an accountant, and one of the principal reasons he had pursued that career was to please her and comply with her wishes.

Masochistic Perversion

Over a year of analysis elapsed before the patient could disclose the details of his sexual perversion. In one extremely tense and dramatic hour, he revealed in a halting, tremulous voice that for over 18 years he had regularly and frequently used prostitutes for sadomasochistic practices. I said little in that hour because he seemed too vulnerable and ashamed to tolerate any intervention; beads of perspiration ran down his face. The general perverse pattern began with Mr. A. giving specific instructions to prostitutes to insult, denigrate, and punish him. Sometimes he had them spank his bare buttocks with a leather belt. Sexual intercourse or masturbation would follow these carefully planned, controlled episodes of punishment and humiliation. The most humiliating and submissive perverse act involved his lying on the floor with the woman squatting above him and urinating on his head.

What are the important meanings of these sadomasochistic practices? Although humiliated and punished during these acts, Mr. A. still controlled the situation because he gave precise instructions to the prostitutes. He would unmercifully berate and scold them if they deviated in any way from what he ordered them to do. The anxiety he experienced in relating his perversion and the need for absolute control over the situation were the important clues I used to understand the unconscious meaning of the perversion: it was an unconscious attempt to master and control traumas the patient had suffered in the relationship with his extremely controlling, cruel mother.

The evidence for the mother's sadistic control of the patient surfaced not only from a reconstruction of past events revived and remembered in the transference situation, but also from the patient's gradual awareness of his mother's current tyrannical oppression of her children, grandchildren, and others. The patient's unconscious need to repeat continually the sadomaso-chistic quality of his early relations with his mother was a manifestation of what Freud (1920) called the ''repetition compulsion''—the unconscious need to repeat traumatic experiences in order to overcome and master them.

Some trauma was specifically sexual. After the death of Mr. A.'s father, the mother had insisted that he sleep in the same bed with her, ''spoon'' fashion, with the son behind the mother. This practice stopped at age 15 when he had an erection. His irate mother accused him of depravity and pushed him out of her bed. From the age of 6 until he left home to attend college, the patient dressed and undressed his mother. His assignments included fastening and unfastening her corset and brassiere and if he did not instantly and correctly obey these assignments, she slapped his face and scolded him.

After considerable analytic work on the sadomasochistic relations with his mother, the patient was able to say, "I was her personal slave." In the third year of analysis, he spontaneously interpreted that his mother had made him her slave just as she, the youngest of a large family, had been enslaved to her own mother for many years.

One crucial difference existed between his ritualized experiences with the prostitutes and the earlier traumatic experiences with his mother. With the prostitutes, he was in control; with his mother, he had been painfully helpless. The traumatized subject became the agent rather than the victim of the unpleasurable activity. Unconsciously, he attempted to master the slave relationship with his mother and the associated feelings of sexual arousal, helplessness, and rage by replicating the sexualized slave relationship with prostitutes. Before analysis, he had no awareness that he repeated with prostitutes the same type of eroticized master-slave experiences he had endured earlier in the relationship with his mother.

The sadomasochistic, master-slave qualities of his perverse sexual practices also occurred in his other relationships. In most interpersonal relationships, he played either the role of the dominating tyrant or the complementary role of the abjectly submissive, obsequious one. He often spoke of trying to "force" or "make" his wife become more emotionally responsive to him and had no awareness that his need to control her actually provoked her withholding and withdrawn behavior.

During our analysis of these early experiences and their relation to his perversion, he had a recurrence of a nightmare he had experienced many times in his adolescence. In the nightmare, he is home alone in his parental family room, hiding because he has done something wrong. Two policemen come to the door of the house to catch him and he awakens from the dream in a state of terror.

The death of the father, the going to bed with the mother, and the punishment dream are, of course, reminiscent of the oedipal situation. I made an oedipal interpretation, stating that he feared punishment for what must have seemed a frightening victory over his father. My interpretation had no impact whatsoever on the patient. His polite and detached response was, "That's a very interesting idea, doctor. I read something like that somewhere." I was obviously on the wrong track, and returned to my hypothesis that his sexual disorder stemmed from his traumatic relations with his mother.[1]

Self-Object and Whole-Object Relations

The major transference configurations during this period of Mr. A.'s analysis involved variations on the master-slave relationship. At moments, he perceived me as the slave, but more frequently the focus of transference interpretations was upon his wishes, fears, and especially unconscious fantasies of being my slave. With the gradual working through in the analytic transference of the master-slave relation, his visits to prostitutes decreased. In the twenty-third month of analysis, he stopped the practice entirely, after having a startling and revealing experience with one of them. Instead of programming a prostitute to carry out his masochistic fantasies, he decided to talk to her. He found that they had common childhood experiences of growing up in the South. This led to what he described as the amazing discovery that she was a real person with thoughts and feelings of her own. Previously, he had denied the personhood of prostitutes and had related to them solely as the depersonalized vehicle of his wishful fantasies (as his mother had so often treated him).

Clinical evidence strongly suggests that perverse masochistic behavior is based on pre-oedipal, or self-object, relationships. Prior to analysis, the patient viewed and treated prostitutes only in terms of sadomasochistic wishes, and any qualities of the prostitute that seemed discordant with his wishes were denied or simply ignored. When he attained a growing capacity for whole-object relatedness through analysis and his conversation with the prostitute, the perverse masochistic desires disappeared.

Homosexuality is also often based on pre-oedipal self-object relationships in which the sexual object is viewed almost entirely as the embodiment of the subject's conscious or unconscious perverse fantasies. During the fourth year of analysis, the patient became obsessed with homosexual fears and fantasies for a brief period. While driving to his office one morning, he picked up an athletic black youth who seemed to epitomize his sexual desires

1. The effects of making oedipal interpretations prematurely have been discussed by Volkan (1976). See also Boyer (1967), Ornstein and Ornstein (1975), and Rosenfeld (1966).

for a young and virile sexual partner. When the young man appeared interested in a sexual affair, the two drove off to a secluded area with a six-pack of beer. While talking with his companion, he noted that his sexual ardor gradually waned. He learned that the young man was the same age as his own son. With intense and mixed feelings of resignation and regret, he realized that his homosexual desire was founded on the fantasy of incorporating through fellatio the imagined masculine strength of the black youth. While thinking over this fantasy, he remembered an interpretation I had made about his wish to incorporate the idealized virility of other men through sexual intercourse. Recognizing the difference between this previously unconscious fantasy and the man beside him led to the collapse of any desire for sexual relations.

The major point of this vignette is the same as the one made earlier about the role of self-object relations in perverse masochistic behavior. Conversation with his companion made him aware of a developmentally higher form of reality testing and he was then able to view the companion as a whole object. The decisive difference between pathological self-object relations and whole-object relations is that the whole object is represented and related to as a person distinguishable from the wish-fulfilling projections of the subject.

Different modes of reality testing are linked with different modes of object relations. In self-object relationships, patients manipulate the external object so that it conforms to their wishes and expectations (Brodey 1965). They do not perceive aspects of behavior that cannot be used to verify their projections.

Mr. A. was both understimulated and overstimulated by his mother. Childhood and adolescent experiences of dressing her and sleeping with her stimulated intense feelings of helplessness and sexual wishes that could not be acknowledged or gratified. Boyer (1956) discussed the relationship between maternal overstimulation and the early development of ego defects. Chronic states of overstimulation were manifested in Mr. A.'s tense hyperactivity and initial difficulties relaxing on the couch. Over time, he developed trust in me and was able to use the couch as a "holding environment" that supported him and made it possible for him to relax. After he learned to use the couch and the analytic situation for relaxing, he observed that he had never before realized how tense and overstimulated he had felt for nearly all his life. The analytic regression to a self-object transference and his trust in me allowed him to gradually relinquish his former pathological dependence on excessive amounts of alcohol and marijuana. Previously, these drugs were the only agents he found useful in relieving his chronic tension states of overstimulation.

Subjective states of understimulation alternated with the states of overstimulation. Episodes of sadomasochistic perversion were often triggered by uneasy feelings of understimulation, such as boredom, loneliness, or depression. In analysis, adult experiences of understimulation could be traced to their childhood antecedents, such as being alone at home after school. His mother worked full time after he was one and a half years old; the patient was often left alone as a child.

The same basic transference issue of trying to control and manipulate me into giving him directives and advice surfaced repeatedly throughout the analysis, albeit in different forms. In the second year of the analysis, when he was again uncertain about whether he should terminate his marriage, he wanted me to tell him what he should do. I told him, "You think of me as having the perfect answers about your marriage, and you wish for me to tell you what you should do." Mr. A. broke down and cried. He said he felt sad that I did not have a magical and perfect answer for him. My interaction revived the still incompletely resolved mourning for his father. After his father's death, he felt all alone, as if there were no one alive who could help him. My response implied that I did not have magical answers for him and temporarily disrupted his idealizing transference.

Conflicts over Separation

In the third year of analysis, Mr. A. seriously planned to drop his treatment and run away to another part of the country. His pressing impulse stemmed partially from fears that he would have to meet my fantasized expectations or face my rejection and abandonment. Living up to my expectations meant that he would have to adopt my rigid, conservative, traditional values. The unconscious fantasy underlying these fears was that I had controlled him and molded him into my slave. This transference reaction involved projecting onto me aspects of the master-slave introject—an introject formed and internalized mainly from his relationship with his mother.

During this crisis, I made several transference interpretations concerning his need to see me as the oppressive, controlling part of himself or his mother. These interventions seemed to have no effect, and he maintained his paranoid attitude that I was secretly intent on controlling and directing his life. The crisis finally passed, and he appeared more comfortable with the analysis. I was puzzled about what had happened and anxiously speculated that the master-slave transference manifestations had simply gone underground, concealed by surface politeness. Was he merely acting compliant and agreeable defensively in order to hide and preserve the unspoken part of how he perceived our relationship?

Several weeks later, while discussing an interaction with his wife, he told me that he had checked himself from giving her a directive about her behavior. He stopped himself when he recalled that a month before I had told him I would not direct him because I would then be depriving him of his rights and capacities to choose his own way of life. He explained that my respect for his freedom had made a profound and lasting impression on him. This surprised me because at the time I made that statement, I had felt that none of my interpretations or interventions had any impact on his paranoid fears about me.

Thereafter, in his interpersonal relations he increasingly adopted the attitude that "everyone has the right to think and decide for himself." He recounted many interactions with others, especially his wife and children, in which he refrained from assuming his former dictatorial and pre-emptory control over their conduct. In the analytic situation, these changes were linked with a new understanding and cautious acceptance of my neutrality. He had not previously understood that my interpretations were intended as useful information; rather, he experienced them as overt or covert directives in which I communicated how he should feel, think, and behave.

Mr. A.'s adoption of my attitude of fostering autonomy is an example of what Giovacchini (1972, 1980) has called the "analytic introject" and what I have referred to as the "analyst introject" (Dorpat 1978). Outside the analytic hours, the patient used fantasies and memories of me to comfort himself and to prevent himself from acting out destructively. The formation and use of the analytic or analyst introject does not in itself instigate permanent ego or superego structural changes; for this to occur, introjection must be followed by identification with the introjected relation with the analyst.

Mr. A. gradually identified with the analyst introject, and integrated these identifications into his improved ego and superego functioning. As a result of the gradual dissolution of the transference configuration, which involved both wishes and fears that I would provide magical directives and advice, he took another step toward autonomy. A new and major theme emerged, one that he called "learning to take care of myself."

One evening, the patient and his three children played pinball at their athletic club. Mr. A. interrupted his game to watch his daughter at a nearby machine. Meanwhile, his 17-year-old son, John, having finished his game, took over his father's pinball machine. The patient mildly protested the intrusion and assumed control of the machine. John launched a tirade of verbal abuse at his father, but Mr. A. stood up to John and finished the game.

The patient was tense while recounting the above episode. I said, "You have been struggling with yourself here over whether or not you have the right to take care of yourself." Pleased, he relaxed on the couch. The idea of taking care of himself and protecting his own interests had not occurred to him before. He explained how he had struggled with two different impulses. Not only had he resisted the impulse to give in to his son and allow him to take over the pinball machine, but he also had restrained himself from becoming overtly enraged and abusive, as had frequently been the case in the past.

During the next analytic hour, he told me how he had set limits on his son's erratic and dangerous driving. John had been arrested several times for driving under the influence of alcohol and speeding. Mr. A. felt unsure and anxious about his capacity to stand up for himself and withstand his son's demands and manipulations. His next associations were to a frightening dream in which a policeman questioned him and accused him of some unspecified crime against a woman in another city. The dream had seemed acutely real to him and had frightened him. Then he recalled the recurrent nightmare of his adolescence in which two policemen came to his door to capture him. He thought that fear of the police might be connected with his adolescent shoplifting.

He recalled the pleasure he had received the preceding weekend by being with his two daughters. He compared the enjoyment he felt when he cooked for them with his father's happiness when he cooked for his family. His father had been an expert cook. He described a conversation with a friend in which he had talked about his sadness over the prospect of missing the children when he divorced his wife. His friend asked him why he had not considered obtaining either partial or full custody of his children, and this prompted him to consider some type of custody of his children for the first time.

I then interpreted the dream in which he was accused of committing a crime as his fear of being punished for looking out for himself. I told him, "It is true that the activities you talked about today—standing up for yourself to your son, wanting to have custody of your children, trying to find a condominium—are not crimes in any usual sense of the word. Still, to you they are crimes because you are doing these things for yourself. In the relationship with your mother, there was an unspoken but powerful rule that you were supposed to take care of her but not of yourself.'' Initially, he was flustered and surprised by my interpretation, but after a few minutes of verbally exploring the validity of my remarks, he stated that there was some truth in them. On the night before his punishment dream, he had gone to bed feeling good about what he had done for himself and his daughters.

About a week later, he anxiously related having lunch with a woman friend who had discussed her marital problems with him. She had held his hand, and he had felt that she wanted a more intimate, sexual relationship with him. He had told her that he liked her but was not sexually attracted to her. I interpreted his anxiety and conflict: ''You have been in conflict between doing what you wanted—taking care of yourself—and another part of you that wanted to please your friend by having a more intimate relationship.'' He replied, ''That's exactly right!'' Again, when I understood and recognized his feelings, Mr. A. felt relieved and immensely gratified.

The theme, ''taking care of myself,'' remained central in the analysis for several months. The notion that he could take care of himself and at the same time respect the rights of others to do the same proved to be novel and liberating for him. At the most basic level, this change represented a further differentiation of the self-representation from the representation of his mother. As always, recognition and gradual appropriation of new and improved ego and superego capacities were not carried out without concomitant interpersonal and psychic (mainly object-relations) conflicts.

In an apologetic and cautious manner, he reported success in a real estate venture. I interpreted his apologetic mode as stemming from his fear that I would appropriate and control his success, as his mother had. He responded with memories of how often he had felt that his achievements at home and school had really belonged to his mother.

In another session, Mr. A. recounted a disturbing encounter with a rude waitress. He was pleased with himself for being neither submissive nor combative with her, stances he had often taken previously in similar situations. His further associations suggested that he felt guilty while telling me about his growing capacity to regulate himself more independently. I told him that he felt guilty because he imagined that I would feel hurt and abandoned by his independent activity. His memories of his mother's desperate hold on him and her use of punishment to discourage his strivings toward autonomy confirmed this interpretation.

He felt guilty and feared punishment because his progressive movements in the analysis toward taking care of himself conflicted with the prohibitions of his introjected representation of his mother against autonomous activity. His normal strivings toward self-caring had broken the implicit rules of the pathological, symbiotic caretaking relation with his mother.

This object-relations conflict contains a specific structure and implicit rules governing the caretaking relation first organized and formed in the mother-child relationship and later displaced to others. The discovery of the structure of this introjected relation with his mother did not surface in a single flash of insight to either the patient or myself. Rather, the analytic reconstruction of this particular object relation was a cumulative and collaborative process in which the pertinent information was obtained more through the analysis of transference and countertransference than through a study of historical events or interpersonal relations outside the analytic situation.

It is both desirable and possible to analyze the structures of object relationships (past or present, actual or imaginary) in terms of the shared rules that regulate specific interpersonal interactions. The sociologist Goffman (1974) and Spruiell (1980) have advanced theories about the rules that govern social interactions. The system of rules defines the frame or structure of the object relation. An important aspect of resistance and transference analysis is the recognition and interpretation of the rules governing childhood object relations which have been unconsciously transferred onto the analyst or the analyst-analysand relationship.

Like other kinds of caretaking relations, the implicit contract between the patient and his mother included the shared rule of reciprocity, an arrangement by which each person would enjoin to take care of the other in return for the other's caretaking. But this mutual caretaking relation differed from more normal ones in that the recipient of the caring was tacitly prohibited from assuming any rights or capacities for self-caring. In the mutual caretaking relation with the mother, there could be only one mind, one center of power, intentionality, and decision, for the dyad. The one being cared for was not represented or recognized by either party as a whole person with rights and capacities for self-caring, self-control, and self-direction. The object of the caring blankly and mindlessly acted out the role projected upon him.

This is reminiscent of mother-infant symbiosis. However, it differs from normal symbiotic relations in that the mother's caretaking frequently was not regulated by the patient's actual needs. At times, he unconsciously lived out the role of being cared for when the role was not congruent with his immediate needs and wishes. For example, the mother would coerce him to accept gifts from her which he did not want or need.

Mr. A. obtained some insight into the unhappy discrepancy between his actual needs and his mother's perceptions of his needs when he remembered what had happened to him and his mother at his father's funeral and afterwards. He recalled how his mother physically had leaned on him at the funeral, ignoring his pressing need for comfort and solace. Afterwards, she had leaned on him in a more figurative sense and, in his words, had treated him more like a "husband" than an adolescent son. In this caretaking relation, the patient and his mother alternated roles, with first one and then the other assuming control and regulation for the other. The mother expected, and sometimes demanded, that he assume duties such as management of the family's finances, which had previously been his father's responsibility. His mother would assume a child-like dependent attitude and look to him for direction, guidance, and leadership.

At the height of the patient's concern and conflict over taking care of himself, he related a dream so frightening that it had awakened him. He dreamed there were two conveyor belts ("the machine") carrying dishes; one belt carried dishes of food from a kitchen, and the other returned the empty dishes. He had to unload the dishes of food quickly, serve them to people seated nearby, and load the emptied dishes onto the belt to return them to the kitchen. Anxiety developed when Mr. A. could not keep up with the machine and accomplish all of the assigned tasks. As a result of his inability to keep up with "the infernal machine," some dishes of food fell on the floor, making a huge mess. Another person, not fully recognizable in the dream (but whom he later identified as me), approached the machine to turn it off. He awoke with a sense of panic over the mess and his inability to serve the seated people.

At various times, I represented the different persons and objects in the dream, including "the infernal machine," but the main and abiding transference element was the vague figure who was going to shut off the machine. The nondescript figure represented the idealized analyst (or idealized parent imago) who would help him gain some relief from his compulsive need to please, take care of, and feed others, primarily his mother.

His dream vividly depicted the essential elements of the introjected caretaking relation with his mother. The machine's actions of rapidly and inexorably carrying dishes to and from the kitchen represented both his and his mother's urgent oral needs and demands. Above all, the impersonal and relentless movement of the Kafkaesque machine replicated early experiences with his unempathic, controlling mother. It represented the coercive pressures she exerted against him to meet her needs. It symbolized the rule that he was to relinquish any concern for his own needs in the service of caring for others. The working through of various meanings of the dream, and particularly the transferential aspects connected with the introjected caretaking relation, were lasting progressive steps made by the patient in taming, if not completely dismantling, the machine within himself.

The patient made several other important changes during his analysis; the most important steps have probably been in the direction of his individuation and gradual emancipation from the pathologic symbiotic relationship with his mother and others. The quality of his interpersonal relations and his capacity for object constancy and object love experienced a solid and enduring gain. He made some headway in transforming narcissistic rage into the nonviolent employment of aggression in the pursuit of personal aims. He gave up his compulsive use of alcohol and marijuana and no longer engaged in sadomasochistically perverse sexual activities. Psychoanalysis helped him to resume his personal development in areas that had been blocked by psychic conflict and trauma.

Object Relations and Masochism

Mr. A.'s punishing relationship with his mother was unconsciously repeated in his masochistic sexual perversion, his interpersonal relations, and his attitudes toward himself. For example, he was punitive toward himself about working. His unstable work pattern varied between loafing or daydreaming and working at a furious pace. When he managed to work productively, he required either conscious or unconscious fantasies of someone forcing or punishing him to initiate and sustain his efforts.

An object-relations perspective explains the self-punishing behaviors of masochistic patients. Freud (1924) distinguished between the self-punishment of masochists and that of obsessional patients. In the latter, the subject turns hostility against the self, but without the attitude of passivity toward another person that occurs in masochism. The masochist's passivity toward another's aggression implies an object relation. In masochistic patients, the need for punishment is linked with either real or imagined relations with an other. In contrast, the self-punishing actions of obsessional and other neurotic patients stems from superego guilt over unconscious forbidden sexual or aggressive wishes.

Psychoanalytic writings often ascribe the self-punishing and self-damaging behaviors of the masochist to a turning of the patient's own sadism upon the self. Although this familiar dynamic is often correct for neurotic patients, it is not a prevalent dynamic pattern in masochistic patients. Rather, in masochistic patients the central dynamic involves the introjection of the parents' sadism. It is not the patient's sadism that is turned against the self, but rather, the sadism of the introjected love object. Berliner (1958) held that the diagnosis of masochism should not be made unless the introjection of another person's sadism is the essential pattern.

Mr. A.'s use of introjects to punish himself and force himself to work developed from his introjection of his mother's punitive attitudes toward him. His need to invoke fantasies of someone punishing him or forcing him to work did not arise from a punitive or cruel superego. The demand that he work as a punishment arose from the introject of his mother, that is, his representation of a controlling authority figure.

In "The Economic Problem of Masochism," Freud (1924) differentiated "erotogenic" and "feminine" masochism from "moral" masochism. All three types of masochism were repeatedly demonstrated by my patient in his daily life and the analytic situation. My clinical observations are in accord with those of Berliner (1958), who believes that there are no sexual masochists who are not also severe moral masochists. The masochistic perversion is a superstructure over a character malformation that the moral masochist and the masochistic pervert share.

Berliner (1940, 1942, 1947, 1958), one of the first to interject object-relations concepts in studies of masochism, linked masochistic phenomena with pathogenic parent-child relationships. He provided clinical evidence for the hypothesis that masochism, in both its sexual and moral forms, constitutes a disturbance of object relations and a pathologic form of loving (Berliner 1958). In his view, masochism means loving a person who gives back hatred and ill-treatment. This was evident in my patient's sexual perversion and interpersonal relations. A frequent transference manifestation of this dynamic was the patient's wish to earn the analyst's love through humiliating and debasing himself.

Some parents of masochistic patients have been outrageously cruel to them as children (Berliner 1958, Bieber 1980, Panken 1973). Another common genetic pattern is that the parents' ambivalence tends more toward hostility, and the child enjoins in the ill-treatment or guilt imposed under the guise of love. Mr. A.'s profound longing for love through suffering stemmed not only from his mother's cruelty to him as a child, but also from the fact that her rare expressions of concern came when he humiliated himself or made himself the object of her pity.

Menaker (1953) also used an object-relations perspective to investigate masochism. She viewed masochistic behaviors as an outcome of traumatic deprivation at the oral level and as a means of perpetuating bonds, however painful, to the mother. My clinical observations support her hypothesis that masochism may be viewed as an adaptive and defensive ego function that is used to maintain a vitally needed love relationship to a primary object.

Bernstein (1957) investigated the role of traumatic early parent-child relations in the pathogenesis of masochism. He found that the ego functions and qualities of such patients were made to serve the narcissistic needs of their parents. Their successes were not their own but their parents', and they were robbed of the gratifications that might have been derived had they been encouraged to accomplish things for themselves. Bernstein described their need to repeat original narcissistic traumas of disappointment, rejection, and humiliation. In adult life, masochistic relationships are repetitive re-enactments of traumatic childhood object relations; they give patients the illusion of actively controlling situations that they once endured passively.

Object-Relations Theory and Conflict

It is necessary to distinguish between psychic and interpersonal conflicts. Psychic conflicts are conflicts between conscious and/or unconscious motives of the subject. Interpersonal conflicts are conflicts between persons.

A hierarchical model of the mind is required for a more integrated understanding of psychic conflict (Dorpat 1976). I constructed such a pattern, following Gedo and Goldberg (1973); I placed the tripartite model at a higher developmental level than the object-relations format. Psychic conflicts were classified into object-relations conflicts and structural conflicts. The object-relations class of psychic conflict covered the pre-oedipal phase of psychic development prior to id-ego-superego differentiation. Object-relations conflicts are psychic conflicts between the subject's wishes and the ideals, injunctions, and prohibitions that are not experienced as his own, but rather, are represented in primary- or secondary-process representations of some (usually parental) authority.

There may not appear to be any difference between an object-relations and a structural conflict, because the content (e.g., wishes, prohibitions, injunctions) of the opposing parts of the conflict may seem the same in both types of conflicts. The crucial difference is that in a structural conflict, the subject experiences (or is capable of experiencing, if part of the conflict is unconscious) the opposing tendencies as aspects of himself. The subject's values, prohibitions, and injunctions conflict with the subject's sexual, aggressive, or other kinds of wishes. In the object-relations conflict, the conflict is between the subject's own strivings and wishes, on the one hand, and the subject's representations (mainly introjects) of another person's injunctions, prohibitions, and values, on the other.

The content of Mr. A.'s guilt was similar to what Modell (1965) described as "separation guilt." Separation guilt, unlike superego guilt, is not experienced as stemming from real or imagined transgressions against one's moral values. The patient did not consider the thoughts, feelings, or overt acts that evoked separation guilt as morally wrong in themselves. Rather, he felt guilty because he believed that his strivings toward self-gratification and individuation would displease his mother. The power of the prohibition against autonomous functioning was subjectively linked with his memories and fantasies of a disapproving mother who rejected his movements toward independence.

Separation and guilt feelings did not arise from structural conflicts (i.e., from real or imagined transgressions against an internalized and impersonal authority). He evoked guilt by feelings, thoughts, and overt actions which he considered displeasing to the introjected representation of his mother. Culpability and wrong-doing were implicitly defined as behaviors opposed to what his mother wanted of him. Guilt and anxiety over psychological separateness from his mother arose from unresolved unconscious object-relations conflicts and fixations at the separation-individuation phase of development. His gradual appropriation of other ego and superego functions in analysis (e.g., establishing ideals and goals, and regulating his self-esteem), were sometimes sources of object-relations conflicts. The most frequent overt indications of such unconscious conflicts were various manifestations of anxiety and guilt over behaving and regulating himself in an autonomous manner.

Transference and Self-Object Relations

Most clinicians view transference as a universal aspect of object relations (Loewald 1960). All human relationships contain an admixture of transference and realistic reactions (Fenichel 1938, p. 72). The analytic situation does not create transference by itself, but provides conditions for transference to emerge into consciousness in order to be understood and worked through.

The major transference reactions that developed in Mr. A.'s analysis were self-object ones. Self-objects are objects experienced as part of the self. Patients who develop predominantly self-object transferences have not fully differentiated their object-representations from their self-representations and, like young children, frequently experience and treat the analyst as an extension of themselves. Self-object relations and transferences should be distinguished from the more highly developed whole-object relations and transferences that are found in psychoneurotic and normal individuals. Whole objects are loved (or at least represented and recognized) for their own qualities, independent of the subject's needs. Wholeness also implies that the subject can sustain both positive and negative feelings for the same object. In contrast, more disturbed patients tend to divide their object-representations into good and bad, weak and strong.

An abiding characteristic of self-object transferences is the subject's need to control the self-object, who is perceived and treated as an extension of the subject's self. This type of omnipotent control is similar to the control 2-year-old children often attempt to exercise over their parents. Patients experience the self-object much as they experience control over their own limbs. Actual or threatened loss of the self-object incurs a sense of helplessness and rage similar to that incurred by loss of a body part or function. The threat of object loss or loss of control over the object triggers a reaction similar in quality, if not always in intensity, to the "catastrophic reaction" described by Goldstein (1939) as a typical emotional reaction of brain-damaged persons. The overwhelming anxiety experienced by brain-damaged persons is connected with their sense of losing a part of themselves, and their helplessness to prevent or defend against the terror evoked by the loss.

Many therapists tend to react adversely to such patients' need for control, and may mistakenly attribute hostile motives to the patient. The need of patients with pre-oedipal fixations to control their self-objects is not always or necessarily fused with hostile or destructive wishes. Viewed from a developmental perspective, their need to control the self-object may be a normal, expected aspect of development. For patients who have not developed more differentiated means of self-regulation, control over the therapist serves the dual purpose of avoiding external traumatic stimulation and maintaining a semblance of internal emotional equilibrium.

Patients with pre-oedipal disorders initially cannot understand or appreciate the psychoanalyst's neutrality and psychological separateness. They tend to perceive the analyst's communications as directives, rather than interpretations. These distortions stem from their unconscious need to project either their ego and superego functions, or the power to co-opt and regulate their own psychic functions onto the analyst. Patients with pre-oedipal disorders commonly project not only sexual and aggressive contents onto the analyst, but also one or more of their psychic functions. Classical literature on transferences involving projection emphasizes the projection of superego elements, but makes little mention of the projection of ego functions, onto the analyst (see Giovacchini 1967, 1975).

Patients with pre-oedipal disorders tend to project their unstable and poorly differentiated ego functions, such as reality testing, decision making, and judgment, onto the analyst far more than do patients with neuroses or neurotic character disorders. One of the most common technical mistakes in the analysis of such patients is the analyst's bending under transference pressures and acting out the role of the idealized parent by providing directives and advice. It is of primary importance that the analyst maintain an attitude and technique of neutrality in such situations (Dorpat 1977).

SUMMARY

An object-relations perspective provides a method for illuminating crucial processes in the pathogenesis and treatment of masochistic patients. In this chapter, I have examined clinical and theoretical differences between structural conflicts and object-relations conflicts. Object-relations conflicts refer to psychic conflicts between the subject's wishes and the ideals, prohibitions, and injunctions contained in introjects of some (usually parental) authority.

In the case example presented here, two critical childhood traumas, the death of the patient's father and a pathological symbiotic relationship with his mother, decisively contributed to the patient's masochism and his developmental fixation at the separation-individuation phase of development. As a child, the patient was compelled to serve as his mother's personal slave. This master-slave relationship was unconsciously replicated in sadomasochistically perverse sexual practices with prostitutes, and then in the transference situation with the analyst.

The patient suffered from intense object-relations conflicts and guilt over functioning independently of his mother. His masochistic perverse behavior was associated with a self-object relation with his sexual partners, who were perceived and treated solely as the embodied projection of his wishes. With the development of a more stable capacity for sustaining whole-object relations, the perverse sexual behavior disappeared.

REFERENCES

Altschul, S. (1968). Denial and ego arrest. *J. Amer. Psychoanal. Assn.* 16: 301–318.

Anderson, C. (1949). Aspects of pathological grief and mourning. *Internat. J. Psycho-Anal.* 30: 48–55.

Berliner, B. (1940). Libido and reality in masochism. *Psychoanal. Q.* 9: 322–333.

———. (1942). The concept of masochism. *Psychoanal. Rev.* 29: 386–400.

———. (1947). On some psychodynamics of masochism. *Psychoanal. Q.* 16: 459–471.

———. (1958). The role of object relations in moral masochism. *Psychoanal. Q.* 27: 38–56.

Bernstein, I. (1957). The role of narcissim in moral masochism. *Psychoanal. Q.* 26.

Bieber, I. (1980). *Cognitive Psychoanalysis.* New York: Aronson.

Boyer, L. B. (1956). On maternal overstimulation and ego defects. *The Psychoanalytic Study of the Child* 11: 236–256.

———. (1967). Office treatment of schizophrenic patients: The use of psychoanalytic therapy with few parameters. In *Psychoanalytic Treatment of Schizophrenic and Characterologic Disorders,* ed. L. B. Boyer and P. L. Giovacchini, pp. 143–188. New York: Science House.

Brodey, W. M. (1965). On the dynamics of narcissism. I. Externalization. *The Psychoanalytic Study of the Child* 20: 165–193.

Dorpat, T. L. (1972). Psychological effects of parental suicide on surviving children. In *Survivors of Suicide,* ed. A. C. Cain, pp. 121–142. Springfield, Ill.: Charles C. Thomas.

———. (1976). Structural conflict and object-relations conflict. *J. Amer. Psychoanal. Assn.* 24: 855–874.

———. (1977). On neutrality. *Internat. J. Psychoanal. Psychother.* 6: 39–64.

———. (1978). Introjection and the idealizing transference. *Internat. J. Psychoanal. Psychother.* 7: 23–54.

Fenichel, O. (1938). *Problems of Psychoanalytic Technique.* Albany, N.Y.: The Psychoanalytic Quarterly, 1939.

Freud, S. (1915). Instincts and their vicissitudes. *Standard Edition* 14: 111–140. London: Hogarth Press, 1955.

———. (1920). Beyond the pleasure principle. *Standard Edition* 18: 7–64. London: Hogarth Press, 1955.

———. (1924). The economic problems of masochism. *Standard Edition* 19: 157–171. London: Hogarth Press, 1955.

Gedo, J. E. and Goldberg, A. (1973). *Models of the Mind*. Chicago and London: University of Chicago Press.

Giovacchini, P. L. (1967). Frustration and externalization. *Psychoanal. Q*. 36: 571–583.

———. (1972). Summing up. In *Tactics and Techniques of Psychoanalytic Therapy*, vol. 1, ed. P. L. Giovacchini, pp. 697–727. New York: Science House.

———. (1975). Various aspects of the psychoanalytic process. In *Tactics and Techniques in Psychoanalytic Therapy*, vol. 2, eds. P. L. Giovacchini et al., pp. 5–95. New York: Aronson.

———. (1980). Epilogue. In *Psychoanalytic Treatment of Schizophrenic, Borderline and Characterological Disorders*, 2d ed., eds. L. B. Boyer and P. L. Giovacchini. New York: Aronson.

Goffman, E. (1974). *Frame Analysis*. Cambridge, Mass.: Harvard University Press.

Goldstein, K. (1939). *The Organism: A Holistic Approach to Biology Derived from Pathological Data on Man*. New York: American Books.

Klein, G. S. (1976). *Psychoanalytic Theory*. New York: International Universities Press.

Krupp, G. (1965). Identification as a defense against anxiety in coping with loss. *Internat. J. Psycho-Anal*. 46: 303–314.

Loewald, H. W. (1960). The therapeutic action of psycho-analysis. *Internat. J. Psycho-Anal*. 41: 16–33.

Menaker, E. (1953). Masochism, a defense reaction. *Psychoanal. Q*. 22: 205–220.

Modell, A. H. (1965). On having the right to a life: An aspect of the superego's development. *Internat. J. Psycho-Anal*. 46: 323–331.

Ornstein, A. and Ornstein, P. H. (1975). On the interpretive process in schizophrenia. *Internat. J. Psychoanal. Psychother*. 4: 219–271.

Panken, S. (1973). *The Joy of Suffering*. New York: Aronson.

Rosenfeld, H. (1966). Discussion of "Office Treatment of Schizophrenia" by L. Bryce Boyer. *Psychoanal. Forum* 1: 351–353.

Spruiell, V. (1980). Classical psychoanalysis and frame theory. Paper presented at the Seattle Psychoanalytic Society, May.

Volkan, V. D. (1976). *Primitive Internalized Object Relations*. New York: International Universities Press. Cited in Donald B. Rinsley, Object relations theory and psychotherapy with particular reference to the self-disordered patient, in *Technical Factors in the Treatment of the Severely Disturbed Patient*, ed. Peter L. Giovacchini and L. Bryce Boyer. New York: Aronson, 1982.

Wolfenstein, M. (1966). How is mourning possible? *The Psychoanalytic Study of the Child* 21: 93–123.

———. (1969). Loss, rage and repetition. *The Psychoanalytic Study of the Child* 24: 432–460.

15. The Narcissistic-Masochistic Character

Arnold M. Cooper

There is an old Chinese curse: "May you live in interesting times." These are analytically interesting times, in which, more than ever before in the history of psychoanalysis, accepted paradigms are being called into question, and a congeries of new and old ideas compete for attention and allegiance. In the history of intellectual thought, such periods of enthusiastic creative ferment have led to the development of new ideas. The great advances in the sciences occur when new techniques lead to new experiments, or when new data contradict old theories, or when new ideas lead to new theories. Since the early 1970s, much of the interesting creative tension in psychoanalysis has focused on the crucial role of preoedipal experiences and the centrality of issues of self or narcissism in character development. In this paper, I propose that masochistic defenses are ubiquitous in preoedipal narcissistic development and that a deeper understanding of the development of masochism may help to clarify a number of clinical problems. I suggest that a full appreciation of the roles of narcissism and masochism in development and in pathology will require that we relinquish whatever remains of what Freud referred to as the "shibboleth" of the centrality of the Oedipus complex in neurosogenesis. I further suggest that masochism and narcissism are so entwined both in development and in clinical presentation that we clarify our clinical work by considering that there is a narcissistic-masochistic character and that neither appears alone.

INTRODUCTION

The problem of reformulating our ideas was foreshadowed as long ago as 1931, almost half a century ago, when Freud (1931), in speaking of the intensity and durations of the little girl's attachment to her mother, said in his paper on "Female Sexuality," "The pre-Oedipus phase in women gains an

Reprinted from Robert A. Glick and Donald I. Meyers, eds., *Masochism: Current Psychoanalytic Perspectives* (Hillsdale, N.J.: Analytic Press, 1988), 117–38 by permission. Copyright© 1988 by the Analytic Press.

importance which we have not attributed to it hitherto. Since this phase allows room for all the fixations and repressions from which we must trace the origin of the neuroses, it would seem as though we must retract the universality of the thesis that the Oedipus complex is the nucleus of neurosis. But if anyone feels reluctant about making this correction, there is no need for him to do so.'' Freud then went on to reveal some of his own difficulties in accepting his new findings by stating that those who are reluctant to make this clearly necessary revision need not do so, if they are willing to accept a redefinition of the Oedipus complex to include earlier events. He said: ''Our insights into this early pre-Oedipus phase in girls comes to us as a surprise like the discovery, in another field, of the Minoan-Mycenean civilization behind the civilization of Greece. Everything in the sphere of the first attachment to the mother seems to be so difficult to grasp in analysis—so gray with age and shadowy, and almost impossible to revivify, that it was as if it has succumbed to an especially inexorable repression.'' Perhaps this is an indication of Freud's and our own difficulty in accepting the breadth of theoretical revision that our data may require. In fact, in his posthumous work, ''The Outline of Psychoanalysis'' (1938), he again stated without reservation that the Oedipus complex is the nucleus of neurosis.

It is questionable whether it was ever the case that most analytic patients presented with primary oedipal pathology. Edward Glover, in his ''Technique of Psychoanalysis'' published in 1955, was already lamenting the scarcity of cases of classical transference neurosis. He referred to ''those mild and mostly favorable cases which incidentally appear all too infrequently in the average analyst's case list'' (p. 205). I suspect that few of us have ever seen many cases of ''classical transference neurosis,'' and yet it has been difficult for us to give up the accompanying clinical idea—so dear to Freud—that the nucleus of neurosis is the Oedipus complex. I in no way depreciate the immensity of the discovery of the Oedipus complex and its vital role in human affairs. But we need not share Freud's reluctance to place the Oedipus complex in perspective as one of a number of crucial developmental epochs—and not necessarily the one most significant for our understanding of narcissistic and masochistic pathology and perhaps not even for understanding neurosis generally.

Heinz Kohut's (1971) development of self psychology represented the most radical attempt to date to address and resolve the various dissonant elements in psychoanalytic developmental research, clinical experience, and general theory. As I have written elsewhere (1983), I believe it is this exposure of some of the major unresolved problems of psychoanalytic work that accounts for much of the passion—positive and negative—that was generated by self psychology. For more than a decade, psychoanalysis has been productively preoccupied with developing a new understanding of narcissism in the light of our newer emphasis on preoedipal events. The scientific and clinical yield of this investigation has been high, and it should prompt us to apply these methods to other of our metapsychological and clinical formulations that are a bit fuzzy. Prominent among these are the concepts of masochism and the masochistic character.

Our major ideas concerning masochism date to an earlier period of psychoanalytic thinking, when the focus was on the Oedipus complex. The cultural climate of psychoanalysis was different then. A reexamination of masochism at this time, using our newer ideas of separation-individuation, self-esteem regulation, the nature of early object relations, etc., might help clarify our understanding of masochistic phenomena. That is the intent of this paper, which has been divided into five parts:

1. An introduction, now completed.
2. A brief review of some of the theories of masochism.
3. A brief statement of the nature of some of the problems and contradictions in our thinking about masochism.
4. An attempt to clarify the theory of masochism by linking it genetically and clinically with our newer knowledge of narcissistic development.
5. A presentation of two clinical vignettes, to demonstrate my thesis that masochistic and narcissistic phenomena are always entwined with each other and that we achieve a conceptual clarification and a clinical advantage by considering that we are always dealing with a narcissistic-masochistic character.

REVIEW OF THEORIES AND DEFINITIONS

The literature is vast, and I will mention only a few salient points. The term *masochism* was coined by Krafft-Ebing in 1895, with reference to Leopold van Sacher-Masoch's novel *Venus in Furs*. The novel described and Krafft-Ebing subsequently referred to a situation of seeking physical and mental torture at the hands of another person through willing submission to experiences of enslavement, passivity, and humiliation. Freud (1920) used Krafft-Ebing's terminology, although in his early writings on masochism he was concerned with perversion masochism with clear sexual pleasure attached to pain. Only later was Freud concerned with the problems of moral masochism, in which humiliation and suffering are sought as part of the character formation and without evident sexual satisfactions. Freud postulated at various times a variety of explanations for these puzzling phenomena:

1. He postulated that it was the nature of physiology that an excess of stimulation in the nervous system automatically led to experiences of both pain and pleasure.
2. He postulated that it was a vicissitude of instinct, Sadism, or aggression—a primary instinct—tended to turn against the self as masochism, a secondary instinctual phenomenon.
3. Masochism was defined as "beyond the pleasure principle"—that is, a primary instinct, a component of the death instinct, a consequence of the repetition compulsion, and thus an independent automatically operating regulatory principle. Masochism as a primary instinct was, in the course of development, directed outward; as a tertiary phenomenon, it was redirected inward, as clinical masochism.
4. He conceived moral masochism as the need for punishment, consequent upon the excessive harshness of the superego. Individuals feeling guilty basically for sexual —generally oedipal—forbidden wishes sought punishment as a means of expiation.
5. He described masochistic suffering as a condition for pleasure not as a source of pleasure—that is, masochists do not enjoy the suffering per se; rather, they willingly endure the pain as an unavoidable guilty ransom for access to forbidden or undeserved pleasures.
6. Masochism seemed related to feminine characteristics and passivity.

I think it is fair to say that Freud struggled throughout his lifetime for a satisfactory explanation of the paradox of pleasure-in-unpleasure. In "Analysis Terminable and Interminable" (1937), he said, "No stronger impression arises from resistances during the work of analysis than of there being a force which is defending itself by every possible means against recovery and which is absolutely resolved to hold on to illness and suffering. One portion of this force has been recognized by us, undoubtedly with justice, as a sense of guilt and need for punishment, and has been localized by us in the ego's relation to the superego. But this is only the portion of it which is, as it were, psychically bound by the superego and thus becomes recognizable; other quotas of the same force, whether bound or free, may be at work in other, unspecified places. If we take into consideration the total picture made up by the phenomena of masochism immanent in so many people, the negative therapeutic reaction and sense of guilt found in so many neurotics, we shall no longer be able to adhere to the belief that mental events are exclusively governed by the desire for pleasure. These phenomena are unmistakable indications of the presence of a power in mental life which we call the instinct of aggression or of destruction according to its aims, and which we trace back to the original death instinct of living matter. It is not a question of an antithesis between an optimistic and pessimistic theory of life. Only by the concurrent or mutually opposing action of the two primal instincts—Eros and the death-instinct—never by one or the other alone, can we explain the rich multiplicity of the phenomena of life'' (p. 242). The death instinct, as we all know, is an idea that never caught on.

The vast subsequent literature on masochism was well summarized by Brenner (1959), and, since I presented a slightly modified version of this paper in 1973, there have been summaries by Stolorow (1975) and by Maleson (1984), as well as a report on a panel of the American Psychoanalytic Association, in which I participated, that appeared in 1981. I will not repeat these summaries, which succinctly convey the large array of functions and etiologies ascribed to masochism. Stolorow's paper deserves special note because he also concerned himself with the narcissistic functions of masochism, pointing out that sadomasochistic development can aid in maintaining a satisfactory self-image. For the remainder of this paper, I intend to confine my discussion to so-called "moral" masochism or, as some have referred to it, "psychic" masochism. I will not be discussing perversion masochism per se, which I believe to be a developmentally separate phenomenon. (See Maleson, 1984, p. 350, for a brief discussion of this issue.)

While many definitions of masochism have been attempted, Brenner's 1959 definition has tended to remain authoritative. He defined masochism as "the seeking of unpleasure, by which is meant physical or mental pain, discomfort or wretchedness, for the sake of *sexual* pleasure, with the qualification that either the seeking or the pleasure or both may often be unconscious rather than conscious" (p. 197). Brenner emphasized that masochism represented an acceptance of a painful penalty for forbidden sexual pleasures associated with the Oedipus complex. He agreed that masochistic phenomena are ubiquitous in normality and pathology and serve multiple psychic functions, including such aims as seduction of the aggressor and maintenance of object-control. Brenner agreed that the genesis of the masochistic character seemed related to excessively frustrating or rejecting parents.

A somewhat different, highly organized, view of masochism was put forth in the voluminous writings of the late Edmund Bergler. Because his theories are relevant to topics that are currently of great interest, because they have influenced my own thinking, and because they are so little referred to in the literature—having been premature in their emphasis on the preoedipal period and narcissism—I will present a brief summary of his work. As long ago as 1949, Bergler had stated in his book *The Basic Neurosis* that masochism was a fundamental aspect of all neurotic behavior, and he linked masochistic phenomena with issues of narcissistic development, or development of self-esteem systems. Bergler described in detail a proposed genetic schema out of which psychic masochism develops as an unavoidable aspect of human development. I will mention only a few elements that are particularly germane to my thesis.

1. Bergler assumed that the preservation of infantile megalomania or infantile omnipotence (today, we would say narcissism) is of prime importance for the reduction of anxiety and as a source of satisfaction—on a par with the maintenance of libidinal satisfactions. This formulation is not dissimilar to Kohut's many years later.

2. Every infant is, by its *own* standards, excessively frustrated, disappointed, refused. These disappointments always have the effect of a narcissistic humiliation because they are an offense to the infant's omnipotent fantasy.

3. The infant responds with fury to this offense to his omnipotent self, but in his helplessness to vent fury on an outer object, the fury is deflected against the self (what Rado [1969] termed retroflexed rage) and eventually contributes to the harshness of the superego.

4. Faced with unavoidable frustration, the danger of aggression against parents who are also needed and loved, and the pain of self-directed aggression, the infant, nonetheless, attempts to maintain essential feelings of omnipotence and self-esteem. In Bergler's terms, the infant "libidinizes" or "sugarcoats" his disappointments. He learns to extract pleasure from displeasure for the sake of the illusion of continuing, total, omnipotent control —both of himself and of the differentiating object. "No one frustrated me against my wishes; I frustrated myself because I like it." It was Bergler's belief that some inborn tendency made it easy and inevitable that a pleasure-in-displeasure pattern would develop. He insisted that this develops at the very earliest stages of object-differentiation and perhaps, I would add, becomes consolidated during the disappointing realization of helplessness that occurs during the rapprochement phase of the separation-individuation process.

According to Bergler, these hypothesized early events of psychic development resulted in the "clinical picture" of psychic masochism, which was characterized by the "oral triad." The oral triad, a phrase Bergler used many years before Bertram Lewin (1950) used the term for a different purpose, consisted of a three-step behavioral sequence that was paradigmatic for masochistic behavior.

Step 1. Through his own behavior or through the misuse of an available external situation, the masochist unconsciously provokes disappointment, refusal, and humiliation. He identifies the outer world with a disappointing, refusing, preoedipal mother. Unconsciously, the rejection provides satisfaction.

Step 2. Consciously, the masochist has repressed his knowledge of his own provocation and reacts in righteous indignation and *seeming* self-defense to the rejection that he consciously perceives as externally delivered. Thus, he responds with "pseudo-aggression," i.e., defensive regression designed to disclaim his responsibility for, and unconscious pleasure in, the defeat he has experienced. Step 2 represents an attempt to appease inner guilt for forbidden unconscious masochistic pleasure.

Step 3. After the subsidence of pseudo-aggression, which, because often ill-dosed or ill-timed, may provoke additional unconsciously wished for defeats, the masochist indulges in conscious self-pity or feelings of "this only happens to me." Unconsciously, he enjoys the masochistic rebuff.

This clinical oral triad—or, as Bergler calls it, the mechanism or "injustice collecting"—is an excellent description of a repetitive sequence of events, observable in almost all neurotic behavior. The term "injustice collector" was coined by Bergler and was later used by Louis Auchincloss (1950) as the title of a collection of stories. In Bergler's view, all human beings have more or less masochistic propensities. The issue of pathology is one of quantity.

THEORETICAL ISSUES

Today there is little disagreement that we can explain masochism in terms of its defensive and adaptive functions, without recourse to the theory of sexual drives. The extraordinary ease with which pleasure-in-displeasure phenomena develop, and their stickiness, suggests a psychic apparatus that is well prepared for the use of such defensive structures; but there is no theoretical need to call upon a primary instinctive masochism.

What is the nature of the pleasure in masochism? The generally accepted formulation that the pleasure is the same as any other pleasure and that the pain is the necessary guilty price has the great merit of preserving the

pleasure principle intact. There has always been a group of analysts, however
—including Rudolf Loewenstein (1957) and Edmund Bergler—who insisted, to quote Loewenstein, that "in the masochistic behavior we observe
an unconscious libidinization of suffering caused by aggression from without
and within" (p. 230). The operating principle would seem to be "if you
can't lick 'em, join 'em." More simply, one may speculate that the infant
claims as his own and endows with as much pleasure as possible whatever is
familiar, whether painful experiences or unempathic mothers. The defensive
capacity to alter the meaning of painful experience so that it is experienced
as ego-syntonic has also been described in certain circumstances in infancy
by Greenacre (1960) and Jacobson (1964). Greenacre reports that as early as
the second half of the first year babies under conditions of extreme distress
will have genital orgastic-like responses and that these early events may
result in ego distortions creating sexual excitation arising from self-directed
aggression. This is similar to Freud's original formulation, and I think we
must leave open the possibility that there is a dialectic here of excessive
quantity changing quality.

From a different point of view, we may ask what are the gratifying and
constructive aspects of pain? We have no difficulty in agreeing with every
mother's observation that painful frustration, disappointment, and injury are
inevitable concomitants of infancy. It is rare that any infant goes through a
twenty-four-hour period without exhibiting what we adults interpret at least
to be screams of discomfort, frustration, and need. The most loving and
competent mother cannot spare the infant these experiences, and there is
good reason to believe that no infant should be spared these experiences in
proper dosage. It seems likely that painful bodily—particularly skin—experiences are important proprioceptive mechanisms that serve not only to avoid
damage but also, developmentally, to provide important components of the
forming body-image and self-image. There are many cases in the literature,
summarized by Stolorow (1975), of persons who experience a relief from
identity diffusion by inflicting pain upon their skin.

A typical pattern for borderline self-mutilators is to cut or otherwise injure
themselves in privacy, experiencing little pain in the process and later exhibiting the injury to the usually surprised caretaking person—be it parent or
physician—with evident satisfaction in the demonstration that they are sick
and suffering and beyond the control of the caretaking person. A prominent
motivation for this behavior is the need to demonstrate autonomy via the
capacity for self-mutilation.

I would suggest that head-banging in infants—a far more common phenomenon than is usually acknowledged and one that is compatible with normal development—is one of the normal, painful ways of achieving necessary and gratifying self-definition. Skin sensations of all kinds, and perhaps moderately painful sensations particularly, are a regular mode of establishing self-boundaries.

Imre Hermann (1976) in his fascinating 1935 paper, published in English as "Clinging-Going-in-Search," stated:

In order to understand masochistic pleasure, one has to recognize that it is quite closely interwoven with the castration complex but behind this link is the reaction-formation to the urge to cling—namely the drive to separate oneself. At this point, we have to go far back to early development. Our guess is that the emergence of the process of separation of the mother and child dual unit constitutes a pre-stage of narcissism and painful masochism; normal separation goes along with "healthy" narcissism. (P. 30)

Hermann then goes on to describe that pain is a necessary concomitant of separation but is a lesser evil than the damage and decay of the self that would result from failure of separation in infancy. He refers to a healing tendency within the psyche and the erotization of pain, which facilitates healing of a damaged psychic area. Hermann views all later self-mutilations, such as self-biting, tearing one's cuticles, pulling hair, tearing scabs, etc., as attempts to reinforce a sense of freedom from the need to cling. "pain arises in connection with the *separation that is striven for,* while its *successful accomplishment* brings pleasure" (p. 30). Hermann views masochistic character traits as a consequence of failure of successful separation with reactive repetition of separation traumas.

Therefore, it is suggested that pain serves the organism's task of self-definition and separation-individuation and is therefore part of a gratifying accomplishment. Mastery—not avoidance—of pain is a major achievement in a course of self-development; mastery may imply the capacity to derive satisfaction and accomplishment from self-induced, self-dosed pain. The tendency for such an achievement to miscarry is self-evident. The pleasurable fatigue of a day's work, the ecstasy of an athlete's exhaustion, the dogged pursuit of distant goals, the willingness to cling to a seemingly absurd ideal —all of these represent constructive uses of pleasure in pain and a source of creative energies.

It is interesting that cultures of all times have set for their members painful tasks—some form of heroism, accomplishment, endurance, or martyrdom. The achievement alone is not valued unless it was fired in pain. No culture chooses to live without inflicting pain on itself; even cultures seemingly devoted to nirvana-type ideals have painful rituals. Rites of passage and experiences of mortification are a means of assuring essential aspects of cultural and individual identity, and their effectiveness may be proportional to their painfulness and sharpness of definition. A circumcision ceremony at puberty is obviously a clearer marker of a stage in self-development and onset of manhood than is a Bar Mitzvah ceremony.

The question of aggression in the induction of masochism is interesting and, I think, not satisfactorily answerable at this time. Regularly in the course of development, aggression is distributed in at least five directions: 1) in legitimate self-assertion; 2) in projection; 3) turned against the self; 4) toward the formation of the superego; and 5) used defensively as "pseudo-aggression." The proportions vary, but in the narcissistic-masochistic character, legitimate self-assertion is in short supply. I will not discuss here the many issues of the relationship of sadism to masochism, of the double identifications with both aggressor and victim, etc. It seems clear that experiences of frustration and the absence of loving care, whether in infant children or infant monkeys, induce self-directed aggression and mutilation. The usual explanations involve ideas of retroflexed rage or failure of instinct fusion. These concepts are convenient but not entirely adequate. I have no better answer, but I would like to mention a rare and extraordinary syndrome called the Lesch-Nyhan syndrome. Due to a specific biochemical genetic defect, children who suffer from this syndrome often show developmental retardation, occasionally spastic cerebral palsy, choreoathetosis, and bizarre self-mutilative behavior, including self-biting, self-hitting, head-banging, and eye-gouging. Dizmang and Cheatham (1970) have suggested a psychobiological basis for masochistic behavior in the postulate of a low threshold for activation of a mechanism that ordinarily controls tendencies toward repetitive compulsive behaviors and self-inflicted aggression.

At what stage of development do the decisive events leading to masochistic character disorder occur? It is clear from what I have been describing that I believe it is now evident that the masochistic conflicts of the Oedipus complex are reworkings of much earlier established masochistic functions. These defenses, by means of the mechanism of secondary autonomy (Hartmann), function as if they were wishes in the later character development.

CLARIFICATION

If even part of what I have been suggesting is correct then masochistic tendencies are a necessary and ubiquitous aspect of narcissistic development. There is convincing evidence that Freud was right—the pleasure principle, as a derivative of libido, is an inadequate explanatory device. If we add an instinct or tendency toward aggression, we still lack heuristic power. Our knowledge of early development and our knowledge derived from the studies of borderline and psychotic disorders make it abundantly clear that a newer theoretical perspective requires that issues of self-development and object relations be accorded their proper weight as crucial factors in early psychological development. Libidinal pleasures and aggressive satisfactions will be sacrificed or distorted if necessary to help prevent the shattering disorganizing anxieties that arise when the self-system is disturbed or the ties to the object disrupted. Whether one refers to Kohut's (1972) narcissistic libido, or Erikson's (1963) basic trust, or Sullivan's (1953) sense of security, or Rado's (1969) basic pride and dependency needs, or Sandler and Joffee's (1969) feelings of safety, or Bergler's (1949) omnipotent fantasy, or Winnicott's (1971) true self—all are ways of addressing the crucial issues of the organism's primary needs for self-definition out of an original symbiotic bond. In fact, Freud, with his unfortunately termed "death instinct," was making the same point. The organism will give up libidinal pleasure for the safety, satisfaction, or pleasure of maintaining a coherent self.

These are the relevant issues:

1. Pain is a necessary and unavoidable concomitant of separation-individuation and the achievement of selfhood. Perhaps *Doleo ergo sum* (I suffer, therefore I am) is one of the precursors of *Sentio ergo sum* (I feel, therefore I am).

2. The frustrations and discomforts of separation-individuation, necessary events in turning us toward the world, are perceived as narcissistic injuries—i.e., they damage the sense of magical omnipotent control and threaten intolerable passivity and helplessness in the face of a perceived external danger. This is the prototype of narcissistic humiliation.

3. Defensively, the infant attempts to restore threatened self-esteem by distorting the nature of his experience. Rather than accept the fact of helplessness, the infant reasserts control by making suffering ego-syntonic. "I am frustrated because I want to be. I force my mother to be cruel." Freud

(1937), of course, often discussed the general human intolerance of passivity and the tendency to assert mastery by converting passively endured experiences into actively sought ones. The mastery of pain is part of normal development, and this always implies a capacity to derive satisfaction from pain.

4. Alternately, one may consider that the infant, out of the need to maintain some vestiges of self-esteem in situations of more than ordinary pain, displeasure, failure of reward, and diminished self-esteem, will still attempt to salvage pleasure by equating the familiar with the pleasurable. Survival in infancy undoubtedly depends on retaining some capacity for receiving pleasurable impressions from the self and object. We may theorize that the infant makes the best adaptation he can—familiar pains may be the best available pleasure.

5. What I am terming narcissistic-masochistic tendencies are compatible with normal development and with loving, although never unambivalent, ties to objects.

6. Where the experience of early narcissistic humiliation is excessive, for external or internal reasons, these mechanisms of repair miscarry. The object is perceived as excessively cruel and refusing, the self is perceived as incapable of genuine self-assertion in the pursuit of gratification, and the gratifications obtained from disappointment take precedence over genuine but unavailable and unfamiliar libidinal, assertive, or ego-functional satisfactions. Being disappointed, or refused, becomes the *preferred* mode of narcissistic assertion to the extent that narcissistic and masochistic distortions dominate the character. Goethe, quoted by Hartmann and Loewenstein (1962), said, "He who despises himself, nevertheless esteems himself thereby as despisor" (p. 59). One can always omnipotently guarantee rejection—love is much chancier. If one can securely enjoy disappointment, it is no longer possible to be disappointed. To the extent that masochistic-narcissistic defenses are used, the aim is not a fantasied reunion with a loving and caring mother; rather, it is fantasied control over a cruel and damaging mother. Original sources of gratification have been degraded, and gratification is secondarily derived from the special sense of suffering.

7. It seems clear that the pleasure sought is not genital—that is, sexual—in origin. Rather, the desired pleasure is preoedipal and is the satisfaction and pride of a more satisfying self-representation—a pleasure in an ego-function, the regulation of self-esteem. Psychic masochism is not a derivative of perversion masochism, although the two are often related. Exhibitionistic

drives, pleasures of self-pity, and many other gratifications play a secondary role.

(8.) Inevitably, when masochistic-narcissistic pathology predominates, superego distortions also occur. The excessive harshness of the superego is, in my view, a feature of all narcissistic and masochistic pathology and often dominates the clinical picture.

9. In any particular case, the presenting clinical picture may seem more narcissistic or more masochistic. The surface may be full of charm, preening, dazzling accomplishment, or ambition. Or the surface may present obvious depression, invitations to humiliation, and feelings of failure. However, only a short period of analysis will reveal that in both instances the patients share the same sense of a deadened capacity to feel, muted pleasure, a hypersensitive self-esteem that alternates between grandiosity and humiliation, and inability to sustain or derive satisfaction from their relationships or their work, a constant sense of envy, an unshakable conviction of being wronged and deprived by those who are supposed to care for them, and an infinite capacity for provocation.

In his brilliant essay "The Fate of Pleasure" (which was based on Freud's "Beyond the Pleasure Principle"), Lionel Trilling (1963) spoke of the change in cultural attitudes from the time of Wordsworth, who wrote of "the grand elementary principle of pleasure" that he said constituted "the named and native dignity of man" and was "the principle by which man knows and feels, and lives, and moves." Trilling refers to a

change in quantity. It has always been true of some men that to pleasure they have preferred unpleasure. They imposed upon themselves difficult and painful tasks, they committed themselves to strange "unnatural" modes of life, they sought after stressing emotions, in order to know psychic energies which are not to be summoned up in felicity. These psychic energies, even when they are experienced in self-destruction, are a means of self-definition and self-affirmation. As such, they have a social reference—the election of unpleasure, however isolated and private the act may be, must refer to society if only because the choice denies the valuation which society in general puts upon pleasure; of course it often receives social approbation of the highest degree, even if at a remove of time: it is the choice of the hero, the saint and martyr, and, in some cultures, the artist. The quantitative change which we have to take account of is: what was once a mode of experience of a few has now become an ideal of experience of many. For reasons which, at least here, must defy speculation, the ideal of pleasure has exhausted itself, almost as if it had been actually realized and had issued in satiety and ennui. In its place or, at least, beside it, there is developing—conceivably at the behest of literature!—an ideal of the experience of those psychic energies which are linked with unpleasure and which are directed towards self-definition and self-affirmation. (P. 85)

For Trilling, the model of this character type is Dostoevsky's "Underground Man"—the provocateur without peer. One could add Melville's Bartleby as the other pole of the masochistic-narcissistic character who dominates through his seeming passivity. Trilling has, with his usual extraordinary perspicacity, described at the level of culture the same shift that we have experienced in psychoanalysis at the level of clinical practice. The new character type Trilling describes is the same one with whom psychoanalysts have been struggling for years—the so-called narcissistic character. Trilling clearly perceives that this character type struggles to achieve self-definition through the experience of unpleasure. When this occurs within socially acceptable limits, we have "normal" masochistic-narcissistic character development. The masochistic-narcissistic character as a pathological type, of varying severity, is marked by the preferential pursuit of suffering rejection with little positive achievement. Every quantitative gradation occurs between normal and severely pathological or borderline. The mildly neurotic "plays" with self-torture, while the borderline or psychotic may cause irreparable self-damage.

CLINICAL EXAMPLES

I will now illustrate this thesis with a clinical vignette and a condensed account of an analysis. In this brief presentation, I will not elaborate on many of the significant elements but will focus instead on only a few relevant to my viewpoint.

Clinical Vignette #1

Miss A., a twenty-six-year-old student, entered treatment with complaints of chronic anxiety and depression, feelings of social isolation, and a series of unfortunate relationships with men. She was the younger by three years of two sisters, who were the children of an aloof, taciturn, successful businessman father and a mother who was widely admired for her beauty and who devoted herself almost full time to the preservation of her beauty. Miss A. recalled as a child having severe temper tantrums that would intimidate the family, but in between tantrums she was an obedient child and an excellent student. Although she always felt cold and distant in her relationships, she recalls that almost up to puberty she continued to make a huge fuss whenever the parents were going out for an evening. She couldn't bear their leaving her alone. When she began to date at the age of fourteen, this middle-class Jewish girl chose lower-class black teenagers for her companions and insisted on bringing them home to meet her parents. As a consequence, she and the father fought and literally did not speak to each other from that time until the father died, when she was sixteen. At the time that she entered treatment, she had repeated several times the following pattern with men: She would become intensely involved with a man who she knew from the start was unsuitable. He might be married, or someone who was intellectually her inferior, or someone she really didn't like. From the beginning of the relationship, she would be aware that this could not last. She would project this feeling and become intensely angry at the man because he, in her view, was unreliable and threatened to leave her. She would, in her fury, become increasingly provocative, finally bringing about the separation she both desired and feared. She would then become depressed and feel abandoned.

The repetition of this pattern was a major element in the transference. She was never late for an appointment, paid her bills on time, and tried hard to be a "good patient," although she found it difficult to talk. She was convinced that I eagerly awaited the end of every session, the break for the weekend, or the start of a holiday because I was delighted to be rid of her, and she felt that she could not survive without me. (She had dreams of floating in space, isolated, and dreams of accidents.) On the surface, her idealization of me was complete, but dreams and other data revealed the anger and devaluation that permeated that seeming idealization. In fact, in the adult idealization in the transference is never pure idealization but is always merged with the hidden rage experienced by the child in the course of separation-individuation. She would never allow herself to take a holiday or miss an appointment, clearly to maintain the clear record that I was the one who did all the abandoning. This was analyzed at length. Midway in the analysis, in the spring of the year, she planned her summer holiday before knowing precisely what my holiday dates would be. We discussed her plan at length, and for the first time she felt confident and pleased about being able to go away on a self-initiated separation. Several weeks later, in the course of a session, I mentioned that the vacation dates had worked out well because in fact my holiday would coincide with hers. She immediately was enraged and self-pitying that I would go away and leave her, and it became utterly unimportant that she had previously made her own arrangements to go away. Several things became apparent in the analysis of this episode.

1. A major portion of her self-esteem and self-knowledge consisted of her representation to herself of herself as an innocent, abandoned martyr.
2. She felt a comfortable familiarity and control of her intimate objects only in the context of her capacity to create a feeling of abandonment or to provoke an actual abandonment by the object. This was at its basic level preoedipal in nature and clearly reflected her sense of being uncared for by her narcissistic mother.
3. Additionally, this constellation represented the repetition of oedipal issues, and in the transference she was also reliving aspects of her oedipal relationship to her father. All preoedipal constellations have another reworking during the oedipal phase, but the latter does not constitute the entirety of recoverable content of the genetic constellation.
4. The intolerable frustration of the original infantile demands for love and union had led to masochistic-narcissistic defenses. What she now sought in her relationships, disguised as an insatiable demand for attention, was the actual repetition of the painful abandonment but with the hidden gratification of narcissistic control and masochistic satisfaction. The demand for love had been given up in favor of the pleasure of rejection.

This is the paradigmatic sequence for masochistic-narcissistic pathology.

Clinical Vignette #2

A forty-year-old, successful, corporate executive entered analysis because he had plunged into a deep depression following an accusation of minor wrong-doing in some financial maneuvers. In fact, he was innocent of the charge, which had arisen out of an equally innocent error committed by one of his assistants. He had been officially cleared of any taint, and the whole matter was minor to begin with. However, this incident was one in a lifelong series of actual, or potentially self-damaging provocations in important situations, which were further characterized by his inappropriate failure to defend himself with sufficient vigor in the face of the attack that followed his provocation. These incidents had regularly been followed by feelings of depression and self-pity, but this time those feelings were particularly severe. He could not rid himself of the feeling that he had shamefully exposed himself to his colleagues, that his entire career would collapse, and that he would turn out to be a laughingstock with fraudulent pretensions to greatness. The presenting symptom thus combined masochistic and provocative self-damage and self-pity with a sense of narcissistic collapse.

I will present here only a few relevant aspects of the history and treatment course and will omit the oedipal material that arose and was interpreted during the course of the analysis. Instead, I will focus on earlier aspects of development. The patient was the youngest of three children, the only boy, and, as he acknowledged only later, clearly the favorite child. He viewed his own childhood with great bitterness. He felt he had received nothing of value from his parents and that they had played no positive role in his life. He regarded himself as a phoenix—born out of himself, his own father and mother. These feelings of bitter deprivation—nobody ever gave me anything —had formed a masochistic current throughout his life.

His mother had been a powerfully narcissistic woman who saw in her son her one opportunity for realizing her ambitions for wealth and status— cravings that she unceasingly berated the father for not satisfying. The patient recalled little affection from his mother and felt she had used him only for her own satisfaction and as an ally against his weak, passive father. His father had been a modest success until the depression hit, when the patient was four, and both he and his business collapsed, never to recover. This probably provided a serious blow to whatever attempts at idealization may have been under way. The parents fought constantly, mother reminded father daily of his failure, and the boy remembers great anxiety that they would separate and he would be abandoned.

The sharp edge of his depression lifted shortly after analysis began, revealing a level of chronic depression and a character of endless injustice-collecting and self-pity, covered by a socially successful facade of charm and joviality. He felt that although many people regarded him as a friend and sought him out, he had no friends and felt no warmth toward anyone. Perhaps he loved his wife and children, but he arranged his work schedule so that he would never have to be near them for any length of time. He felt isolated and lived with a constant dread each day that some disaster would befall him. The incident that precipitated his depression bothered him partly because he felt he was being hauled down by something trivial rather than an episode fittingly grandiose. He battled endlessly with his associates in business and made wildly unreasonable demands. He then felt unjustly treated when those demands were not met. At the same time, he maintained a killing work pace and never asked for the readily available help that might have reduced his work load. He had a mechanically adequate sex life with his wife and fantasied endlessly about the beautiful women he wanted to sleep with. In fact, he was convinced that he would be impotent with anyone except his wife and never dared to attempt an affair.

Early in the treatment, he expressed two major concerns with regard to me. First, that it was my goal to make him "like everyone else." "I couldn't bear to live if I thought I was like everyone else. I'd rather be bad or dead than not be a somebody. Before I give up the feeling of awful things happening to me, I want to be sure I won't be giving up my sense of being special." Secondly, he was convinced that I had no interest in him and saw him only because I wanted the fee. That suited him because he had no interest in me, but it worried him that I might not need the fee badly enough so that he could count on my availability for as long as he might want me. Interestingly, convinced then that I only saw him for the money, he was regularly late in paying his bills, would worry about the consequences, but not mention it himself. When I would bring up his tardiness, he would then feel a combination of terror—I was now going to be angry with him and throw him out—and fury—I had the nerve to dun him for money, when everyone knew he was an honest man. From that point on the transference quickly developed a variety of narcissistic and masochistic themes.

The early transference combined both idealizing and mirror forms. These narcissistic transferences are, in my view, always equally masochistic, since they are regularly suffused with rage and the expectation of disappointment. The idealization is often the facade for constructing larger, later disappointments. As adults, masochistic-narcissistic characters no longer have genuine expectations that their grandiose fantasies will be fulfilled. In fact, grandiose fantasies are occasions for the reenactment of unconsciously gratifying disappointments. The seeming insatiability of so many of these patients is not due to excessive need. Rather, it represents their raising the demand for love, time, attention, or whatever, to a level where they are sure their demands cannot be met. This man, for example, seemed to look forward to our sessions, was friendly, felt that my most obvious remarks were brilliant, and seemed happy to attribute to me all of the intelligent ideas that he had contributed during analysis. The other side of the coin, however, was his angry conviction that I used my intelligence totally on my own behalf and had no interest in helping him. He felt that all the work in analysis was being done by himself. A typical dream was of himself and a guide scaling a high mountain, making remarkable progress but never speaking, with him in the lead. In discussing this dream, he said, "All you do here is nudge me along.

Why don't you help me more? The work is all mine. I can't bear the thought that anyone else has a part in anything I do.'' Fantasies of this sort have the double purpose of maintaining a grandiose, omnipotent image of himself and of maintaining an image of a totally refusing mother. The narcissistic portion of the fantasy requires the masochistic portion. ''I give myself everything; my mother gives me nothing.'' A sense of grandiosity and a sense of self-pitying deprivation paradoxically are sides of the same coin; neither can exist without the other. The narcissistic grandiose self as viewed in the adult can never be the original germ of narcissism but is always tempered by the experiences of frustration that then become part and parcel of the narcissistic fantasy. ''I am a great person because I overcome the malice of my refusing mother.''

At a later stage of treatment, when I insistently brought up the issue of his feelings about me, he reacted fiercely, saying, ''This is a process, not a human relationship. You are not here. You are not. There is just a disembodied voice sitting behind me.'' As I persisted and discussed how difficult it was for him to acknowledge that he received something from me and felt something for me, he reported, ''I feel creepy. I have a physical reaction to this discussion.'' He was experiencing mild depersonalization, related to the disturbance of self and narcissistic stability, which resulted from the revival of remnants of the repressed affectionate bond toward his mother. The acknowledgment of this bond immediately induced feelings of terrifying weakness—a feeling of being passively at the mercy of a malicious giant. On the other hand, this masochistic, passive, victimized relationship to a maliciously perceived mother was an unconscious source of narcissistic gratification (I never yield to her) and masochistic gratification (I enjoy suffering at the hands of a monster). One could see much of this man's life as an attempt at narcissistic denial of underlying, passive masochistic wishes.

As further memories were recovered of affectionate interactions with his mother, he began to weep and became depressed. He dreamed that I was pulling a big black thing out of the middle of him, a cancer that wouldn't come out but which would kill him if it did come out. The analysis, which had been pleasant for him before, now became extremely painful. He insisted that I was deliberately humiliating him by forcing him to reveal his stupidity because I knew the answers to all the questions that I was raising with him and he did not. I enjoyed making a helpless fool out of him. He dreamed he was in a psychiatrist's office in Brooklyn, which for him was a term of derogation, and was receiving a special form of treatment. ''I was hypnotized and totally helpless. People are ridiculing me, screaming guffaws like a fun house. Then I run down a hill through a big garage antique shop.'' In another dream at this time he was driving a huge, shiny antique 1928 Cadillac in perfect condition. "As I am driving, the steering wheel comes apart, the right half of it comes off in my hand, then the big, black, shiny hood is gone, then the radiator cap is gone." He was born in 1928. At this time he also developed a transitory symptom of retarded ejaculation, which was a form of actively withholding the milk that he insisted was being withheld from him.

The revival of repressed positive ties to his mother threatened his major masochistic and narcissistic characterological defenses. His entire sense of being exceptional depended on his pride in having suffered unusual deprivation at the hands of mother, and his entire experience of being loved and favored by his mother had been perceived by him as a threat of passive submission to a superior malicious force. He perceived this turn in the treatment as endangering his life of narcissistic and masochistic satisfactions and exposing him to the hazards of intimacy, mutual dependence, and a genuine recognition of the extent of his unconsciously sought-for bittersweet pleasure in self-damage and self-deprivation. The increasing recognition of a bond to me was accompanied by an exacerbation of the fantasy that I was the all-powerful withholding mother and that he was the victimized child. Loewenstein (1957) has remarked, "Masochism is the weapon of the weak—of every child—faced with the danger of human aggression." I would only emphasize that every child, in his own perception, faces the danger of human aggression.

At this stage of the treatment the patient's injustice-collecting surged to new refinements. Frequent requests for appointment changes, the presentation of complicated dreams to which I did not have magical, brilliant interpretations, the fact that he was not already cured, my insistence that sessions had to be paid for—all of these were proof of my malicious withholding and of his innocent victimization. The injustice-collecting, partly a result of fragile and fragmented self and object representation, is also a guilt-relieving, rage-empowering reinforcement of masochistic and narcissistic defenses. These patients are indeed singled out for mistreatment by especially powerful figures to whom they have a special painful attachment.

After a great deal of working through, two incidents occurred that signaled a change in the transference. The first was that I had made an error in noting the date of an appointment that he had canceled. Instead of his usual reaction of outrage and indignation, he sat bolt upright on the couch, looked at me as if this were the first mistake I had ever made, and said, "You mean, you make mistakes too?" The second incident occurred a few weeks later. After a particularly resistant session, I said, "I wish we could better understand your relationship to your mother." He was again startled and said, "You mean you really don't know the answer?" I assured him that I did not and that we would have to work it out together. He now began to acknowledge my reality as a human being, fallible and yet concerned for his welfare. From this point on, the case increasingly tended to resemble that of a classical neurosis, although with many detours to deep masochistic and narcissistic issues.

One could further discuss the nature of the Oedipus complex in this type of patient, from this point of view, but that is beyond the scope of this chapter.

SUMMARY

On the basis of genetic hypotheses and clinical data, I have suggested that the themes of narcissism and masochism, which are crucial in all human psychic development, achieve their particular individual character at preoedipal stages of development. Furthermore, narcissistic tendencies and masochistic defenses are intimately and inevitably interwoven in the course of development. In fact, they are so interwoven that I further suggest that the narcissistic character and the masochistic character are one and the same. I believe that the vast literature on these entities may become more coherent when considered from the point of view of a single nosological entity—the narcissistic-masochistic character.

In any particular individual either the narcissistic or masochistic qualities may be more apparent in the lifestyle, as a result of internal and external contingencies that may be traced and clarified in the course of analysis. A closer examination, however, will reveal the structural unity and mutual support of the two characterologic modes, despite the surface distinctions. Neither can exist without the other. Interpreting masochistic behavior produces narcissistic mortification, and interpreting narcissistic defenses produces feelings of masochistic victimization, self-pity, and humiliation.

The analysis of the narcissistic-masochistic character is always a difficult task. I hope that our changing frame of reference and the beginning elucidation of the genetic and clinical unity of these seemingly disparate pathologies may help to make our efforts more consistent, coherent, and successful.

REFERENCES

Auchincloss, L. 1950. *The Injustice Collector*. Boston: Houghton-Mifflin.

Bergler, E. 1949. *The Basic Neurosis, Oral Regression and Psychic Masochism*. New York: Grune & Stratton.

————. 1961. *Curable and Incurable Neurotics*. New York: Liveright Publishing.

Brenner, C. 1959. The masochistic character: genesis and treatment. *J. Amer. Psychoanal. Assn.* 7: 197–226.

Cooper, A. 1983. Psychoanalytic inquiry and new knowledge. In *Reflections on Self Psychology*, eds. J. Lichtenberg and S. Kaplan. Hillsdale, N.J.: The Analytic Press.

Dizmang, L., and Cheatham, C. 1970. The Lesch-Nyhan syndrome. *Amer. J. Psychiatry* 127(5): 131–37.

Erikson, E. 1963. *Childhood and Society*. New York: W. W. Norton.

Freud, S. 1914. On the history of psychoanalytic movement. *Standard Edition*, 14: 226.

————. 1920. Beyond the pleasure principle. *Standard Edition*, 18: 3–66.

————. 1931. Female sexuality. *Standard Edition*, 21: 223–46.

————. 1937. Analysis terminable and interminable. *Standard Edition*, 23.

————. 1938. An outline of psychoanalysis. *Standard Edition*, 23: 141–208.

Glover, E. 1955. *Technique of Psychoanalysis*. New York: International Universities Press.

Greenacre, P. 1960. Regression and fixation: Considerations concerning the development of the ego. *J. Amer. Psychoanal. Assn.* 8: 703–23.

Hartmann, H., and Loewenstein, R. M. 1962. Notes on the superego. In *Psychoanalytic Study of the Child*, vol. 17. New York: International Universities Press, 42–81.

Hermann, I. 1976. Clinging-going-in-search. *Psychoanalytic Quarterly* 54: 30.

Jacobson, E. 1964. *The Self and the Object World*. New York: International Universities Press.

Kohut, H. 1971. *The Analysis of the Self*. New York: International Universities Press.

————. 1972. Thoughts on narcissism and narcissistic rage. *Psychoanalytic Study of the Child* 27: 360–400. New Haven: Yale University Press.

Krafft-Ebing, R. F. 1895. *Psychopathia Sexualis*. London: F. A. Davis.

Lewin, B. 1950. *Psychoanalysis of Elation*. New York: W. W. Norton.

Loewenstein, R. 1957. A contribution of the psychoanalytic theory of masochism. *J. Amer. Psychoanal. Assn.* 5: 197–234.

Mahler, M. 1972. Rapprochement subphase of the separation-individuation process. *Psychoanalytic Quarterly* 51: 487–506.

Maleson, F. 1984. The multiple meanings of masochism in psychoanalytic discourse. *J. Amer. Psychoanal. Assn.* 32: 325–56.

Rado, S. 1969. *Adaptational Psychodynamics*. New York: Science House.

Sandler, J., and Joffee, W. G. 1969. Towards a basic psychoanalytic model. *Int. J. Psychoanal.* 50: 79–90.

Stolorow, R. D. 1975. The narcissistic function of masochism and sadism. *Int. J. Psychoanal.* 56(4): 441–48.

Sullivan, H. S. 1953. *The Interpersonal Theory of Psychiatry*. New York: W. W. Norton.

Trilling, L. 1963. *Beyond Culture*. New York: Viking.

Winnicott, D. W. 1971. *Playing and Reality*. New York: Basic Books.

16. The Role of Internalization in the Development of Certain Aspects of Female Masochism: Ego Psychological Considerations

Ruth F. Lax

I

Aspects of masochistic behaviour in women have been regarded from many different points of view. Freud (1924, 1931, 1932, 1937), Bonaparte (1949), Deutsch (1930, 1944), Lampl-de Groot (1965), Reik (1941) among many others have emphasized constitutional, economic, moral and psychodynamic factors. I shall not review these findings since they are well known and have been investigated extensively. I shall focus my discussion of self-defeat in women on specific kinds of internalization[1] processes and on ensuing identifications which typically occur within the framework of certain object-relation constellations. Further, I shall attempt to indicate how these lead to the subsequent formation of deviant ego and superego structures. Discussion of developmental phases will be limited to those aspects which contribute to the formation of the pathological ego features to be examined.

My patients suffered from a predominantly obsessive character neurosis with hysteroid, narcissistic and depressive features. Each of them, upon analytic scrutiny, seemed strangely 'at odds with herself'. Namely, though each appeared to be driving assertively towards the fulfillment of her goals, each failed repeatedly for reasons beyond her comprehension. They all identified with progressive causes, appeared to have good, though somewhat competitive relations with both sexes, were physically attractive, 'free' in their love life and sought self-fulfilment.

Analytic investigation, however, disclosed that their assertive, achieving behaviour and conscious convictions corresponded to only one aspect of their personality. The other revealed itself via unconsciously provoked failures which led to patterns of self-defeat. These, like a leitmotiv, ran through their

Reprinted from the *International Journal of Psycho-Analysis* 58 (1977): 289–300 by permission. Copyright © Institute of Psycho-Analysis.

lives resulting in narcissistic mortifications which eventually led to a lasting depletion of their self-esteem. These narcissistic hurts evoked feelings of depression and worthlessness, unending ruminations and a growing sense of perplexity which eventually brought these women to therapy.

I shall attempt by the following vignettes to illustrate some manifestations of these patients' pathology.

II. CLINICAL VIGNETTES

Case 1

Mrs Y., a much sought-after lawyer, who specialized in family law and civil liberties cases, entered treatment after 24 years in a marriage which she experienced as demeaning. Her husband did not regard her as his peer. He believed it was the man's prerogative to concern himself exclusively with professional activities while it was her duty to take care of the domestic, financial and social responsibilities he considered chores. Mrs Y. complied 'for the sake of harmony'. Eventually, however, her husband's attitude activated old childhood conflicts and Mrs Y. came to feel denigrated. She became extremely angry about her 'lot in life', but continued to fulfil her marital role, rationalizing that she was doing so 'for the sake of the children'.

Analysis revealed that, at the unconscious level, Mrs Y. experienced her marital situation in terms of the childhood paradigm. She had a much older brother who had been held in high esteem by both mother and father. Nothing was ever permitted to interfere with brother's intellectual pursuits. Mother served father and brother 'hand and foot', and expected her daughter to do likewise. As a child, Mrs Y. had felt that her intellectual achievements, which equalled her brother's, were of no real significance to her parents. She felt that brother also treated her as an inferior. Since neither parent took issue with his attitude, Mrs Y. concluded that they concurred. Mrs Y. had also noticed that mother's status in the family's 'pecking order' did not equal that of father or brother and she therefore thought of mother as inferior. Mother's obvious preference for brother and her catering to him confirmed Mrs Y.'s feelings of inferiority.

For her unconscious, Mrs Y.'s husband represented a combined father-brother image. She was hurt and angered by her husband just as she had been by her father and brother in the past. Yet she was unable to directly oppose him, in spite of being successfully assertive in her professional life. The reason for this inhibition became clear when it was understood that Mrs Y. unconsciously equated her husband's love for her with the love bestowed on mother by father and brother. In her unconscious, father, brother and husband were merged into the desired, idealized oedipal object, whose love she sought unconditionally. Mrs Y.'s unconscious identification with mother as an inferior became clear both from her submissive attitude towards her husband and from her contrasting attitudes toward her own son and daughter. Mrs Y. repeated in her relationship to her children the pattern that had been established by her mother; thus Mrs Y. continued to act out her unconscious identification with her image of the debased and debasing mother.

Case 2

Mrs G., a successful travel agent, suffered from a chronic depression. She considered her husband's repeated and prolonged love affairs, which had begun approximately one year after the birth of their child, the precipitating factor. Prior to that, their marriage could have been considered conventionally 'happy'. After the birth of their child, however, their sexual contact decreased. As Mr G.'s love affairs took on increased importance, he withdrew all sexual interest from his wife. Mrs G. responded to this with extreme mortification. As Mrs G.'s sense of stagnation in the marriage grew, professional success, rich enduring friendships and varied extra-professional interests lost all significance for her. She spent hours imagining her husband's love life. She also brooded about her inability to divorce him. Mr G. was a rather superficial, callous and emotionally unavailable person; Mrs G. did not really love him. Her inability to leave him in spite of her professional and financial independence resulted in a further loss of self-esteem.

After several years of analysis Mrs G. was finally able to reveal the following masturbation fantasy, which she had had since adolescence.

A sultan with a great harem had a first wife whom he no longer desired, but by whom he wanted to have children. It was his custom, while he was engaging in sex play with a current favourite mistress, to have the first wife at the same time in his bed, tied in such a way as to be available to him for impregnation. The mistress would excite him and he would fondle her and sexually gratify her. Finally, at the very last minute, he would impregnate his wife.

Associations connected this fantasy with her parents and linked it to conflicts of the oedipal phase. Mrs G. recalled that during adolescence she had overheard mother reading to a friend a fragment of a letter in which father had referred to himself as a sultan and said that 'even if he had a hundred wives, she (mother) would always be his first wife'. Mother had felt complimented and honoured by this, but the patient had felt humiliated and appalled for two reasons: she experienced father's remarks as a denigration of women's status and was horrified that any woman could feel honoured by it. Mortified, Mrs G. admitted that her masturbation fantasy started shortly after this incident.

Upon analysis, Mrs G. realized that she identified in her own marital situation with the 'first-wife-mother' of the masturbation fantasy. This realization was facilitated by the fact that the patient now was herself a mother and that she experienced her sexual deprivation as due to her husband's involvement with his mistress.

Further analysis revealed, however, that the patient also identified with the mistress of the masturbation fantasy. This identification had several meanings. It signified that the patient accepted mother as father's prime love object, but it also expressed the patient's vengeful fantasies—namely her wish to deprive mother of the sexual gratification she (mother) received from father. The patient had thus attempted, via the masturbation fantasy, to resolve the conflicting feelings she had experienced towards mother during the oedipal phase. In the fantasy, the patient had accorded mother the superior position of 'first wife–procreation vessel', but simultaneously had deprived mother of sexual gratification, which the patient desired for herself.

The point in the fantasy at which orgasm was reached, varied. Sometimes it took place when the wife was impregnated, and sometimes when mistress was excited to the utmost. Further analysis indicated that the patient also identified with the sultan, who misused both women for his pleasure. The fantasy thus served as a compromise solution for the negative and positive aspects of the oedipal conflict. Elaboration of the meaning of identification with the sultan revealed profound feelings of self-debasement, which seemed to go beyond the parents' jointly-held attitude regarding women's 'inferior' status.

The detailed analysis of this masturbation fantasy contributed to the understanding of the causes which had led to Mrs G.'s difficulty in leaving her husband. The unhappy marital situation, in which she was sexually deprived, represented for Mrs G.'s unconscious the oedipal triangle in which she had identified primarily with the humiliated yet elevated 'mother-first-wife'. Mrs G. had become immobilized in her painful and frustrating marriage because its specific constellation masochistically gratified all the repressed oedipal wishes.

Acting out the unconscious identification with the bound 'mother-first-wife', the passive receptor for the paternal phallus, Mrs G. inhibited all her assertiveness and became masochistically tied to her husband, who represented for her unconscious the father-sultan. The vicious cycle of reality frustration and unconscious gratification perpetuated the marriage. It led to increased self-destructive behaviour, depression, and eventually seriously affected Mrs G.'s professional and social life.

Case 3

Ms V. was an account executive in her early thirties, successful and respected by her firm. She was known for her assertiveness and capabilities in dealing with business executives, and was usually given difficult accounts to handle. However, in spite of her successes, Ms V. had an erratic work history, which seemed puzzling. Thus Ms V. would start a job enthusiastically, work for months with great diligence and devotion, and then suddenly, when a promotion was in the offing, begin slackening in her efforts: she would get to work late, do her assignments at the last minute, become unpredictable in her dealings with clients, etc.

Careful scrutiny indicated that this change in her functioning usually coincided with an upheaval in her love life. It would occur when Ms V. felt 'deeply in love' and wished her lover to 'take care of her'. At such times Ms V. would fantasize becoming pregnant and having a baby. She would declare in moments of sexual ecstasy that her lover could do with her anything he wished—even kill her.

The men Ms V. picked as lovers, although highly gifted and of unusual intelligence were, for a variety of reasons, unable to meet her dependency needs. In spite of this, Ms V. would for a long time continue to devote herself to them and to their needs, even though her analytic sessions were filled with complaints about them. Though she was usually very independent and enjoyed flirting with many men, Ms V. wanted at such times to be asked by her lover to become his wife; she would turn her back on her hitherto cherished independence and agonize over the fact that she was still unmarried. She saw this as a sign of her 'worthlessness'. Ms V. would become excessively self-critical and self-doubting.

During such periods of personal upheaval, Ms V. would endanger her position in the firm by various subtle and unconscious provocations. As a consequence, Ms V. would either be threatened with dismissal or fired outright. Distraught, she would turn to her lover for support. In her fantasy the lover at this point assumed complete care of her. This fantasy, however, was never fulfilled. Disappointed, disillusioned and angry, Ms V. would eventually turn against the lover, openly find fault with him and finally break off the relationship. Whether on her old job or a new one, Ms V. would return to work full of enthusiasm. Since Ms V. was very attractive and charming, she would very soon find a new lover and the entire cycle would start again.

Ms V. suffered from an obsessive character neurosis with hysterical, depressive and narcissistic trends. She had had several abortions following so-called 'accidental' pregnancies. The following is the terrifying dream she had while coming out of anaesthesia following a D.C.:

She was a small part of an elaborate scientific 'instrumentation system, consisting of pipes, tubes and U-shaped vials, all connected and in motion'. She was 'at the bottom of the U'. She could do nothing to stop what was going on; she was immobilized by it. She could not express her needs or desires.

She woke up in a state of panic. The dream had haunted her ever since.

In time Ms V. recognized that her repeated provocations at work were unconsciously motivated and that a connexion existed between the upheavals in her business and her love life.

The patient was very embarrassed to admit that she masturbated by rubbing against the corner of the mattress, 'in a humped position like a man'. She was reluctant to consider the possible implications of this manner of masturbation and seemed intent on dropping the subject altogether. As if at random, Ms V. began to speak about the certainty with which her parents had anticipated the birth of a boy while mother was pregnant with her. She added sadly: 'They even bought cigars and liquor in advance of the bris. No one ever drank the liquor or smoked the cigars.'

She had slept in the parental bedroom until the age of 12. Slowly her understanding of the sexual interaction between the parents became clear. She felt mother did not want sex and father imposed it. 'Mother gave in for the sake of peace, to get rid of his nagging and to have it over with. Mother had no choice: she just had to.' The patient reported the following recurring masturbation fantasy: 'I am in bondage in a concentration camp, tied up and being whipped. The assailants are nondescript and the cause for the punishment unspecified.' In association the patient recalled sex play when she was 8 or 9 years old. She said: 'It was a cowboys-and-Indians game. I was the Indian. I would let the cowboys catch me and tie me up, then they would tickle me in the genitals, especially the clitoris. At first I directed them "how and where". This was the "torture".' The patient maintained that she never 'did it' to anyone else and admitted that she wanted 'it done' to herself.

Analysis revealed that the patient identified in fantasy with both the tortured and the torturer. She envied the male and identified with him, yet she also identified with the woman. She was both. She had been made aware since early childhood of the greater importance of men. She said with a sigh: 'In my house, the man was boss, the woman catered to his every need, even if she did not like it.' She always wished she had been a boy. In many ways she acted like one. During latency and early adolescence she hated every maturational aspect which forced her to recognize her femininity. However, as she matured, Ms V. became a beautiful woman, aware of and able to use her beauty.

The presence of two trends was brought to light in the patient which varied in intensity during different periods of her life and which were always in conflict with each other. Thus, in addition to her envy of the boy-man she wanted to be, Ms V., because of her unconscious oedipal longings, also wanted to be the most beautiful and feminine of all women. Her ideas, however, of what constituted 'femininity' were confused, since they were founded on her conception of mother's debased role.[2] Ms V. complained: 'Why are women masochists? Why was mother a slave?'

The masochistic relationship of the slave-woman to the sadistic male, depicted by Ms V. in her masturbation fantasies, had its intrapsychic parallel in the sadomasochistic interaction between the patient's ego and superego (Schafer, 1960).

III. RELEVANT OBJECT-RELATIONS CONSTELLATIONS

In this section I shall attempt to present in outline form the childhood histories of these patients, emphasizing factors which reappeared in each case and which had a pathognomonic significance for the development of the syndrome under consideration. I shall focus on the importance of internalizations which occurred within the framework of the specific libidinal and aggressive object-relation constellation, crucial for the development of the character neurosis of these patients.

I hope to demonstrate that in my cases the unconsciously provoked defeats were related to distortions in the structure of the ego, reflecting structuralized derivatives of object relations which in turn influenced the patients' object relations. Thus, ego deviations caused by these specific developmental vicissitudes were the most significant factor determining the pathology.

The patients came from middle-class families with a pronounced patriarchal structure and a definite bias in favour of the male. The parents loved one another within the framework of a Victorian relationship.

The threats to the narcissistic cathexis of the self, which exist from the moment of birth and stem from the interaction of the child's libidinal and aggressive drives with the demands, frustrations and gratifications of the real world, were affected in a unique way by the familial constellation into which these patients were born. Thus, although these patients believed their parents had wanted children, they did not feel themselves to be as valued as they might have been, had they been boys.[3] Further, though the birth of a daughter was a disappointment to both parents, it appears to have been more painful to mother than to father (Freud, 1932). Thus the patients experienced the phallocentric orientation more strongly in their relationship with mother than with father.

The investigations by Benedek (1959) and by Coleman, Kris & Provence (1953) indicate the extent of cultural and individual variations in parental attitudes. They illustrate the significance and variety of unconscious meanings which a particular child may have for a parent. For the mothers of my patients, the birth of a daughter was an upsetting experience. It is likely that the acceptance of phallocentric values accentuated these mothers' unconscious longing for a penis, which might have been gratified via identification with a male child. Thus the birth of a daughter may have even re-emphasized these mothers' unconscious feelings of being castrated and deprived.

The mothers of my patients were unable to develop a genuine 'maternal preoccupation' (Winnicott, 1956) because their infant daughters did not represent the embodiment of their 'fantasy child' (Lax, 1972). Thus the infants were cared for but not nurtured and consequently lacked a sense of being cherished, which stems from mother's narcissistic valuations. These patients felt 'needy' throughout their life.

Jacobson (1954) points out that 'the affective identification between mother and baby results in the inducement of mother's affects in the infant.' Thus, the conscious and unconscious displeasure on the part of these mothers had been experienced and internalized by their infant girls. Giovacchini (1972) states that such trauma in the symbiotic phase leads the child to develop a sense of identity that incorporates mother's devaluing attitudes which are subsequently directed towards the developing self. As a result, the self is experienced as being unlovable, worthless and inadequate. Consequently, self-esteem is lacking and vulnerability becomes excessive. During the anal and phallic phases these early internalized feelings became merged in my patients with the affects related to the conflicts specific for these periods. Feelings of denigration stemming from all these sources were primarily directed towards the self, but also in part towards the mother who thus became devalued.

These mothers were unable to provide the 'refuelling' necessary for successful mastery of the *rapprochement* subphase (Mahler, 1968). Consequently, complete separation and individuation could not be achieved. Thus, unconscious aspects of the symbiotic child–mother linkage persisted, affecting these patients' internalization of maternal attitudes and facilitating specific identifications with her.

The patients' recollections indicate that as children they sought out father rather than mother because they experienced him as more accepting. They felt father liked to be with them and play with them. These circumstances, as well as the high esteem in which father was held by the entire household, led to his idealization and lent impetus to the wish of these girls to identify with him.

As is generally the case, mother, experienced at the oral and anal levels as unloving and depriving, was also blamed for the deprivations experienced at the phallic stage. Following the discovery of genital differences, an extremely stormy period of interaction with mother ensued. Since mother rejected them because they were girls, they had great difficulty accepting their femininity. It is understandable therefore that analysis brought to light long periods during which they had denied their lack of a penis, and even longer periods during which, after they finally acknowledged their so called 'defect', they simultaneously expressed a desire that the hoped-for penis would eventually grow. These little girls identified with and even exaggerated the phallocentric attitudes of their parents. They thus experienced mother's wish to 'keep them in their place' and 'make of them little mothers and ladies', with pain and rebelled against it.

Mother's rejecting attitude, experienced and incorporated from the symbiotic level onward, fuelled a vicious cycle in which the girl, feeling rejected by mother because of her supposed 'defect', rejected and profoundly depreciated mother for the same reason, and finally reintrojected these feelings and turned them against herself. Further, this experiential complex was influenced in a specific way by the attitudes of both parents towards women and by father's special attitude towards his daughter. These girls considered themselves 'exceptions' because their fathers had accorded them a special, privileged position by exempting them from the status to which women generally were relegated. Since father's attitude was not based on an erotized relationship with daughter, the child felt accepted in spite of her sex. The daughters, at times and to varying degrees, became the fathers' companions, in contradistinction to the mothers who simply 'went along' with their husbands. Ongoing psychic processes of this nature led to an intensification of the girls' identification with father's valued attributes.

In the early years of these patients' analyses the hostile affect towards mother predominated. It was related to the patients' feeling that mother was 'unappreciative' and lacked understanding. Most important, however, was their complaint that, regardless of what they did, they never were accepted as 'good enough' by mother. This led in the middle years of the analyses to the surfacing of feelings of pervasive depression, helplessness, hopelessness and loss. The patients held the conviction that 'mother had really not wanted them and nothing could be done about it'.

The relationship with father was experienced as loving, often understanding, supportive and sometimes even nurturing. Though father was considered to have been much more demanding, he was regarded as more accepting. These patients 'knew where they stood' with father: they were accepted, provided they fulfilled father's demands. They consequently moulded their behaviour to do so and became successful in areas meaningful to father. Although the conditional acceptance by father also resulted in unconscious feelings of depression, it did not evoke the same feeling of helplessness that had been associated with feelings related to mother. Since father made demands which the girls could and did fulfil, their feelings towards him became linked with active strivings towards mastery and a sense of hope; whereas the feelings related to mother were linked with a sense of *a priori* defeat, possibly accounting for the suicidal element of some of these patients. Though father possessed the virtues and values the little girls cherished and he was the idealized and greatly admired parent, he did not become their ideal of a man.

The devalued view of woman with which these patients grew up had a profound and devastating effect on the development of their self-image during each psychosexual phase. Since they never felt fully accepted by either of their parents, their self-image was cathected with an insufficient amount of narcissism. Real self-acceptance consequently became almost impossible. During the pre-oedipal and early oedipal phases, the patients identified unconsciously with their image of the devalued mother, while at the same time consciously aspiring with equal intensity to become like father.

Indications were present in each case that both phases of the oedipal conflict were experienced. The positive oedipal feelings, however, predominated. Characteristic for these patients was the fact that, during the oedipal phase, each one of them had displaced her erotic feelings, usually directed towards father, on to a male relative or a close family friend. The affectionate relationship with this surrogate was highly charged: it involved a lot of kissing, lap-sitting and hand-holding. Evidence suggests that these relationships were overstimulating and resulted in sexual excitement and sexual frustration.[4]

The oedipal period was relatively long and dissolved slowly. The relationship with father did not undergo any marked changes. Mother emerged during this period and thereafter triumphantly as father's undisputed love object, admired and envied by the girl for her beauty, gracefulness, charm and femininity. Thus, the mother imago combined both coveted and devalued aspects. The girl who felt rejected by mother, unconsciously felt enraged by father's love for mother which, to her, was an enigma. The little girl also recognized that mother derived power from father's love for her and this was an additional cause for envy. None of these patients recalled any kind of seductive behaviour towards father. They believed they never competed for his erotic love towards mother and felt they would have failed had they done so. They remembered, however, feeling jealous and possessive about the erotic feelings of the object of their displaced oedipal longings. It appears that the displacement of their oedipal feelings had defensive functions. It kept unconscious their real rivalry with mother and protected the 'companionship' quality of their relationship with father.

Analysis did not result in the recall of any direct erotic feelings towards mother. Daydreams and fantasies indicate that the latent homosexual component in these women was relatively weak. It was related, as is usually the case, to the negative oedipal phase and an identification with father. The unconscious desire—even though displaced—to be, or become father's erotic love object predominated during the oedipal phase. This became clear during the course of treatment. While struggling with intensely self-deprecatory feelings, the patients confessed, with inappropriate shame, that as children they had admired mother's beauty and had wished to become as beautiful as she was when they grew up.

Analysis of the feeling of mortification associated with the 'admission' of this deeply guarded secret, revealed a complex of emotions related to the core of these patients' psychic problems. It led to the uncovering of an unconscious identification with an exalted and denigrated maternal imago conceived as a slave, a sexual object used for pleasure and gratification of desire, debased, mistreated, beautiful, adored and thus wanted and loved by father.[5] The internalization of this disparaged imago and the unconscious identification with it, had profound consequences for the formation of these patients' self-image and wishful self-image.[6] The existence of this unconscious identification was corroborated by the themes of repetitive sadomasochistic masturbation fantasies which had persisted in these patients from early adolescence into adulthood.

Intense narcissistic mortification was associated with the recounting of these masturbation fantasies. This was due in part to the extreme contrast between the avowed ideals and goals to which these patients were consciously committed, and the manifest content of the masturbation fantasies which culminated in orgastic gratification. Even though the patients were completely unaware of the latent significance of their masturbation fantasies and of their unconscious identifications, the mere recognition that they were able to engage in and enjoy sadomasochistic fantasies filled them with self-disgust.

During latency and early adolescence the patients were tomboys. They played almost exclusively with boys, engaged and often excelled in the games and pursuits of boys and dressed by preference like boys. These girls frequently had a particular boy as a 'special' friend. Such a relationship had a predominantly narcissistic character inasmuch as the girl identified with the boy who in part represented her ego ideal (Reich, 1953).

The relationship with mother worsened during this period since mother made strong objections to the girl's tomboyishness. Father, however, either encouraged or condoned it. A further detachment from mother followed, associated sometimes with an intensification of the 'companionship' with father. Analysis revealed that on the unconscious level father's acceptance signified his approval of their goals and wishes to be forceful, active, independent and assertive; wishes that were considered masculine in these phallocentric families. Mother's disapproval was experienced as an attempt to curtail these strivings. For the unconscious of these girls this meant that mother wanted to 'subjugate' them, to 'make them like she was', an idea which filled them disgust.

During adolescence these patients developed a narcissistic pride in their 'inner values', their moral integrity, the high level of their standards, and in the relentless strength of their ideals (values which Jacobson, 1964, pp. 113–4, describes as the feminine ego ideal and which, according to her, represent an unconscious 'inner penis'). They felt accepted and admired only for their character and achievements, their intellect and their ethical and moral values. These young women denied the significance of their attractiveness and charm even though they were often complimented for them. They appeared to be somewhat haughty even though they were in fact gracious. They were unusually efficient, decisive, and seemed very independent. They knew that they appeared 'strong and able to others' and this behaviour fitted in with their standards. These women, however, were also aware of having dependency longings and needs which they sometimes expressed to their close friends and lovers.

Severe mood swings, frequent periods of despair, depression and a sense of hopelessness and futility had characterized these patients since adolescence. The vulnerability of their self-esteem indicated that the libidinal and aggressive cathexis of their self representation had never been sufficiently neutralized. The disturbances in the regulation of these patients' self-esteem reflected the pathology inherent in their self representation.[7]

IV. DISCUSSION AND THEORETICAL CONSIDERATIONS

Freud examined the phenomenon of splitting from different points of view. He recognized as early as 1923 that incompatible object identifications may lead to disruption of the ego (1923a, pp. 20–31). Subsequently (Freud, 1923b) he asserted that splitting of the ego may follow as a consequence of disavowal. His final conceptualizations (Freud, 1937, section v; 1940a, ch. 8; 1940b) regarding the causes and effects of splitting, stress topographic and structural differences which occur in different pathological conditions. Freud implies in his discussion that as a result of splitting, two consequences may arise. In the neurosis proper, where the psychopathology is less severe, the disavowed aspect is repressed but continues to have the kind of influence typical for the repressed and which, in Freud's words, leads to 'psychical complications'. However, when the pathology is more severe, splitting of the ego results in the coexistence of two contrary dispositions throughout life which by implication are—or can be—conscious and which do not appear to modify each other.

Freud's formulations regarding developmental processes leading to structural ego distortions have been elaborated further by the findings of child psychoanalysis and the contributions of psychoanalytic ego psychology. Kernberg (1966) clarifies what is being split in splitting when he states: 'splitting . . . can pathologically persist at higher levels of ego organization and characteristically then affects the self, and ego identity in general'. He conceptualizes a 'dynamic unconscious as a system composed of rejected introjections and identification systems'. When considering lack of impulse control, Kernberg (1967) speaks of

the emergence into consciousness of a dissociated identification system . . . which is ego syntonic during the time this impulse behavior lasts . . . and which is characterized by its repetitive nature . . . and by the lack of emotional contact between that part of the patient's personality and the rest of the self-experience . . . (p. 661).

The specific genetic constellations experienced by my patients resulted in developmental vicissitudes which led to the formation of a conscious and an unconscious identification system.[8] The former was paternally and the latter maternally derived. These two identification systems did not become fused. Their existence and interaction affected the structuralization and the characteristics of these patients' self-image, wished-for self-image, ego ideal and superego.

The divergent attitudes of these girls towards father and mother, combined with the differences in attitude exhibited by each parent towards the child, led to the formation of separate mother and father object representations which were not subsequently fused in the structure of the superego and the ego ideal. The patients had created, on the one hand, an idealized grandiose image of a powerful and loving father and, on the other hand, an image of a rejecting mother who was a powerful 'depriver', beautiful, loved, and yet devalued because she was a woman.

Aetiological factors described in Section III led to the development of a specific form of self representation, characteristic of these patients. Thus, based on the identification with father and interaction with him, the patients developed a self-image characterized by assertion, striving and a recognition that active mastery was indeed possible. This self-image was invested primarily with libidinal feelings experienced by the girls in their interaction with father and with neutralized libidinal cathexis withdrawn from the paternal imago. The patients' avowed standard of aspiration was derived from the internalized paternal model. These factors contributed significantly to the structure and content of these patients' *conscious, wishful self-image*[9] which in its derivation could be considered masculine.[10]

Analysis demonstrated, however, that only one aspect of these patients' self representation was revealed by their behaviour patterned on the paternal identification. My patients, due to the specific constellation of object relations existing during their childhood, developed two identification systems simultaneously. The self-image maternally derived was invested primarily with feelings of rejection experienced as coming from mother, and secondarily with aggressive feelings first projected on to mother and subsequently reintrojected and directed towards the self. As has been indicated, concurrently with the process of identification with father, these patients during the oedipal phase also wished, as all little girls do, to become father's love object. These oedipal longings spurred their wish to become as they perceived mother to be. Thus, the girls' sense of biological identity with mother and the residual feelings of oral and anal dependency on her, fuelled their identification with the introjected, devalued maternal imago[11] which became the basis for the formation of what could be considered as these patients' maternally derived *feminine wishful self-image*. It was cathected predominantly with self-deprecatory feelings.

These patients thus had two separate wishful self-images each based on different internalizations. These wishful self-images were antithetical to each other and differently cathected. They persisted in the ego as permanent substructures. The feminine wishful self-image may have had a degree of consciousness during some part of the oedipal phase but subsequently became totally repressed. It continued, however, to manifest itself via the seemingly inexplicable masochistic masturbation fantasies as well as by the unconsciously provoked and thus perplexing self-defeating behaviour patterns. Sandler & Rosenblatt (1962) and Sandler, Holder & Meers (1963) have found that the changing character and shape of the self-image is normal during childhood. However, as maturation progresses, a more stable and integrated self-image should evolve. The absence of such development in these patients represents a specific aspect of their pathology. Their self representation had a faulty structure because it contained two diverse, yet permanent self-images which were split-off from one another and therefore could not modify each other.

The maternally derived wishful self-image was ego-alien, since it conflicted with those aspects of the wishful self-image which had become the avowed level of aspiration. Assertion, excellence, mastery, a desire for autonomy and certain ethical principles became narcissistically significant values which were embodied in the conscious aspects of the wishful self-image. This structure had become during the process of maturation sufficiently depersonified to function as a partial ego ideal. However, the existence and disruptive effects of the unconscious wishful self-image interfered with the development of a complete and harmonious ego ideal necessary for integrated, cohesive character formation.

The study of the vicissitudes of interaction between the split-off self-images and the conscious and unconscious wishful self-images was most significant for the understanding of these patients' pathology, since the dissociated identification system affected their behaviour and came to the fore under specific circumstances. Currently significant goals related to one of the wishful self-images at times activated these patients' behavior. However, most of the time these women tried to satisfy simultaneously the aims of both their wishful self-images. This led to intrasystemic conflict (Hartmann, 1950). A state of almost continuous psychic discord which manifested itself by contradictory and self-defeating behaviour was concomitant in these patients with a sense of helplessness and dejection.

When erotic impulses prevailed, the split-off self-image, cathected mostly with aggression turned against the self, became activated. Longings to become like the maternally derived wishful self-image predominated. Swayed by love, they acted out in accordance with their understanding of the oedipal model. Thus, though their tendencies toward self-debasement and self-defeat manifested themselves in many different ways, specific object relations were most frequently utilized for the enactment of these conflicts, probably because this area lends itself most effectively to the re-creation of oedipal conflicts. In such an object relationship, experiencing the devaluation that is unconsciously interpreted as a manifestation of love, can easily be provoked. These women chose for their love object men who in many ways resembled the unconscious image of their aggrandized phallic father rather than men who embodied the characteristics of their idealized male imago. Since these choices were unconsciously motivated, they remained perplexing to the patients who complained that love is 'irrational'. Analysis disclosed that in these relationships, which soon after inception repeatedly became sadomaso-chistic, the patients unconsciously identified with the loved yet denigrated maternal imago and their love object represented the oedipal father.

These patients' masturbation fantasies were elaborations of oedipal themes contaminated by anal, urethral and phallic preoccupations about power and love. Though the fantasied abuse of the woman may have also been a gesture of atonement towards the harsh superego for incestuous wishes, the main function of the fantasies was the attainment of the unconscious gratification through the total enactment of the parental interaction as perceived by the child. Since these patients' unconscious wishful self-image was embodied in the identification with the fantasied 'slave-woman' who represented the intro-jected devalued mother, their predominant erotic gratification unconsciously was linked with debasement. This theme was compulsively repeated during masturbation.

The fantasies, however, also gratified other unconscious impulses (Waelder, 1936). Thus analysis indicated that these patients identified with the male who enjoyed the woman's debasement, while they at the same time wished to castrate him and usurp his power. These impulses were usually expressed in latent content of fantasies which also contained lesbian wishes. The following is an example of such a fantasy: 'Women with artificial penises trained young girls to become "experts" in giving sexual pleasure to their future male masters. These women were cruel and demanding. They were the real rulers of the harem.'

When strivings to become like the conscious wishful self-image predomi-nated, these patients were active, assertive achievers, moulding their behav-iour in accordance with their aspirations and attaining their ego-syntonic goals. During such periods the patients experienced, at least temporarily, a sense of accomplishment and an increase in self-esteem, probably related to the presence of more abundant narcissistic supplies. Yet, even during such periods of relative well-being, the insidious effect of the unconscious wishful self-image persisted and was experienced as a vague sense of inner dissatis-faction. Though with lesser frequency, self-defeating behaviour also occurred in these patients' professional lives. It most frequently took the form of 'inexplicable' failure in the course of apparently successful attempts for the attainment of a leadership position. Prolonged analysis revealed that these failures were caused by an unconscious conflict. Typically, the patient uncon-sciously feared that success would preclude the possibility of being 'really

loved' by the oedipal father, whose acceptance and recognition she si
neously sought by excelling and achieving. Such a conflict resulted in «
behaviour, inconsistency and mood swings: factors which interfered
business success.

The chronic subliminal depression of these patients intensified at times
when their impulses and behaviour approximated the characteristics of the
unconscious wishful self-image.[12] It is likely that during such periods narcissistic libido was withdrawn from the psychic self representation, followed by
an increase in aggressive cathexis. The patients' feelings of mortification
increased.

The patients in moments of greatest despair, felt they had a 'rotten core'
which they believed could not be eradicated. Such a feeling is understandable
since the deepest genetic roots of their depression stem from their conviction
that they were not acceptable to mother. Their awareness that father's acceptance and love was only conditional further aggravated their sense of hopeless
worthlessness.

From the life histories of these patients it appeared that they were doomed
to feel pain, no matter what they did. If they succeeded in the attainment of
their avowed goals, they felt unloved as women; if they gratified their
libidinal impulse patterned on the oedipal model, they became involved in
object relationships that were essentially sadomasochistic and unsatisfactory.
The psychic contradictions inherent in the pathology of these women's ego
structure manifested themselves in the oscillation of their behaviour and in
the oft-repeated patterns of masochistic self-defeat.

Conflicts and misunderstandings on the oedipal level superimposed upon
unresolved conflicts about passivity and activity, aggression, submission and
dominance, contributed to the persistence and predominance of the harsh,
sadistic and primitive elements in the superego.

SUMMARY

An attempt has been made via several vignettes and relevant genetic material
to describe the deviant ego structure of masochistic women who unconsciously provoke their self-defeat. It has been found that two wishful self-
images developed concomitantly: one related to the maternal internalizations
which became unconscious, and one related to the paternal internalizations
which became the core of the patients' conscious avowed standard of aspira-

tions. Their self representation was split. It contained two self-images: one maternally and one paternally derived. Fusion of these substructures could not occur because of the permanence of the ego split. Subsequently, superego and ego-ideal development became deviant. Intrasystemic conflict led to pathological behaviour patterns.

For valuable suggestions and thoughtful criticism of an earlier version of this paper, thanks are extended to Drs W. Grossman, E. Jacobson, L. and D. Kaplan, O. Kernberg, D. Milrod, S. Tuttman, M. Zimmerman; and my discussants Drs G. Blanck and Z. O. Fliegel.

NOTES

1. Throughout this paper the terms 'internalization', 'incorporation', 'introjections', 'identification', 'self-image', 'self representation' and 'object representation' are used according to the definitions in Moore & Fine (1968).
2. The effect of oedipal jealousy colouring Ms V.'s interpretation of mother's reaction to coitus was explored and analysed.
3. A report by the *New York Times* (5 April 1974, p. 47) of a study conducted by the National Fertility Ass. in 1970, indicates a preference ratio of 189 boys to 100 girls with regard to the sex of the first-born.
4. Masturbation fantasies recalled as belonging to this phase all had as their conscious theme, excitement, frustration and deprivation of urinary discharge. The frequent confusion between sexual excitement and urinary need has been fully discussed by Greenacre (1950).
5. There can be no doubt that the formation of such a maternal imago stemmed in large measure from these patients' envious, hostile and sadistic impulses towards her.
6. These terms are used throughout the paper as defined and described by Jacobson (1954, 1964).
7. Jacobson (1954) states: 'Self-esteem is the ideational and specially emotional expression of self-evaluation and of the corresponding more or less neutralized libidinous and aggressive cathexis of the self-representations.'
8. As defined by Kernberg (1966).
9. It is likely that the concept of the 'conscious wishful self-image' corresponds in many respects with the concept of the 'ideal self-image' discussed by Sandler *et al.* (1963).
10. These patients were aware that by the standards of our society many of their personality characteristics were considered 'masculine'. They believed that such an appraisal was biased, reflecting the attitude that active and assertive, goal-orientated activity is the prerogative of the male.
11. The exaggerated devaluation of mother, no doubt, was also based on the child's wish to take revenge on her for the infantile helpless dependency which had not been experienced as a loving interaction. Similar views of factors leading to maternal denigration have been expressed by Lerner (1974) and Chasseguet-Smirgel (1976).

12. Similar observations were made by Kaplan & Whitman (1965) in their discussion of behaviour that approximated what they described as 'negative ego ideal'.

REFERENCES

Benedek, T. (1959). Parenthood as a developmental phase: a contribution to the libido theory. *J. Am. Psychoanal. Ass.* 7, 389–417.

Bonaparte, M. (1949). *Female Sexuality*. New York: Int. Univ. Press, 1953.

Chasseguet-Smirgel, J. (1976). Freud and female sexuality: the considerations of some blind spots in the exploration of the 'Dark Continent'. *Int. J. Psycho-Anal.* 57, 275–286.

Coleman, R. W., Kris, E. & Provence, S. (1953). The study of variations of early parental attitudes: a preliminary report. *Psychoanal. Study Child* 8.

Deutsch, H. (1930). The significance of masochism in the mental life of women. *Int. J. Psycho-Anal.* 11, 48–60.

———. (1944). *The Psychology of Women*, vol. 1. New York: Grune & Stratton.

Freud, S. (1923a). The ego and the id. *S.E.* 19.

———. (1923b). The infantile genital organization. *S.E.* 19.

———. (1924). The economic problem of masochism. *S.E.* 19.

———. (1927). Fetishism. *S.E.* 21.

———. (1931). Female sexuality. *S.E.* 21.

———. (1932). New introductory lectures on psychoanalysis: Lecture 33. *S.E.* 22.

———. (1937). Analysis terminable and interminable. *S.E.* 23.

———. (1940a). An outline of psychoanalysis. *S.E.* 23.

———. (1940b). Splitting of the ego in the process of defence. *S.E.* 23.

Giovacchini, P. L. (1972). The symbiotic phase. In P. L. Giovacchini (ed.), *Tactics and Techniques in Psychoanalytic Therapy*. New York: Science House.

Greenacre, P. (1950). Special problems of early female sexual development. *Psychoanal. Study Child* 5.

Hartmann, H. (1950). Comments on the psychoanalytic theory of the ego. In *Essays on Ego Psychology*. New York: Int. Univ. Press, 1964.

Jacobson, E. (1954). The self and the object world. *Psychoanal. Study Child* 9.

———. (1964). *The Self and the Object World*. New York: Int. Univ. Press.

Kaplan, S. M. & Whitman, R. M. (1965). The negative ego-ideal. *Int. J. Psycho-Anal.* 46, 183–187.

Kernberg, O. (1966). Structural derivatives of object relationships. *Int. J. Psycho-Anal.* 47, 236–253.

———. (1967). Borderline personality organization. *J. Am. Psychoanal. Ass.* 15, 641–685.

Lampl-de Groot, J. (1965). *The Development of the Mind*. (Ch. 1, 2, 14, 24, 26.) New York: Int. Univ. Press.

Lax, R. (1972). Some aspects of the interaction between mother and impaired child: mother's narcissistic trauma. *Int. J. Psycho-Anal.* 53, 339–344.

Lerner, H. E. (1974). Early origins of envy and devaluation of women: implications for sex role stereotypes. *Bull. Menninger Clin.* 38, 538–553.

Mahler, M. (1968). *On Human Symbiosis and the Vicissitudes of Individuation*. New York: Int. Univ. Press.

Moore, B. E. & Fine, B. D. (eds.) (1968). *A Glossary of Psychoanalytic Terms and Concepts*, 2d ed. New York: Am. Psychoanal. Ass.

Reich, A. (1953). Narcissistic object choice in women. *J. Am. Psychoanal. Ass.* 1, 22–44.

Reik, T. (1941). *Masochism in Modern Man.* New York: Farrar, Straus.

Sandler, J., Holder, A. & Meers, D. (1963). The ego ideal and the ideal self. *Psychoanal. Study Child* 18.

Sandler, J. & Rosenblatt, B. (1962). The concept of the representational world. *Psychoanal. Study Child* 17.

Schafer, R. (1960). The loving and beloved superego in Freud's structural theory. *Psychoanal. Study Child* 15.

Waelder, R. (1936). The principle of multiple function. *Psychoanal. Q.* 5, 45–62.

Winnicott, D. W. (1956). Primary maternal preoccupation. In *Collected Papers.* New York: Basic Books, 1958.

17. A Consideration of Treatment Techniques in Relation to the Functions of Masochism

Helen Meyers

The treatment of masochistic character problems has long been considered one of the more difficult analytic challenges. The fixity of masochistic trends and their self-defeating nature in life and treatment, as well as the related countertransference reactions, are major constituents of this difficulty. But a part is also played by the complexity of the genesis and the variety of the functions of masochism. Thus, the very differences among the many contributions to the theory of masochism rather than obscuring and contradicting each other (Maleson, 1984) add valuable components to the whole picture. Each contribution is clinically valid and addresses a different function of masochism derived genetically from a different developmental level. Each adds another piece to the puzzle, enriching and filling in the theoretical understanding that informs our clinical interventions. Each piece is necessary for completion of the puzzle. The relative dominance of a particular meaning or function may vary from patient to patient, but often all the pieces play a part and need to be addressed in the same treatment at different times.

Treatment considerations of masochistic features seem of particular importance to me, since I believe that some degree of masochism is universal as long as there is a superego, helplessness and frustration in childhood, a need for object relatedness and self-definition, a need for separation and individuation, and a need for repair of the loss of infantile omnipotence. The difference, of course, is one of degree and quality of maladaptation. I recall no analytic treatment during which masochistic issues did not arise. Certainly in every treatment, resistance to recovery contains masochistic goals as well. This resistance is exemplified *par excellence* in the masochist in the "negative therapeutic reaction," where the patient gets worse instead of better as a result of a "correct interpretation" or after some longed-for success. In a way, all defenses have a masochistic aspect in that they cling to a miscarried

Reprinted from Robert A. Glick and Donald I. Meyers, eds., *Masochism: Current Psychoanalytic Perspectives* (Hillsdale, N.J.: Analytic Press, 1988), 175–88 by permission. Copyright © 1988 by The Analytic Press.

repair (Rado, 1969). Masochistic features appear in the treatment of all character pathologies; however, in the masochistic character disorders, masochistic compromise formations predominate.

THE TREATMENT OF CHARACTER TRAITS IN GENERAL

In this essay, I will address characterologic masochistic problems, masochistic character traits, and their treatment. Before focusing on masochism per se, a few words are in order on the treatment of character traits in general, with its inherent difficulties and complexities. Whether we argue that character is synonomous with the ego or the ego ideal, or is one of its functions, or is a supraordinate concept synonymous with psychic structure as a whole, character results from compromise formations involving identifications and counteridentifications, early endowment, and conflict solution. Character is consolidated in late adolescence. It has been defined as the habitual mode of bringing into harmony the tasks that are presented by internal demands and by the external world, the habitual way of achieving synthesis and integration —involving id, ego, and superego pressures and identifications and internal object relations. Although originating to a significant degree in conflict, character is removed from conflict by its codification of conflict solution and patterned fixity—fixity being represented by distinctive traits or qualities and by typical ways of conducting oneself. The function of character is the maintenance of psychosomatic homeostasis, patterned self-esteem regulation, stabilization of ego identity, and automatization of threshold and barrier levels—with both levels shifting in accordance with the intensity of internal and external stimuli (Blos, 1968). Character traits are consciously ego syntonic but not necessarily adaptive or ''healthy.'' What makes us consider a character trait as pathological is its degree of rigidity and its compulsory nature, the resultant degree of constriction, and the interference with desired function and gratification. While the character trait is developmentally the best compromise solution available under the circumstances, its current use is maladaptive.

Character traits are difficult to change in treatment because of the multiple determinants that reinforce them and contribute to their relative fixity. Letting go of the traits means giving up the secondary gain inherent in the traits, as well as the primary gain involved in the original compromise formation or conflict solution. For the person this may mean giving up a mode of functioning that provided early approval, self-esteem, and self-definition. It may even mean the loss of an idealized introject—as well as facing the original danger. This ego syntonicity, the relative distance from conflict, and the relative efficacy in protecting from anxiety lessens the person's motivation for change and increases the resistance to change. In the masochistic character, we may have a small ally—in that, although there is pleasure in pain, there also is pain.

Turning to the analytic situation, some authors have distinguished between characterologic defenses—that is, those inherent in character traits—as non-specific defenses against the establishment and recognition of transference in general, particularly early in treatment, and the specific resistances that appear in the transference during treatment—that is, the transference resistances. This differentiation has led to a technical debate between those who suggest an approach to character analysis of first "breaking through the character armor" in order to get to the analysis (Reich, 1953) and those who recommend waiting until later stages to analyze character traits—and then only if those traits serve resistance. However, the distinction between character resistance and transference resistance is somewhat misleading. Characterologic defenses continue to appear as resistance against further transference throughout treatment. And the resistances, as they appear in specific transferences, are apt to use the same defense mechanisms as the character defenses. Both use the same armamentarium of available ego techniques to deal with the patient's infantile drive pressures, infantile object relations and superego identifications, and infantile conflict solutions, which have been transferred in a somewhat altered form to the present treatment relationship. Of course, as regression proceeds, earlier constellations are uncovered, and more primitive defenses may come into play. After working through, it is hoped that new, more adaptive and flexible defensive compromises will replace the old, pathologic, rigid characterologic ones. Thus, just as character traits first have to become ego dystonic in order to be analyzed before being interpreted, all resistances first need to be isolated, to be confronted by the observing ego, and to be clarified.

THE MEANING OF MASOCHISM

A number of authors contend that the concept of masochism has become too broad to be meaningful. They have advocated a return to a more limited definition of masochism as states of suffering with a clear linkage to conscious or unconscious sexual (genital) pleasure. I, however, see much merit in the broader concept, which I find extraordinarily useful both clinically and theoretically. The broader concept embraces phenomena that are found throughout our clinical experience and defines a constellation that has specific clinical manifestations and implications and an essential core mechanism. That we recognize this constellation to be multidetermined, and to serve different defensive and narcissistic functions arising from different developmental levels, adds to our ability to understand and deal with it clinically.

The essence of masochism is the intimate connection between pain and pleasure. Masochism has been defined as pleasure in pain. It is the seeking or pursuit of psychic or physical pain, discomfort, or humiliation, where the unpleasure becomes gratifying or pleasurable. Either the seeking or the pleasure or both may be unconscious. Indeed, the masochist, unaware of his or her own agency and satisfaction, frequently is conscious only of the suffering that is experienced as imposed from the outside by fate or by others, who are angrily blamed for the pain. And yet, often there is no mistaking the evident satisfaction in the sufferer's voice, or the gleam in the sufferer's eyes, as he or she asserts yet another failure or humiliation, as defeat is snatched out of the jaws of victory. Only after much work does the sufferer comprehend his or her part in the painful play. There is pursuit of the "pain"—that is, pleasure in the "pain"—because it is unconsciously considered the indispensable condition for need satisfaction or "pleasure." The "pain" then becomes inextricably associated with the "pleasure."

But the gratification need not be only sexual. There are other pleasures and excitements. It may indeed be the gratification of sexual or aggressive drives or their derivatives. Or it may be an ego gratification, such as maintenance of object relations, or self-definition, or self-esteem enhancement. The gratification may be appeasement of the sadistic superego's need to punish. In the compromise formation of masochism, the price of pain pays for gratification and avoids attendant anxiety and dangers of damage, object loss, or loss of self-esteem or identity. Whether the pain itself also is experienced as pleasure, by libidinalization of the destructive instinct or based on the physiologic prototype of excitement associated with any strong stimulus (Freud's, 1924, "erotogenic masochism"), or whether the pain is only the prerequisite for pleasure is still a matter of debate. But it is close enough for the pursuit of pain to become an apparent end in itself. Of course, in life not all pain or humiliation is masochistic. Pain may be inflicted from outside without choice, or unavoidable discomfort may be consciously accepted for the sake of an ideal or conscious goal. It is the motivation of *seeking of the unpleasure* and the satisfaction in it that are key. Compare one war hero's acceptance of danger to achieve a vital objective with another's repetitive seeking out of life-threatening situations for their own sake. Or compare a woman's tolerance of labor pains in order to have a desired child with seeking the pain of labor as the goal and taking pleasure in its severity. It is not masochistic if a mother enjoys her child's pleasure in eating the last piece of chocolate cake; it is masochistic if the enjoyment is heightened because of her own deprivation.

THE FUNCTIONS OF MASOCHISM AND TREATMENT APPROACHES

Masochism is a complex configuration that is multiply determined from different developmental levels and serves various functions. In this motivational hierarchy, one or another of these components may have played a dominant part in the formation of a particular masochistic phenomenon in a particular patient. However, the other components are likely to have been engaged as well, although only in a minor way. Ultimately, it is our understanding of the fact that pain serves an unconscious function in achieving some need satisfaction that gives us our therapeutic leverage to uncover this continued unconscious purpose and its genesis. In treatment, any one of these functions may take center stage or may dominate at any given point in the transference. Sooner or later, however, the other functions will have to be dealt with as well, and sometimes all are operating together in a condensed fashion. Understanding this will determine the timing and content of our interpretations and other interventions.

The following outline is an attempt to relate various technical emphases to our understanding of each function of masochism. Clearly, these points are overlapping and cannot be neatly separated, but the outline should provide a theoretical structure.

(A) Masochism and Guilt

The pain and suffering of masochism are payment for forbidden, unacceptable oedipal desires and aggression, to avoid danger of retaliation—damage and abandonment. The sadistic superego needs to punish, and the masochistic ego submits to punishment out of an excessive unconscious sense of guilt (Freud, 1924). The pain and humiliation unconsciously serve as both payment and permission for further transgression—that is, "pay as you go"

(Rado, 1969). The self-directed aggression is libidinalized. The sadistic superego is appeased and feels pride in its punishing, and the ego feels pleasure in its suffering-moral masochism. At the same time, aggression is directed outward as the masochist provokes and invites hurt and anger from others and with the pain seeks to play on their guilt. In this context, one meaning of a negative therapeutic reaction during treatment is the patient's guilty refusal to accept anything good or to have pleasure without pain. The patient needs to defeat both himself and the analyst.

Insofar as we are addressing this dynamic, the relevant classical technique involves: (1) confrontation of the unconscious active seeking of unpleasure in and out of the transference, a quest that is often consciously misperceived as a search for pleasure that failed; (2) clarification of the projection of this destructive activity onto the outside world—analyst or other—in a kind of "injustice-collecting"; and (3) interpretation of the motivation of the unconscious sense of guilt in its reconstructed genetic context and its current transference manifestations. Here, then, we focus on the oedipal conflict and the role of guilt. The mechanism for change involves mutative interpretation, with a lessening of the severity of the superego. Clearly, it is mainly the third step—the content of the interpretations and reconstructions—that will vary with the elucidation of other functions of masochism; but to some degree the relative reliance on other mechanisms for change also will differ.

(B) Maintenance of Object Relations

Maintenance of object relations is, of course, involved in the oedipal conflict as well, but I would like to focus here on preoedipal issues. Preoedipal aggression against mother in the face of infantile helplessness and frustration is turned against the self (Bergler's [1961] "psychic masochism") to gratify aggression yet avoid retaliation. But here the emphasis is on the maintenance of the all-important object relationship with mother—that is, appeasing the aggressor mother and buying her love with suffering. This has been referred to as "seduction of the aggressor" in childhood (Loewenstein's, [1957] "protomasochism"). As a result of traumatic fixation in this period, for the masochist pain and discomfort continue to be the mode for maintaining vital object relations (Berliner, 1958). Unconsciously, the masochist continues to "seduce" the internalized, critical, maternal object and repetitively reenacts in current relationships and in the transference the old scenario learned at mother's knee. It is a poor way of getting love, but the masochist knows not, nor trusts, another way. Unconsciously, the masochist is convinced that he or she will get love only by submitting to pain and humiliation and will lose his objects if he stops suffering. In this context, a negative therapeutic reaction in treatment also represents the patient's fear that getting better would mean the loss of a vital object relationship.

In addressing this dynamic the relevant technique includes the same three steps as described in the previous section, except that the interpretations and reconstructions would focus on preoedipal issues of helplessness, aggression, and maintenance of object relations. But it involves more: namely the fact that, in the analysis, the relationship does not stop in the face of each success or with each sign of pleasure on the patient's part; nor is the relationship destroyed by the patient's aggression. This new experience provides for the patient a temporary base of trust on which to build. The patient is then able to try out further steps toward a different adaptation without the threat of object loss. Confidence in the continuity of a relationship is, of course, also a factor in working out the oedipal transgressions discussed earlier. Indeed, it is a factor in all analyses, though of relatively different importance. This is not a "corrective emotional experience" stance but the result of the analytic posture and situation.

The maintenance of object relations is of particular importance in masochism in the presence of more severe pathology. Excessive frustration and aggression due to an early experience with a primitive or narcissistic, nonempathic mother may lead to relatively impaired internal object relations and self-images. Defensively, to keep the bad from destroying the good, the bad is split off from the object image, which, for survival, must be maintained as all good, while the self becomes all bad—in a kind of "identification with the aggressor." Aggression and punishment are then directed against the bad self. The defensively idealized, omnipotent, all-good object or self-object is necessary to merge with and shore up the defective or bad self. When masochism serves this function, the two sides of the treatment mechanism described previously assume added importance. The aggression and defensive split must be addressed vigorously by interpretation. Eventually the split must be healed, and the defensive all-good and all-bad images replaced by more complete and stable self and object images. On the other hand, in order to make these interventions work, the patient must first experience a different object relationship in the treatment, contact with an empathic, accepting analyst who validates the patient's feelings and perceptions of earlier experiences. This will lead to the establishment of the necessary trust to permit the patient's internalization of different object and self representations (Berliner, 1958; Stolorow, 1975). Thus, in addition to interpretations in the transference and reconstructions, the added mutative mechanism here is in the diatrophic patient-therapist relationship (Loewald, 1960) and in the empathic self-object function of the analyst, who accepts both the anger and pleasure of the patient.

(C) Masochism and Self-Esteem

Implied in the concept of psychic masochism is a narcissistic function of masochism. In the face of unavoidable frustration, helplessness, and loss of magical infantile omnipotence, the child attempts to repair this injury to self-esteem by asserting some sense of control. The child cannot gratify his own needs or control the environment, but he can pain himself. By turning passive into active, the child can assume responsibility for disappointments and can provoke rejection and extract some pleasure from that: "No one frustrates me against my wishes; I frustrate myself because I like it." This narcissistic function of masochism may be consolidated during separation-individuation with its attendant frustrations and pain (Cooper, this volume, chap. 15). If being disappointed and pained becomes the preferred mode of gratification, the adult masochist feels pride in his or her own agency and sense of control in creating his or her own displeasures—that is, "victory in defeat" (Reik, 1941). This narcissistic investment in masochism comes from various developmental levels. There is pride in undoing early helplessness; in being in control; in manipulating others into sadistic, guilty, or helpless responses; and in being in charge of the desired degree of discomfort (Smirnoff's [1969] "masochistic contract"). There is superego pride in the ability to control one's instincts, in self-abnegation, and in the mastery of pain. There is pride in pursuing one's own course, even if it is painful. There is pride in being special as a victim of fate: "I am in control. I want to be pained. I asked for it. I enjoy it. I can handle it. I have more discomfort than anyone."

In relation to the narcissistic function of masochism, certain technical directions are indicated. Step 1 in the previously described sequence, i.e., confrontation of the patient with his own activity in unconsciously but purposefully seeking unpleasure, assumes special importance. Done tactfully, this approach enhances the patient's self-esteem by underlining his control, rather than his helplessness and victimization by external forces (Eidelberg, 1959). Of course, this intervention also involves the other steps of clarification and interpretation so that by understanding the infantile reasons and origins for the search for and pleasure in pain, the patient will not feel helplessly victimized from within either. The patient can then use this sense of control and understanding to obtain more direct and more fulfilling gratification—pleasure without pain—with a now more mature and competent ego.

At the same time, care must be taken to protect the patient's narcissistic vulnerability. Such interventions must be done with tact and empathy. Otherwise, confrontations of the patient's aggression may be experienced as further proof of worthlessness and badness by the masochist (already burdened by a severe superego) and would represent a further support for the critical internalized object, leading to further masochistic submission. Indeed, these patients often react with increased *mea culpa* after such an interpretation. Or such a confrontation may be experienced by the patient as a sadistic assault by the analyst—a reaction indeed frequently provoked in others by the masochist. This elicits further anger and guilt and further masochistic behavior in the patient.

Insofar as masochism is a component of the narcissistic personality disorder as such, an additional function of the negative therapeutic reaction (Kernberg, 1975) has to be considered. The good object and self representations—the ego ideal—are defensively condensed with the real self images to bolster the real self and form the grandiose self, while the internalized objects are left fragmented and with only a negative valence. This defensive balance is maintained by narcissistic withdrawal, entitlement, and devaluation, which prevent the punitive objects from being effective but also prevent the internalized objects from being invested with anything good. If these objects were to be seen as good it would upset the balance, increase the sense of badness of the self, and lead to further intolerable envy and greed—the basic archaic affects that needed to be defended against in the first place. Thus, the narcissist cannot permit anything "good" in the object. In the transference, the patient must destroy the "good analyst" and reject a good or helpful interpretation. Instead, the patient has to get worse. This is a self-defeating move that is destructive to himself but it also succeeds in destroying the good within the object—thus satisfying the patient's aggression as well as his defensive need to maintain his grandiose self and sense of control. In treatment, this has to be interpreted, as the role of primitive aggression, greed, and envy is confronted and worked on, and the defensive nature of the grandiose self is analyzed.

(D) Masochism and Self-Definition

Frustration and unpleasure are necessary aids in an infant's self-other differentiation and in the establishment of boundaries during the separation-individuation process. The child's need for separateness is tied to the unpleasurable feelings of loss, anger, and guilt toward the "mother of separation" during rapprochement. The "no" of the two-year-old toddler helps him define himself, even when it involves getting into trouble. Unpleasure is experienced as a necessary accompaniment, or condition, for the pleasure in and drive for separateness and individuation. The adult masochist's "I will, too, be self-destructive, and you can't stop me" asserts his control but also defines him as an independent agent—separate, autonomous, and individuated. "I am the sufferer" defines his identity, although it is a negative one. The masochist needs to "do his own painful thing" to feel individuated. Thus, masochistic phenomena appear at various treatment stages in the transference at times in the service of a need for separateness. In patients who must struggle against their wish for and fear of merger masochistic features are seen throughout treatment; in other patients masochism is employed in the pursuit of separation from the therapist only toward the end of treatment. Of course, in certain patients with very early pathology, pain itself can serve the function of self-definition and self-reality.

Technically, masochism in the service of separation-individuation requires interpretation in the transference and genetic reconstruction—although early reconstruction to that phase of separation-individuation may be difficult. But at times, despite all interpretive efforts, the patient seems to have to act out painfully in order to establish a sense of autonomy, even though it may be a self-defeating, masochistic act. This may be difficult for the therapist. However, it may be necessary for the patient to fail on his own, before he can give up this masochistic stance without fear of merger.

Case Illustration. The patient was a bright, good-looking, talented young public-interest lawyer who was pursuing her goal of "serving those in need." She was married to a successful journalist, whom she "loved" and idealized but with whom she was engaged in a painful sadomasochistic relationship in which he abused her physically in frequent fights, humiliated her publicly with frequent affairs, and generally neglected her. It quickly became clear how she masochistically provoked these attacks, knowing just how to stir up this vulnerable man whom she had unconsciously selected in the first place for his narcissistic and sadistic aspects. However, it took some time and much work for her to accept her active part in this pursuit of pain—rather than experiencing herself as the victim. She used this insight into her activity, of course, to further flagellate herself emotionally. As treatment progressed, guilt over oedipal conflicts emerged as the dominant theme in her masochism. She had been her admiring, seductive father's "golden girl," in angry competition with her "sexy" mother, who preferred her brother. She had fled from (yet acted out) this conflict early by moving into several sexual escapades with unacceptable partners, which led to several guilt-filled abortions. One of these partners became her husband.

At this point during treatment, interpretation of oedipal issues was the main tool. She improved and lessened her provocations. The husband first reacted by ceasing to abuse her physically, then stopped his affairs. Things were going better. The patient followed with a series of new provocations and an orgy of self-defeating, humiliating behavior both in relation to her husband and at work. She reported each episode triumphantly with tears and anger. These episodes were multiply determined: Guiltily she could not tolerate success and felt she did not deserve anything good. In the transference, she expressed her rage against her mother-therapist and tried to provoke her by failing and defeating the therapist's efforts—mother was revealed as narcissistic and distant, yet competitive. The patient asserted her control and independence by not getting better. As these issues were worked through, she slowly revealed her conviction that she needed to suffer to seduce her analyst in order to maintain this important sustaining relationship, as she had appeased her critical mother with her painful failures. When neither the aggression nor her slow improvement seemed to interrupt the treatment relationship, the patient permitted herself less pain and more pleasure. When the husband entered his own treatment, which she had dearly hoped for, she acted out self-defeating sabotage by initiating a move to California. As the plan neared completion, analysis revealed that she had felt she needed to fail once again to retain her identity and prove her separateness from the analyst. This was again interpreted, and treatment proceeded to a relatively good termination.

This case, while predominantly oedipal, involved many preoedipal issues as well. The masochism was multiply determined and served various functions. At times, one or another function was dominant in the transference. At times, they all operated simultaneously. The analysis of all of the functions with relevant interventions helped in bringing this case to a fairly successful conclusion.

MASOCHISM AND GENDER

There can be no discussion of the treatment of masochism without some mention of masochism in women, as different from that in men. The theoretical understanding of masochism in women obviously can affect their treatment. If, for instance, women are assumed to be normally masochistic, then a particular masochistic trait in a particular female patient might not be addressed in treatment. On the other hand, a particular behavior in a woman not experienced as masochistic by the woman—for instance, her devotion to a child—might be viewed as masochistic by a male therapist and treated as pathological.

Freud postulated a special feminine masochism. In his view, this type of masochism was an expression of intrinsic feminine nature, linking passivity, submission, masochism, and femininity. This was supposedly based on (1) drive endowment, a constitutional tendency in women toward internalization of aggression; (2) anatomical sex differences, the discovery of which turns the girl from active to passive, and from mother to father, to achieve satisfaction by submission to father in order to get the penis-child; and (3) on oedipal fantasies. This conceptualization was expanded on and supported by Helene Deutsch (1944), who felt that the truly feminine (erotic) woman was one who joyfully embraced the pain of defloration, penetration, menstruation, childbirth, and motherhood. Deutsch postulated masochism, passivity, and narcissism as the three basic feminine traits.

No evidence has been found that women have a greater endowment for deriving pleasure from pain, and the theories of feminine development based on defect have been by now largely discarded (Blum, 1977). Any greater frequency of masochism in women, as evidenced by masochistic sexual fantasies and general masochistic behavior, has been attributed to other factors relating to early development, child rearing, and socialization, such as ego ideal factors involving identification with a mother's masochistic self-representation; parental attitudes toward boys and girls, and internalization of a dependent, passive, childlike, or devalued female gender role image learned from mother or father; superego aspects involving greater prohibition against, and therefore greater guilt around, sexual activity in girls; and the realities of greater male power and privilege in our culture. These factors lead to the "seduction of the aggressor," with masochism being the "weapon of the weak."

Actually it is my thesis that there is no more masochism among women than among men. Perhaps it surfaces in different areas because of the different value systems and content of the male and female superego and ego ideal. But I am not even sure of that. Some behavior considered masochistic in women may be seen as such only by men but not experienced as such by women. Maternal devotion, for example, or faithful support of a partner is likely to be the pleasurable gratification of a loving feeling and should not be confused with masochistic renunciation, enslavement, or guilt over aggression. Of course, some masochistic women do choose the arena of maternal or marital relations to express their masochism. In the case discussed earlier, the presenting problem was a masochistic relationship with a man.

Is this picture of masochistic interpersonal relationships then what we see predominantly in masochistic women, as differentiated from masochistic men? Hardly. The literature is rich with examples of men whose behavior repetitively provokes painful rejection or deprivation from women—the very thing they presumably do not want—and men who masochistically tie themselves to ungiving, abusive, or exploitative women—one need think only of Somerset Maugham's *Of Human Bondage* for an example. Our clinical experience is also rich with such examples. Nor are early developmental issues of narcissistic repair for lost omnipotence or of the separation and self-delineation functions of masochism found less frequently in men than in women. It may be that the issue of men's masochistic relationships to women often emerges only later in the analysis of men—after some regression has taken place and after some of the more obvious self-defeating, success-fearing, guilt-ridden patterns in relation to work and career have been worked through, such as painful overwork, repetitive professional failure, and being "wrecked by success." In the analysis of men, issues about relationships to women are sometimes presented in terms of lack of intimacy, distance, or potency disturbances to start with rather than in terms of pain-dependent attachment. This is perhaps still a reflection of the difference in male and female ego ideal content. Lack of relatedness may still be more acceptable than submission as a part of the male gender role.

This raises the question: How does the analyst's gender influence the clinical process? Can it be that certain masochistic patterns in both men and women are more prevalent or apparent in treatment with a female therapist, who may more easily be experienced transferentially as the preoedipal mother

TYPES OF CHARACTER PATHOLOGY AND TREATMENT TECHNIQUES

(or, of course, with a male therapist who is aware of and permits a preoedipal maternal transference to develop)? For instance, masochism, when equated with passivity, might be more admittable in front of mother. Or, analysis with a woman may be more easily equated with submission to the preoedipal mother and thus reveal early masochistic defenses. The regression to a "seduction-of-the-aggressor" mechanism may emerge more readily in the transference to the preoedipal mother, as a way of dealing with aggression and avoidance of punishment as well as a plea for love. The need for separateness to protect against the wish for and fear of remerger with mother during the reworking of the rapprochement phase of separation-individuation may be in sharper relief in the transference to a female therapist; thus, the issue of pain and guilt in relation to self-definition and self-object differentiation might be more evident.

In my experience (Meyers, 1986), the analyst's gender may influence the sequence of certain transference reactions, their intensity and inescapability, and their temporary displacement to extratransference objects; but the work of the analysis of the multiple dimensions of masochism remains.

REFERENCES

Bergler, E. 1961. *Curable and Incurable Neurotics,* 15–124. New York: Liveright.

Berliner, B. 1958. The role of object relations in moral masochism. *Psychoanal. Q.* 27:38–56.

Blos, P. 1968. Character formation in adolescence. *The Psychoanalytic Study of the Child* 23:245–63.

Blum, H. P. 1977. Masochism, the ego ideal, and psychology of women. *J. Amer. Psychoanal. Assn.* 24:157–91.

Deutsch, H. 1944. *Psychology of Women,* vol. 1. New York: Stratton.

Eidelberg, L. 1959. Humiliation and masochism. *J. Amer. Psychoanal. Assn.* 7:274–83.

Freud, S. 1924. The economic problem of masochism. *Standard Edition,* 19:159–70. London: Hogarth Press, 1961.

Kernberg, O. 1975. *Borderline Conditions and Pathological Narcissism.* New York: Jason Aronson.

Loewald, H. 1960. On the therapeutic action of psychoanalysis. *Int. J. Psycho-Anal.* 41:16–33.

Loewenstein, R. M. 1957. A contribution to the psychoanalytic theory on masochism. *J. Amer. Psychoanal. Assn.* 5:197–234.

Maleson, F. 1984. The multiple meanings of masochism in psychoanalytic discourse. *J. Amer. Psychoanal. Assn.* 32:325–57.

Meyers, H. 1986. Analytic work by and with women: The complexity and the challenge. In *Between Analyst and Patient: New Dimensions in Countertransference and Transference,* ed. H. Meyers. Hillsdale, N.J.: Analytic Press.

Rado, S. 1969. Development of conscience. In *Adaptational Psychodynamics,* 128–37. New York: Science House.

Reich, W. 1953. *Character Analysis*. New York: Orgone Institute Press.

Reik, T. 1941. *Masochism and Modern Man*. New York: Farrar and Straus.

Smirnoff, V. M. 1969. The masochistic contract. *Internat. J. Psycho-Anal*. 50:665–72.

Stolorow, R. D. 1975. The narcissistic function of masochism (and sadism). *Int. J. Psycho-Anal*. 56:441–48.

18. The Rotten Core: A Defect in the Formation of the Self During the Rapprochement Subphase

Ruth F. Lax

A MYTHIC EXPRESSION OF IDENTIFICATION WITH THE AGGRESSOR

The Balinese myth about Rangda, the blood-thirsty, child-eating demon queen (Covarrubias 1974, Hoefer 1974), illustrates the universality of certain early mother-child interactions, and highlights the vicissitudes of identification with the aggressor, which results in a split of the self.

In one version of this story the queen, Dewi Kunti, for reasons unknown, had to sacrifice Sadewa, one of her sons, to Rangda. This made Dewi Kunti very sad since she was a good and loving mother. She could not bring herself to sacrifice her son. However, when the witch, Rangda, entered into Dewi Kunti, she became bewitched and transformed into an angry Fury. In this state Dewi Kunti commanded her Prime Minister to take Sadewa to Rangda's forest. The Prime Minister, who loved Sadewa, did not want to sacrifice him and was saddened by this terrible command. However, the witch, Rangda, also entered into him. This transformed the Prime Minister, and he became angry and violent. He took Sadewa to the forest, tied the boy to a tree in front of Rangda's abode and abandoned him.

Shiwa, the most powerful of all the gods, took pity on Sadewa and gave him immortality. When Rangda arrived, eager to kill and eat Sadewa, she was unable to do so. Admitting her defeat, Rangda asked Sadewa for redemption so she could go to heaven. Sadewa granted her wish and killed her, thus enabling her to go to paradise.

Rangda's most important disciple, Kalika, begged for a fate identical to

Reprinted from Ruth F. Lax, Sheldon Bach, and J. Alexis Burland, eds., *Rapprochement: The Critical Subphase of Separation and Individuation* (New York: Jason Aronson, 1980), 439–56 by permission of Jason Aronson, Inc.

that of her mistress. Sadewa, however, refused. In the ensuing battle Kalika was twice defeated, but when Kalika transformed herself into the powerful Rangda, Sadewa could no longer vanquish her.

In the dance-drama enactment of this story[1] the dagger dancers attack Rangda. The attack, however, fails. Rangda, the embodiment of evil, cannot be destroyed. Finally, to give vent to their anger and, I believe, helpless despair, the Kris dancers turn their daggers upon themselves and in a frenzy repeatedly stab themselves.

Vicissitudes of the child's early fantasy and reality interactions with mother and father are dramatically depicted in this tale. The different personages in the story represent split-off good and bad objects. The destructive element predominates, changing the good mother and also the good father into raging, unfeeling demons. Mother, however, is seen as the prime evil-doer since she — as Rangda (the bad mother) — not only demands the sacrifice of the child, but also as Dewi Kunti (the seemingly good mother) sacrifices him. Expression is thus given to the early *experiential* struggle in which mother is perceived as the potential destroyer. Father — as Prime Minister — at first is seen as weaker than mother. However, as Shiwa, he subsequently becomes the rescuing all-powerful figure onto whom the child projects his omnipotence, which he then reintrojects as the gift of immortality. Made invulnerable, the child's fury at mother and his wish for revenge find expression in Sadewa's killing of Rangda.

The changes in Sadewa's attitude toward killing Rangda can only be understood when one realizes that the plot condenses various versions of the same act, thus reflecting the changing dynamic balance of psychic forces. In the tale different fantasy elements are combined and allowance is made for the conflicting attitudes of the child. Thus:

—the mother is killed but the murder undone by her redemption and immortality in paradise;
—no guilt need belong to the child for it is mother who asks to be killed as an act of atonement for her wrong-doing toward the child;
—the child's unforgiving, vindictive and destructive anger, disguised in the killing of Rangda at her own behest, is apparent in the savage interaction with Kalika, who is killed twice and denied salvation;
—Kalika's final transformation into Rangda, who cannot be defeated, represents the child's awareness of the ''bad'' mother as an ever-present threat.

1. The Barong and Kris dance. A Kris is a dagger often having magical powers. A Kris dancer is a man in a ritual trance.

The myth describes the intensely affect-laden, internalized object relations of early childhood as they are experienced, projected, and expressed primarily in interaction with mother. The Kris dancers who turn their daggers against themselves because they are unable to vanquish Rangda, the "bad" mother, depict one possible resolution of such mother-child strife. They represent the child whose fury has merged with mother's experienced rage and who, having succumbed in the futile struggle with mother, also identified with the self-destructive elements in her (Rangda pleading to be killed). Thus, the Kris dancers dramatically portray the ultimate consequence of an identification with the aggressor (A. Freud 1936).

I suggest that the turning of aggression against the self (as victim) is based on an identification not only with the aggressive but also with the self-destructive elements in the aggressor (mother).

THE ROTTEN CORE: CLINICAL EXAMPLES

Every discussion of a specific aspect of pathology constitutes a delimitation which results in an artifact since it is an exploration of but one strand from the interwoven fabric comprising the harmonious and discordant elements of the human psyche. Mindful of such qualifications, I shall nonetheless make use of this method to highlight a specific form of self-pathology, which is central and gravely disturbing in some personalities.

The women to be described presented a puzzling picture. Each sought treatment after one or two previous therapeutic experiences, and each complained of great suffering in spite of leading an apparently adaptive social and professional life and even enjoying at least partially gratifying object relations.

As far as I could ascertain, there was no uniformity in the causes which brought these patients into treatment initially. On the basis of my work with these women, I did surmise that their previous therapeutic experience was partially successful. It did not enable them, however, to resolve the underlying cause of their recurrent, deep depressions, nor did it enable them to overcome their feeling of discontent with themselves.

In the course of treatment with me, though pained by anxiety, depression, and physical symptoms, each of these patients insisted that the real cause of her suffering stemmed from "something rotten within her" which comprised her innermost self and which filled her with a pervasive sense of doom. One patient said: "It is the sensation of something bad within which makes me feel bad.'' The patients were convinced that nothing they could do or become would change this fundamental fact. The "rottenness" was their essence and made it impossible for them to like and accept themselves.

The patients felt as if they had two selves, thus experiencing a sense of duality. In contrast, outsiders only perceived their well-functioning capable self. The patients sometimes responded to such an appraisal with a modicum of pleasure and sometimes with a feeling of being a "fake." Though the patients enjoyed their achievements they frequently looked upon them as a "way to survive." In general, achievements, accomplishments, and love were only a solace. They mitigated the anguish but did not change its fundamental nature. Good feelings and praise expressed by love objects were appreciated, sometimes even sought actively. They filled these patients with surprise, made them sad and ready to cry. The patients explained these reactions as due to their awareness that good feelings expressed by others neither depicted nor related to their "real self," that is, to their "inner rottenness."

The analyses of these patients' "outer self," which they considered a sham, did not reveal any significant pathology. Were it not for their reported suffering, it would appear that one was dealing with individuals functioning autonomously in a chosen sphere of ego interests, interacting quite adequately with others, and obtaining narcissistic gratification from goals syntonic with their conscious wishful self-image. Ego strength seemed sufficient for the achievement of well-sublimated aims pursued energetically. These patients even appeared to experience pleasure from their achievements. Such gratification, however, was short-lasting. Without any apparent cause, these women again and again would become depressed, filled with suffering, and complain, ascribing their pain to a "bad feeling." The patients insisted that a feeling of inner rottenness interfered with their having a sense of well-being.

I have observed this type of pathology, though it may have differed in degree of severity, in quite a number of patients. Analytic reconstructions indicate that it develops as a consequence of a specific form of interaction with a mother who becomes severely depressed during the patient's toddlerhood.

In the last ten years, chance had it that I worked with four patients whose mothers suffered from a severe reactive depression while their daughters were in the rapprochement subphase. Family anecdotes acquainted my patients with this historical material which they claim to have known all their lives. They told it to me as a bit of life history, in a manner which indicated that it was totally isolated or split-off from their conscious emotions or psychic reactions. I stress this point to emphasize that the patients initially had no conscious awareness of their reactions to mother's depression, nor did they recognize that it had any effect on them. The consequences of their childhood interactions with the depressed mother only became apparent in the later phases of treatment from the analyses of dreams, fantasies, and specific transference manifestations. Analytic work also revealed that the selection of specific types of object relations was unconsciously motivated by this mother-child paradigm.

In my patients, the sense of inner rottenness became a focal aspect of their pathology. The analyses of this malformation led to the understanding of the processes by which it developed and the consequences to which it led.

I have chosen to discuss three of these cases to illustrate, via ''extreme'' examples, the dynamic interactions following maternal libidinal unavailability due to severe depression, and to demonstrate how such mother-child interaction leads to the development of self-pathology.

I do not mean to imply by presenting these three cases that such pathology develops only when mother's depression is reactive. It is also possible that the trauma which evoked mother's reactive depression triggered a latent chronic state. I did observe, however, that the self-pathology which manifested itself by a profound sense of inner rottenness varied in severity depending on the extent of mother's unavailability due to her depression.

The following vignettes will serve to illustrate some of these points, and throw light on specific genetic factors and developmental malformations.

Case 1

Nina, a very successful kindergarten teacher, married and with many friends, could neither accept nor emotionally integrate the love and esteem in which she was held. She would frequently say: ''I am 'hatable' because mother hated me. Since it was mother who had these feelings, they must be correct. I always feel I somehow fool all who love me, only mother knew the truth.''

When Nina was 18 months old, her grandmother, a daily visitor in the parental household, suddenly died of a stroke. Mother, as Nina learned from family anecdotes, became deeply depressed following this event.

Nina pictured her mother as angry and morbid, a compulsive cleaner and housekeeper. Mother accused the family of making her into a workhorse and slave. Nina was a special target of mother's endless accusations. She felt that mother favored her younger sister and looked upon her as a Cinderella. Nina could not become reconciled to mother's lack of loving feelings toward her; she recalled long hours spent in her room tearfully reassuring and consoling herself that, nonetheless, mother really did love her.

Nina was fortunate to have had, and been able to make use of the love she experienced from her maternal grandfather, aunts and uncles. She contrasted their attitudes and lives with the hell she experienced at home. It is not surprising that in her early teens Nina decided that "mother was crazy." She stood alone in this belief, however, since mother capably pretended to the world that "all was well, and she was loving and reasonable." No one but Nina recognized mother's false facade, and even Nina wavered in her conviction.

The feeling of craziness, however, did not apply to mother only. There were times when Nina felt she also was "crazy inside and hid behind the pretense of an outer normal shell." She kept saying, "I feel like a freak. I raised myself to look normal but inside I am crazy. Others tell me I handle things well but this is not how I experience it. I feel I know nothing." These convictions about herself were so powerful that Nina refused to have children. She feared that in her relationship with her child she would reenact the hateful interaction experienced by her with mother. She feared she would curse her child to reexperience her own fate.

The patient said: "I cannot believe I am okay because I was not okay with mother. I am very angry but I learned to cover it up. I sometimes have a feeling of not being there while I smile and talk and everything goes on. That is how I survived my childhood: by not being there so that what mother did and said would not hurt. I feel everything is wrong with me though everyone praises me. Now all of them say I do such a wonderful job, but mother humiliated, ridiculed and destroyed me. I feel sometimes the 'I of me' no longer exists. I feel, most of the time, that the praise I now receive does not relate to me. I can't relate to it and enjoy it. I devalue it."

The patient had broken off contact with mother in her mid-twenties and had not seen her for many years when she started her analysis.

Case 2

Professionally successful, married, and the mother of four, Irene was an anthropologist associated with a leading university. Though she seemed to enjoy life, she complained about a sense of doom and a belief that she was damned to eternal hell. She acknowledged these ideas as irrational but could not free herself of their effect. Irene looked on her personal and professional achievements as not related to her real self. Her depression was well-hidden from the outside world but she was fully aware of it, reporting the onset at about age 5 when she began to pray for death at 100. The ensuing long life span seemed to reassure her; it seemed like eternity. As a child Irene felt guilty though she did not know her crime. Irene grew up to be self-righteous. She had an almost compulsive need to rescue those in distress.

Mother was a beautiful, self-absorbed, empty woman. Though middle class, Irene remembers her as an avid practitioner of preventive voodoo, engaged in rituals to "undo the evil eye." She recalls mother scrupulously collecting her nail parings and cut-off hair, packing them into little bundles and making sure they were completely burned. This procedure was necessary —so Irene learned—to prevent evil-doers from causing her harm. Irene, in spite of her seemingly secure environment, grew up always having a sense of foreboding. Her attempts in later life to refute mother's warnings of an evil around her did not free her of an inner sense that it was always present.

Irene recalled many days of her childhood when mother was silent, distant, and ignored her. On those days Irene felt that mother's behavior was her fault, proof of her wrong-doing. There were other days when mother would clutch her and hold her tight; such behavior made Irene want to get away from mother. Yet, when she succeeded, the sensation that something terrible was going to happen would intensify and overcome Irene. She would feel evil. She would run back to mother only to find her once again distant and silent.

Since late adolescence Irene knew that, during the eleven years following her birth, mother miscarried five times. The first of these miscarriages occurred when Irene was about 22 months old. The significance of these facts, however, only became clear during treatment. Analysis of dreams, memories, and free associations made the specific mother-child interaction more understandable. Via reconstructions it became clear how these events, so traumatic for her mother, incomprehensible to Irene as a child, contributed to her sense of foreboding and doom. Following each miscarriage and intensifying as the years passed, mother expressed her ambivalence on the one hand by possessively holding onto her only living child, and on the other hand, by ignoring her for long periods of time. Mother seemingly became more and more depressed and could not stop mourning for her lost babies. This supposition was confirmed by the fact that Irene recalls that the feelings of foreboding and the sense of being evil intensified as she grew older.

Irene described her self-feelings when she came for treatment as follows: "A time came when nothing good about me felt real. All I knew was the pain of never feeling well. When I made good, kind and friendly gestures to which others responded by grateful, loving acceptance, it did not make me feel good. I knew that I was only propitiating and warding off their evil intents. I did not extend the good gesture out of love but rather out of fear of their evil, to placate them, to buy their good intent, perhaps even love. Thus, the success of my gesture did not ameliorate my sense of inner evil. The knowing, doing, succeeding belongs to the outer part of me. It does not change the rotten core inside. However, as an adult I no longer feel that my rotten core causes others evil, rather it seems to be sapping my life."

Familiar with analytic theory, the patient added: "The evil my mother projected into the world and then tried to undo with her rituals got into me anyhow. It was her hatred."

Case 3

Anna, a Hindu social worker, came to New York from India as a scholarship student to obtain an advanced degree. Extreme anxiety, however, soon interfered with her ability to study. The patient complained about loneliness; analytic work indicated she had difficulty tolerating her separation from mother.

Anna's father had developed Hodgkins disease when she was almost 2. Though her mother was acclaimed to have special healing powers,[2] father refused her help. Mother's anxious depression apparently started at that time.

Mother wanted to make sure that Anna, at least, was protected. To forestall all possible dangers to her daughter, mother purged Anna once a week with a mixture of herbal laxatives. During these sessions a struggle would ensue. Anna would try to run away, but in vain. Mother always triumphed. Anna, exhausted by the ordeal, finally would crawl onto mother's lap. She would feel mother's body enfolding her, "like a spider's web: safe and suffocating." She would fall asleep.

These experiences contributed to the conviction Anna developed that there was something rotten within her. She believed the purgings must have been

2. Mother was a respected homeopathic practitioner.

to "cleanse her from within." Anna said: "I am stuck with it, and there is nothing that can touch it, this feeling of 'I am rotten'. No matter what happens on the outside, I still feel this way. It is like a homunculus in me, black and in flame. I should go to a sorcerer so he could exorcise it and expurgate it. That is what mother tried to do with the purgatives she gave me. It did not work, it is still in me."

DISCUSSION

The term *rotten core* evolved to denote my patients' awareness of an aspect of their psyche which simultaneously is a part of, and yet also is alien to, their self. Grossman and Simon (1969) discuss the causes which lead to the description of inner experiences in anthropomorphic terms. The rotten core should be understood along these lines of reasoning, as a metaphor depicting a specific inner feeling, "a sense of rottenness," known to my patients throughout their lives.

I have used this term in two ways: to provide a phenomenological description of a certain group of observable psychic data and, also, to categorize them. In this latter sense, the term is employed as a hypothetical construct on a level of abstraction corresponding to, but not identical with, such concepts as the bad or good introject and the self-image. Consistent with the structural delineation of the psychic apparatus, the rotten core, along with other self-images, can be conceived as one of the components of the self-representation.

Balint's description of the *basic fault,* as well as Winnicott's observations regarding the *true* and *false self,* will be mentioned briefly since, phenomenologically, patients suffering from each of these deviations appear to have certain similarities with patients manifesting rotten core pathology.

Commenting on the basic fault, Balint (1968) states: "The patient feels there is a fault within him that must be put right. The fault is something wrong with the mind, a kind of deficiency" (p. 21). "A basic fault can perhaps be merely healed provided the deficient ingredients can be found; and even then it may amount only to a healing with defect, like a simple, painless scar." According to Balint, the origin of the basic fault lies in the "lack of fit" between the biopsychological infant needs and the physical, psychological and affectionate care he receives (p. 22).

According to Winnicott (1956, 1960), the origin of the split into true and false self takes place in early infancy. Differences in the degree of this type of pathology are determined by the stage of development at which the greatest pressure for conformity occurred. Winnicott claims that the true self which arises from the vital, creative, subjectively genuine aspects of the individual rooted in the biological givens, becomes stilted, distorted, or completely obliterated, depending on the extent to which the infant is deprived of a "holding" environment provided by "good enough" mothering necessary for unencumbered growth.

Thus the false self develops in proportion to the absence of such mothering and results from premature accommodations to the demands of external reality. It is serviceable in terms of adjustment but internally unsuccessful since it is primarily reactive, the outgrowth of object pressure (usually maternal) and therefore defensive.

The pathology of the self from which my patients suffered resulted from a specific form of identification with the aggressor which occurred at a crucial time in the development of the self. The description of rotten core pathology is an attempt to conceptualize the formation and consequences of a specific split in the self-representation which gave my patients the subjective awareness of a duality of their selves. They described an outer self, the shell or persona which they frequently regarded as "phoney," and a real self, the rotten core. Though the split of the self-representation predominated as the central problem, derivatives of conflicts from various developmental stages were present and combined into different characterological pictures for each patient. However, typical for all these patients was a superego with many primitive sadistic elements experienced by them as a harsh conscience and an ego-ideal containing nonmetabolized grandiose and overidealized elements. A well-developed and wide conflict-free sphere accounted for excellent functioning in many areas of secondary autonomy. Ego functioning was related to a strongly developed conscious wishful self-image (Milrod 1977).

The pathological mother-child interaction affected the nature and quality of the object representation. It partly reinforced the infantile tendency to split the maternal imago and led to a corresponding splitting of the self-representation. The persistence of the splitting process interfered with the consolidating effect of the synthetic function of the ego. As a consequence of these two factors, the achievement of complete self-constancy and libidinal object constancy remained tenuous. Regressive pulls easily eroded this attainment whenever the libidinal object assumed an unconscious, pathogenic maternal significance. When this occurred, like in the instance of a lover's criticism, the ensuing ambivalence triggered splitting with consequent patterns of idealization and devaluation. These patients on the one hand longed to fuse with the idealized object, and on the other acted self-righteously toward the devalued one. Frequently, both these feelings were directed at different times toward the same person. These patients also had a tendency to choose objects onto whom they could project their unconscious devalued self (Lax 1975), as well as objects toward whom they could act out an idealized maternal role.

The patients' pathology, to which there may have been precursors stemming from earlier phases of development, crystallized as a reaction to a specific constellation of internalized object relations (Kernberg 1966, 1976) directly as a response to the consequences of mother's depression. The patients were at that time in the rapprochement subphase. This, as is well known from the studies of Mahler, is a relatively difficult period in the life of the toddler (Mahler, Pine, and Bergman 1975). The "practicing" subphase (Mahler 1968, 1971, 1974), characterized by feelings of exuberance and power which found expression in the "love affair with the world," comes to an end. Typically, these developmental sequelae upset the child's emotional equilibrium. Toilet training brings about further tensions which, at least temporarily, may stimulate aggressive impulses. Omnipotent fantasies, related to anal negativism (whether retentive or projective), are sometimes held onto defensively. In more complicated cases, anal submission may lead to various forms of masochism.

"Shadowing" and "darting-away" behavior patterns are indications of the conflict between the wish for reunion with mother and the fear of engulfment by her. This is the time when the child's increasing awareness of growing separateness stimulates an increased need for mother's love and an increased wish to share with her. As is well known, the intensity of the toddler's wooing behavior can be used as an indicator of the magnitude of the rapprochement crisis.

Only mother's loving acceptance of the child with its ambivalence, as well as her encouragement, provides the necessary ambience for further autonomous growth (Mahler 1971) and leads to normal resolutions of the rapprochement crisis.

Analytic work with my patients made it clear that their mothers could not respond to these typical, phase-specific conflicts and longings. Dreams and transference patterns provided evidence indicating that the mother's psychic equilibrium was seriously disrupted as a result of the trauma she experienced. This manifested itself in several ways.

As illustrated by the case of Irene, mother's behavior became inconsistent.

This was especially significant for the toddler, to whose spurts toward independence mother responded unpredictably, at times with seemingly angry behavior and at other times with possessive holding-on. It is likely that this "clutching," experienced by the child as an invasion of its body autonomy and an interference with "darting-away" behavior, was an expression of mother's reactivated symbiotic needs. Such maternal behavior, however, seems to have intensified the child's age-specific negativism and led to increased power struggles and outbursts of rage.

Nina's case suggests that the quality of her mother's relating also appears to have changed. The child was now seen much more frequently as either good or bad, possibly indicating a breakdown in mother's libidinal object constancy.

Apparent in every case and of foremost significance, however, was mother's depression, which made her emotionally unavailable to the child. Her withdrawal was interpreted by the toddler as anger. This maternal attitude evoked a "hostile dependency" in the child who eventually developed a "basic depressive mood" (Mahler 1966).

Since a toddler is unable to comprehend the objective origins of mother's depression, he regards his own aggressive as well as libidinal strivings as the causes of her moods. A child may thus come to regard mother's emotional unavailability as a punishment. Such an attitude also interferes with the normal progression of separation and individuation processes. This is especially true if the toddler, due to identification with mother, begins to regard his impulses toward autonomy with the disapproval he ascribes to her.

Margaret Mahler (1971) points out that a stormy separation-individuation process results in the development of

an unassimilated foreign body, a "bad" introject in the intrapsychic emotional economy. In the effort to eject this "bad" introject, derivatives of the aggressive drive come into play and there seems to develop an increased proclivity to identify with, or to confuse, the self-representation with the "bad" introject. If this situation prevails during the rapprochement subphase, then aggression may be unleashed in such a way as to inundate or sweep away the "good" object, and with it the "good" self-representation [p. 412, italics mine].

Following such a conflagration, a defensive regression to the stage when object and self are less clearly differentiated and are split into a "good" and "bad" self-object, may occur.

I suggest that the prevalence of such an intrapsychic conflict state may lead to the formation of the rotten core which on the most primitive level represents the fusion of the "bad" (angry-rejecting) maternal introject with the "bad" (rejected) aspects of the self. Subsequently experienced maternal anger fused with the child's projected anger becomes turned against the self. Under the impact of intensified separation anxiety, a regression may occur, and annihilation anxiety may become reactivated. Such a condition leads to further defensive splitting in an attempt to preserve the "good" object and the corresponding "good" self (Kernberg 1966, Mahler 1971, Giovacchini 1972). As a consequence, not only the object representation but also the self-representation remains (or becomes) divided. The rotten core represents that part of the self which was "hatable" to mother. Continued identification with the aggressor (A. Freud 1936) contributes to the establishment of the rotten core as a permanent substructure. Two aspects of this process can be recognized, each reenforcing the existing split in the self-representation.

First, the identification with the maternal attitude toward the child fosters in the child an *identical* attitude toward his self. Thus, maternal aggression becomes self-aggression, and the self becomes the victimized object. Further, aspects unacceptable to the aggressor-mother also become rejected by the child merging with the primitive rotten core toward which the combined mother-child hatred has been directed.

The second aspect of the process of identification with the aggressor arises from the wish to obtain mother's love and to participate in her power. Identifications so motivated augment early introjections and the fusion with the "good" mother and her beloved aspects. They contribute to the formation of the "good" self and its loved aspects.

The rotten core and "good" self are formed at a developmental stage during which polarization and splitting still prevail (Kernberg 1966, 1971, Mahler 1971). A preponderance of hostility in the vicissitudes of mother-child interaction prevents subsequent merging of these psychic substructures into a consolidated and integrated self-representation.

Internalization of mother's self-destructive tendencies, of her depression, hopelessness and helplessness represents a further aspect of these children's identification with the aggressor. The dynamic continuation of these processes was indicated in the treatment situation by a conviction these patients held that change was not possible. The patients frequently felt desperate.

These patients' adaptive functioning in their capacity to make use of their resources led me to the assumption that mother-infant-toddler interaction preceding mother's trauma was sufficiently good to result in the formation of a "good" introject. This provided the basis for the unconscious identification

with loved, admired and even envied aspects of the maternal imago. In later
years, selective identifications consonant with the conscious wishful self-
image eventuated in satisfactory autonomous ego functioning in circumscribed areas. Mahler's finding (1966), which indicates that autonomous ego
functioning can remain unimpaired in children in spite of intense psychic
conflicts, supports my observations and conclusions.

The self to which these patients referred as the "persona" or "outer shell"
combined all the "good" identifications. However, an apparent insufficiency
of neutralized libido and aggression interfered with the development of an
optimal narcissistic cathexis of this self. Thus, adequate self-esteem was
lacking. Harmonious interaction between ego, superego, and ego-ideal remained impeded. The self-representation remained split because it contained
the nonmetabolized rotten core.

I recognized early in my work with this type of patient the cleavage in
their self-representation. I remained puzzled, however, by the apparent complete lack of malleability of the rotten core. Its poisonous effect continued in
spite of the narcissistically gratifying attainments of the "outer self." Some
answers to this enigma were provided by the analyses of the transference and
also by the patients' continued and current relationships to their mothers.
Thus, in spite of an ungratifying and frustrating interaction, these patients
persisted in their tenacious demandingness and holding-on. Likewise, behavior in the transference was demanding, pleading, and provocative.

Analysis of these patterns of relating revealed an unconscious fantasy in
which mother was idealized as the good fairy able to gratify the child in
every conceivable way, no doubt representing the good symbiotic mother
(Mahler 1971). The intensity of longing for this fairy-mother grew depending
on the extent of the mother's libidinal unavailabiity in the child's reality and
the painful frustration this evoked. This fantasy persisted into adulthood
because the reality of mother's behavior was unconsciously justified by a
corresponding unconscious conviction that it was caused by an inability to
evoke her goodness. Transgressions in fantasy and reality were used to
explain mother's anger, aggression, and hatred. These patients felt mother
hated them because they were "rotten." The uncovering and analysis of this
fantasy also elucidated the reasons for these patients' openly provocative
childhood behavior: it served to change what seemed like mother's incomprehensible anger into an understandable reaction.

Bound up with the rotten core, emanating from the "bad" introject and
reinforced by subsequent identifications with the aggressor, the self-turned,

hateful anger remained unrelieved in these patients in spite of the gratifications related to the functioning of the "outer self." Their continuous "pain
of living" (a patient's phrase) and the identification with the self-destructive
elements in the aggressor led to intense suicidal wishes. However, the fantasy
belief that sufficient suffering would bring atonement and with it the rescue
by the good mother kept these patients in their pervasive self-torture and
prevented them from actually committing suicide. Nonetheless, the wish for
relief brought by death was great. Expressed in the idiom of the Balinese
myth, Rangda, who could not be vanquished, made those fighting her turn
their daggers against themselves.

I have observed the rotten core with its related pathological character
formation primarily in women. I do not wish to imply, however, that this
pathology is prevalent in women only or primarily. Colleagues have reported
on similar character constellations in men.

I have not discussed the father since he did not seem to have a direct role
in the formation of the rotten core. He was, however, very significant for my
patients in their childhood, both in his role as rescuer (Abelin 1971), and as
a model for identification (Lax 1977). Frequently the relationship with father
was prematurely intense, complicating the subsequent oedipal involvement.

SUMMARY

The formation of a psychic substructure, the *rotten core,* which originates as
a reaction to a depressed mother's lack of libidinal availability to the child
during the rapprochement subphase, is described as a specific type of self-
pathology. The child perceives and experiences such a mother as rejecting.
The internalization of the interaction with her results in a specific kind of
identification with the aggressor. This identification leads to the formation of
a rotten core which on the most primitive level represents a fusion of the
"bad" (angry-rejecting) maternal introject with the "bad" (rejected) aspects
of the self. In patients with such a pathology, the rotten core and the "good"
self do not merge into a consolidated and integrated self-representation. This
is due to the preponderance of hostility in the mother/child interaction which
accounts for the persistence of defensive splitting.

The description of rotten core pathology is an attempt to conceptualize the
formation and consequences of the specific split in the self-representation
which gives these patients the subjective awareness of a duality of their

selves. Developmental consequences of this pathology are discussed. Three clinical vignettes are presented.

REFERENCES

Abelin, E. L. (1971). The role of the father in the separation-individuation process. In *Separation-Individuation: Essays in Honor of Margaret S. Mahler*, eds. J. B. McDevitt and C. F. Settlage, pp. 229–253. New York: International Universities Press.

Balint, M. (1968). *The Basic Fault: Therapeutic Aspects of Regression*. London: Tavistock.

Covarrubias, M. (1974). *Island of Bali*. Kuala Lumpur: Oxford University Press.

Freud, A. (1936). *The Ego and the Mechanisms of Defense*. New York: International Universities Press.

Giovacchini, P. L. (1972). The symbiotic phase. In *Tactics and Techniques in Psychoanalytic Therapy*, ed. P. L. Giovacchini, pp. 137–169. New York: Jason Aronson.

Grossman, W. I., and Simon, B. (1969). Anthropomorphism: motive, meaning, and causality in psychoanalytic theory. *Psychoanalytic Study of the Child* 24:78–111. New York: International Universities Press.

Hoefer, H. (ed.) (1974). *Guide to Bali*. Singapore: Apa Productions.

Kernberg, O. (1966). Structural derivatives of object relationships. *International Journal of Psycho-Analysis* 47:236–253.

———. (1971). Prognostic considerations regarding borderline personality organization. *Journal of the American Psychoanalytic Association* 19:595–635.

———. (1976). *Object-Relations Theory and Clinical Psychoanalysis*. New York: Jason Aronson.

Lax, R. (1975). Some comments on the narcissistic aspects of self-righteousness: defensive and structural considerations. *International Journal of Psycho-Analysis* 56:283–292.

———. (1977). The role of internalization in the development of certain aspects of female masochism: Ego psychological considerations. *International Journal of Psycho-Analysis* 58:289–300.

Mahler, M. S. (1966). Notes on the development of basic moods. In *Psychoanalysis a General Psychology*, eds. R. M. Loewenstein et al., pp. 152–168. New York: International Universities Press. Reprinted in *The Selected Papers of Margaret S. Mahler*, vol. 2, ch. 5. New York: Jason Aronson, 1979.

———. (1968). *On Human Symbiosis and the Vicissitudes of Individuation, volume I: Infantile Psychosis*. In collaboration with M. Furer. New York: International Universities Press.

———. (1971). A study of the separation-individuation process and its possible application to borderline phenomena in the psychoanalytic situation. *Psychoanalytic Study of the Child* 26:403–424. New York: International Universities Press. Reprinted in *Selected Papers*, op. cit., ch. 11.

———. (1974). Symbiosis and individuation: The psychological birth of the human infant. *Psychoanalytic Study of the Child* 29:89–106. Reprinted in *Selected Papers*, op. cit., ch. 10.

Mahler, M. S., Pine, F., and Bergman, A. (1975). *The Psychological Birth of the Human Infant: Symbiosis and Individuation*. New York: Basic Books.

Milrod, D. (1977). The wished-for self-image. Unpublished manuscript.

Winnicott, D. W. (1954). The depressive position in normal emotional development. In *Collected Papers*, pp. 262–277. New York: Basic Books, 1958.

———. (1956). Primary maternal preoccupation. In *Collected Papers*, op. cit., pp. 300–305.

———. (1960). Ego distortion in terms of true and false self. In *The Maturational Processes and the Facilitating Environment*, pp. 158–165. New York: International Universities Press, 1965.

19. The Anti-Analysand in Analysis

Joyce McDougall

In this chapter I shall trace the portrait of a certain kind of analytic patient who is becoming more frequent in today's practice. I hope to delineate characteristic features which may be recognized by other analysts as belonging to a specific clinical "family." The patient I have in mind appears well motivated to undertake an analysis. Filled with good intentions, he adapts readily to the analytic *situation*—in contradistinction to the analytic *process* —and accepts with apparent ease the formal aspects of the analytic protocol. This patient comes to sessions regularly, fills the silent spaces of the analytic hour with clear and continuous associations, pays the fees at the end of the month—and that is all. After several weeks of listening to him, you begin to realize that nothing is happening, either in the context of his discourse or between him and yourself. No transference feelings are expressed with regard to the present; as to the past, his stock of childhood memories remains static, divorced from present-day reference, and lacking in affect. Such a patient shows a preference for recounting daily events in which, though irritation may be expressed, there is little trace of anxiety or depression. Limited tenderness toward others is displayed, and one often has the impression that "love is just a four-letter word." This analysand rarely seeks within himself the factors that might contribute to his conflicts with others, yet he is far from happy and totally unsatisfied with his life. In spite of his diligence— and your own—the analytic process never quite gets started.

You may have noticed in this description that this patient in no way resembles those considered as "counterindications" for a classical analysis: that is, patients who do not tolerate the frustration imposed by the analytic situation with its customary austerity, who take flight at the first awakening of transference feelings, who act out in ways that may be disastrous for themselves or others, or who lose contact with reality and seek escape in psychotic fantasies. The analytic experience makes an overwhelming impact on the psychic equilibrium of such patients, and one must be careful not to

Permission granted from the *Revue Française de Psychanalyse* (1972). Originally published in English in 1980.

engage them too rapidly in full-scale analysis. In contrast, the patients I am trying to describe appear unmoved by the impact of the analytic relationship, do not regard it as frustrating, do not lose for one moment their firm grip on reality, do not act out either within or outside the analysis (unless one considers their whole way of life as a continual acting out). Finally, it is important to emphasize that these analysands do not in any large measure display that particular form of acting out manifested in psychosomatic illness. That unexpressed emotional conflict is not somatized is of specific interest in that these patients reveal many of the characteristics of the mental functioning of so-called "psychosomatic" patients, and in particular, the phenomenon which Marty and de M'Uzan (1963) have named "operational thinking." I shall return to this point later.

It is tempting to name the subjects of my study the "robot analysands." Indeed I shall sometimes refer to them in this way since they give the impression of moving through the world of people and things like automatons, their thoughts appearing to be programmed along accepted channels. For many this also affects their manner of speaking, a robot language impregnated with clichés. However, the term "robot" carries with it a suggestion of passivity which would be erroneous. By choosing instead the term "anti-analysand" I hope to convey the impression of force as implied in the concept of anti-matter, a massive strength that is only revealed through its negative effect, its opposition to the functions of cohesion and liaison. In the psychic economy, such a force mitigates against the formation of all the creative links that allow a psychoanalytic treatment to become what Strachey (1934) called a "mutative" experience. In a certain sense these patients might be said to be engaged in "anti-analysis" which requires a measure of forceful and continued activity, but whose effects are only discernible through the absence of psychic change: a negative force of antiliaison which at the same time petrifies all that has been split, foreclosed, or otherwise ejected from inner psychic reality. Such a patient does not speak in an incomprehensible or distorted fashion. He talks of people, and of things, but rarely of *the relation between people or between things*. In listening to his analytic discourse we do not clearly detect behind the manifest communication a vitally important latent one. Nor do we have any inkling of who we are or what we represent for the patient at different moments in the session. Nor do we witness that interpenetration of primary-and secondary-process thinking, the intermingling of dream imagery, fantasy and conscious thought that so often opens the way to an intuitive understanding of what the patient is struggling to communicate. The unconscious inner theater never reveals itself. We slowly come to realize that certain essential linking thoughts, which normally give depth of meaning to the analytic discourse, are missing. These may be links in time between past and present events, links in the content of associations, or affective links with others having libidinal or narcissistic importance for the patient—and last but not least, there is little evidence of transference ties to the analyst or to the analytic adventure. The primordial tendency of human beings toward object-relating which gives to the transference relationship its blind instinctual quality (and makes life itself a worthwhile adventure) is perhaps the most conspicuous lack. What phenomena are we engaged in observing?

The outstanding scientific observer Konrad Lorenz once remarked that the most difficult and often the most important observations are those that detect that an object is *missing,* that an action *fails to occur,* that an anticipated phenomenon is absent. In psychoanalysis, which is also an observational science, it is equally essential, and difficult, to ''see'' what is missing from the analytic scene or from the patient's communications. We owe to the French psychoanalysts, Marty and de M'Uzan (1963), a series of observations of this kind, which I would readily compare with those of Lorenz, that led to the discovery of a missing dimension in the recorded verbal communications of patients with psychosomatic illness in an interview situation. As with these patients, the style of speech of the anti-analysands tends to be flat, lacking in nuance, meager in the use of metaphor. As to content, there is in both cases an apparent poverty of imagination and a difficulty in understanding other people. Added to the restriction in the content of thought and the quality of communicating is a noticeable lack of affect. An impoverishment in the communication of ideas as well as of emotion cannot but limit severely the field of analytic observation. But since the analyst is also a trained observer of his own thoughts and emotions, he is usually quick to detect his countertransference affects and to turn them to account in order to understand more profoundly what is occurring in the analytic relationship. It is largely through studying my countertransference feelings (insofar as they are conscious) that I have become aware of the clinical picture I am describing and have arrived at certain theoretical deductions regarding the psychic structure and functioning of these patients.

Although interesting and different from normal-neurotic patients, these analysands do not always afford us much pleasure in the exercise of our analytic function. Not only do they engender in us a feeling of helplessness;

in addition, they make us feel guilty! So they are something of a challenge. After all, it seems inadmissible to say of a patient who comes regularly to his sessions month after month, who follows as best he can the basic rule of saying all that comes to his mind during the session, and who clings tenaciously to the belief that psychoanalysis is a valuable experience and one that he wishes to possess, that this diligent patient is unanalyzable! Unless we ourselves, like him, are insulated against self-criticism, we can scarcely avoid feeling that something must be wrong with our analytic work. Before blaming him for his incapacity to profit from what we are offering him we must first question our decision that led to his being in analysis. Are we in the wrong for having judged him to be analyzable and having thus accepted him? Is his true symptom the fact that he continues to be in analysis? These and other harassing questions form the basis of a searching inner dialogue.

I am also beset, as time goes on, by the countertransference queries that graft themselves onto those already mentioned. The patient lying on my couch is offering me today a series of associations that in no way differ from those he brought to his first analytic sessions some four years ago! Is it a resistance on my part to grasp the underlying significance of what he recounts? Over the years, in my seminars for young analysts on the phenomena of transference and countertransference, I have steadily maintained that everything the analysand says has some reference to the analytic situation or relationship; that no thought, no fantasy, is ever entirely gratuitous. If I have been unable, in spite of my concern and my varied attempts to communicate something which would produce some change in this analysis, have I been unimaginative with him? Should I have made more "Kleinian" interpretations of increasingly archaic material, overlooking his constant refusal to accept any interpretation as worthy of attention? Should I have adopted an aggressive "Reichian" approach and attacked with force his characterological "armor-planting"? Yet, when I come to think of it, over the four years I have elaborated many hypotheses, tried many an innovation, made interpretations of Kleinian, Reichian, Winnicottian and Lacanian inspiration as well as some special ones of my own—to no avail. Experience has taught me that to remark on the feelings of emptiness and dissatisfaction (for the analysand is quite as unhappy as the analyst in these situations), or to propose fantasies of one's own, which might be linked to the endlessly factual narrative, can only lead such a patient to the conclusion that *his analyst has a problem.* "But I say everything that comes into my head and you are not satisfied. What do *you* want me to talk about?" Should I throw away the structured analytic situation? Have him sit up and face me? Invite him for a drink? Anything to shake him up. I become aware that, even if my analysand shows no trace of conscious fantasy, I on the contrary am filled with odd ideas, with a wish to act out, change something, anything to get us out of the rut. But then if I were to act upon these ideas I in turn would become an *anti-analyst!* The structured protocol that protects my patient from my violence toward him also keeps me in my role of analyst. Thus I resist the temptation to throw away the analytic relationship—but what next? I must also resist the temptation to fall asleep!

At this point, I admit that most of what I have written above was noted down during a recent session of Mr. X. He is a typical robot analysand. I consider my work with this patient as a complete and spectacular failure. And he is no more satisfied than I with this fruitless partnership. Architect, forty-four years old, married, with two children, Mr. X comes from a milieu in which analysis is highly esteemed, wherein many friends and even family members have had analysis. These latter details are also typical features of my anti-analysands; they are not specific to Mr. X.

In the beginning I saw X four times a week. After two years of seeming stalemate, I tactfully reduced him to three, then to two weekly sessions. X was not fooled. He told me he was well aware that his analysis was not progressing. This opinion was further supported by the fact that a friend told him an analysis lasts four years—and here we were in the fifth! He wondered whether I might have bungled his case. I seized the occasion to tell him that I had been asking myself the same question, and suggested we might consider a change of analyst. But Mr. X would not hear of it. Denying my intervention to the effect that he felt rejected, he requested I return the two sessions that had been taken away. He seemed prepared to settle in for another four-year siege, as though he were not truly suffering from the sense of stagnation. I was and could not feel optimistic about the value of continuing. These countertransference feelings should have been useful to me and should have provided the basis for future interpretations, but I did not hold such expectations in this case. Even though my affective reactions have given me valuable insight into the psychic functioning of patients like Mr. X, this did not produce any significant change.

I could take at random any of X's sessions to demonstrate the atmosphere generated by his associations. On the day on which these lines were written he was complaining, as he had often in the past, of his children's constant and inexplicable demand to be always at his side. He loved them, naturally, but enough was enough! Without transition, he went on to describe a sort of cupboard he was building in his country cottage. He complained bitterly of his wife's lack of interest in the cupboard. After twenty minutes, like his wife, I too lost interest in it. The sole difference was that I felt guilty about it. Yet I knew in advance that for X a cupboard would never be accepted as a symbol; there was no significance to be found in this choice of topic. I could, of course, suggest that he was trying to find out if I was more interested in his cupboard than his wife. He would most certainly reply: "Do you think so?" and proceed to give me the measurements. Refusing to let slip my analytic mask of benevolent neutrality—which otherwise might have led me to say, "Ah, how you bore me, you and your cupboard"—I beat a narcissistic retreat. Embedded in my own thoughts and fantasies, I suddenly realized I had stopped listening.

What went on in Mr. X that led him to cling so tenaciously to this nonanalysis we were doing together? And *why* did nothing ever happen between us that might turn this laborious partnership into a truly constructive analytic experience?

Before attempting to answer these questions I should first comment on my reasons for having accepted X as an analytic patient. I had no lack of patients; indeed, he was obliged to wait nearly a year before beginning his analysis— a delay he accepted cheerfully, although he expressed considerable disappointment at not beginning immediately. X had been referred to me by a senior colleague who knew the family well and, having talked with X about his analytic prospects, considered him a "good analytic case." But this did not in any way make me feel I had to take him. The truth of the matter was, having interviewed X myself and having weighed his reasons for wanting analysis, I too was convinced that he was an excellent "case." Like the other patients who resemble him, he was intelligent, showed a cultural acquaintance with psychoanalytic ideas, knew several people (including his own wife) whom he considered to have benefited considerably from analysis. Among the different reasons he advanced for seeking analysis the first was that his wife had brought up the question of divorce, an eventuality to which he was bitterly opposed. He was to tell me many months later that he was opposed to divorce as such because it was not consistent with moral standards. "Normal" people did not divorce and that was that. The fact that his wife might have been unhappy in the marriage, or that he himself might have felt emotionally attached to her, did not enter into his approach to the problem. In this initial interview, however, he offered a more promising insight into his wife's demand. He confided that all his relationships seemed unsatisfactory, in particular that which he maintained with his wife. He even went so far as to question whether something in his own character might have led his wife to wish to leave him. In saying this he was trying to give me what he considered to be a good "analytic" explanation for the inexplicable; this in no way meant that he believed it or intended to explore such an idea. X then went on to offer, as others like him had done, a sprinkling of neurotic symptoms: a hindering phobia, some professional inhibitions, and a recurrent sexual symptom. I was to discover to my dismay that these symptoms did not interest him in the slightest. He talked to me also about the early death of his brother when he was ten, of his weak and philandering father, and of his pious and stern mother—promising internal objects such as a "good neurotic" might be expected to harbor. Not only was he in search of self-knowledge, he was convinced that analysis could help him to find it, and was prepared to devote time and money to this end. What more could I want? Alas, I did not know that Mr. X had never failed an examination in his life —and that he was little likely to fail his initial interviews with the psychoanalyst. I am tempted to say that X "fooled" me, which in fact he did, but this would imply that he acted in bad faith, which was not the case. He revealed everything he considered it his duty to show me in order to justify his request for analysis. In the bottom of his heart he held his wife responsible for all that was wrong between them, and where she could not be held to blame the world in general was considered at fault. These were articles of faith that could neither be put in question nor modified; they formed an integral part of his character and were essential to the maintenance of his feeling of identity.

Patients like Mr. X have all developed such pivotal keys to explain their problems and dissatisfaction with life. If for Mr. X the cause of his discontent was the existence of his wife, his children, and his colleagues, for Mrs. O, a young professor in her thirties, married, with two little girls, all misery stemmed from the fact that she was a woman. The following fragment of her analysis comes from a session in the third year of our work. "You say I never talk about my childhood. Well now I was born in L. . . . and my cousin also, the boy who was two years younger than I was. We lived there until my mother's death. My father preferred my cousin, that was only normal. My mother tried to show no preference, but of course she was pretty disappointed to have had a girl. But I've told you all this before." "Yes, but you have never explored the question of how painful this must have been for you." "Nonsense. I won't buy that. Why those were the happiest years of my life.'' ''It might not have been easy feeling that both your parents preferred the boy. You may have wondered why?'' ''Naturally I would have preferred to be a boy—but who wouldn't?'' Having gone into this question with Mrs. O from every conceivable point of view, I tried on this occasion to elicit a new fantasy. I told her that some men envied women because of their ability to create children, or to attract the father sexually. ''Then they must be nuts!'' replied Mrs. O vehemently. The implication once more was that my continuing attempts to find an underlying meaning to her pain and fury about being a woman obviously meant I had a problem, since her position was the only sane one. Perhaps she was right in considering this to be my problem, since I could clearly remember that one of my principal reasons for accepting her in analysis was that she had sobbed bitterly when I told her that from all she said I felt she had problems about being a woman. Through her tears she had whispered she ''lacked femininity.'' What I had not grasped was that she felt convinced I would see the dilemma of being a woman in the same light. My effort to find an explanation for her intense bitterness only served to exasperate her. If I had not had the courage to point out that, even after analysis, she would still be a woman, it was because I truly believed she wanted to understand her pain and find a creative solution to it. Instead she wanted to convince me of the grave injustice she had suffered from birth, and stick to her simplified solution. There is no doubt she had suffered from hurtful parental words concerning her sexuality and her femininity, but the neurotic symptoms to which these had given rise evoked no interest in her. Her total frigidity, a severe phobia about being touched, even by her husband and children, seemed to her to warrant no exploration. ''It's like that and that's all there is to it!'' Later she confided to me that her therapeutic goal was to have completed ''a thousand analytic hours.'' This figure had been proffered by a psychoanalyst friend as being the right number.

Here briefly are the clinical features of my anti-analysands:

—This type of patient presents himself with a convincing and acceptable set of problems from the usual analytic point of view with regard to suitability for analysis. His robotlike character structure enables him somehow to be correctly ''programmed'' in advance for his project.

—Once installed in the analytic situation (whose conditions he accepts without ado) he begins a detailed and intelligible recital but the language he employs is striking by reason of its lack of imagery and affectivity. In spite of better than average intelligence, the patient is capable of displaying a banality of thought akin to mental retardation. The affectless quality of his object relations recalls those of children who have suffered early object loss. Where events of loss or abandonment have actually existed, these are recalled without emotion, and treated like inevitable injustices. There is no reliving of such events in the transference, nor interest in exploring the loss.

—His neurotic problems, as well as those of others, arouse no curiosity in him.

—With the exception of a few fixed memories, he lives firmly rooted in the present; like journalists, he seems to live for the events of a single day. Though his past or present be filled with dramatic events, he seems to devitalize these, making them appear banal.

—His emotional links to the people important to his life are presented as flattened, lacking in warmth. He nevertheless frequently expresses dissatisfaction rising sometimes to heights of considerable anger against his close friends and family, or directed to the human condition in general. In spite of this the patient maintains stable object relations and in no way seeks to be separated from the objects of his wrath and rancor.

—The transference carries the same feeling of affective emptiness; even the aggressive feelings readily expressed against the entourage are stifled in the analytic context. The analyst may have the impression of being *a condition rather than an object for the analysand*. I would readily describe this as an "operational" transference. It in no way resembles the *transference resistance* noted by Bouvet (1967) as characteristic of obsessional patients. The anti-analysand does not maintain an optimal safe distance from the analyst as does the obsessional neurotic: instead, he appears to deny that any distance exists, thus denying the analyst any individual psychic reality. This way of apprehending the analyst is repeated with people in the everyday world. To this extent, it may be considered a sort of "transference" from an habitual relationship pattern, but its roots in the infantile past are difficult to discern since the world of internal objects is also somewhat delibidinized.

The course of the analysis does not reveal massive repression—which otherwise might have found some transference expression or revealed itself in dreams, symptoms, and sublimations. Rare dreams do, however, reveal evidence of primitive psychic conflict. A vast chasm seems to separate the anti-analysand from his instinctual roots, giving the impression that he is also out of contact with *himself,* that this is not restricted to his inner and outer objects. There is thus an overall impression of an ill-defined transference from the past in which the small child of former times urgently had to create a void between himself and others, wiping out their psychic existence and so stifling intolerable mental pain. The distance between subject and object is then reduced to nothing, but *without any recovery of the decathected object in either its loved or hated aspects.* Where the object should have found a place either as part of the subject's own ego or as an object of his ego, there is a blank. Such patients do not therefore get lost in their contact with others or merge in psychotic fashion with parts of other people. It would be more exact to say that others have become lost somewhere inside them. These are children who have never mastered the spool and the peekaboo games which inspired such profound reflection in Freud. Refusing to admit other people's psychic reality, refuting the trauma of separation, these patients dispense with many aspects of identification because Others have become exact copies of themselves. Instead of seeking to know their psychic reality they offer their own. It is no doubt for this reason that the analyst's interventions and interpretations elicit only marginal interest and have little impact. When the patient finds himself forced to recognize difference and separate existence, whether this becomes evident through serious differences of opinion or a mere difference in matters of taste, he is quite likely to react with excessive hostility. But in general Otherness does not threaten him in that he disavows its possible influence.

Since the same phenomena appear in the transference, with consequent denial of the analyst's separate psychic reality, little affect is projected into this psychic space. As a result, hypotheses and anxiety about what the analyst thinks of him do not unduly preoccupy the analysand and do not propel him to fear criticism or to seek approval or to question his desires and relationships, nor even his symptoms. If the analyst persists in trying to *analyze* different aspects of the patient's associations, thoughts, and feelings, or to interpret fleeting transference manifestations—in other words if through these means the analyst reveals himself as *Another* by searching for underlying meanings in his analysand's discourse—the patient is liable to feel persecuted, unless he comes to the conclusion that the analyst is disturbed in some way.

What holds this psychic structure together? Such denial of certain cardinal aspects of the external world would suggest the danger of psychotic symptoms. This disavowal of difference more closely resembles a radical rejection from the psyche of all that threatens the individual than it does a fantasy construction that has simply been repressed from consciousness. There is thus created a sterile void between the subject and others, across which no threatening feelings or ideas risk to invade him. Yet disavowal and denial of reality form part of the fundamental mechanisms that structure the human psyche from babyhood onward, and thus continue to function in limited areas in everybody. The important factor is the way in which such eliminations from the psychic sphere are recovered or otherwise compensated for. The denial of reality and difference is more simple to follow at the level of the phallic phase and the denial of the difference between the sexes than at this more global level of the difference between one human being and another. In previous chapters I traced the successive variations that might result from the disavowal of the primal scene and from attempts to deal with all the fears that are subsumed under the concept of the castration complex such as neuroses, perversions, and sublimations, which are different ways of recovering what is lost from psychic content through repression and denial. However, the defense mechanisms I am attempting to delineate here are of an all-encompassing kind. They correspond to what Freud called "repudiation from the ego" (*Verwerfung*). This might no doubt be considered as a prototypic form of castration anxiety—centered around archaic fears of separation, disintegration, and death—and which no doubt underlies the more sophisticated problems of sexual identity, oedipal rivalry, and forbidden sexual wishes. The prototypic anxiety concerns the dawning of psychic life and the beginning of subjective identity.

Our robot analysands, faced with what one might presume to have been overwhelming psychic trauma in early childhood have been unable to fill the gap left by the absence of the Other, a gap that might otherwise have been constructed by lively inner object fantasy or identification (in the service of maintaining ego identity and autonomy), by fantasies of a forbidden nature destined to be repressed (nuclei for future neuroses), or by the creation of a delusional system to compensate for the violent "repudiation" (such as Freud described in the Schreber case). Neither repression nor pathological projective identification predominate in this defensive system. Instead, these patients would appear to have constructed a sort of reinforced concrete wall to mask the primary separation on which human subjectivity is founded—an opaque structure that impedes free circulation both in inner psychic reality and between the internal and the external world. This approaches what Winnicott called the *false self* construction, in which an attempt is made to keep alive a sensitive inner self that dares not move, while an outer shell is maintained to adapt to all that the world is felt to demand. The patients I am describing maintain their existence in the world of others by following a set of strict conduct rules in an immutable system. This system appears to be detached from any inner object reference of either a superego or ego-ideal kind, and reflects a dimension of what Abraham called "sphincter morality." In settling problems, these analysands appear to know the "rules" without understanding the "law" that underlies them, and thus tend to make their own laws while being careful not to break rules that might lead to sanction. An example comes to mind.

Mrs. O, of whom I spoke earlier, believed that all men despised women and that all motorists despised pedestrians. One day she arrived in a triumphant mood for her session, having just killed two birds with one stone: A few minutes earlier she had been preparing to cross a little-frequented street, when a man in a sportscar passed right in front of her. Without a second's thought she brandished her umbrella, like a vengeful phallus, in such a way as to score a deep scratch the whole length of the little red car. The man, enraged, sprang from his seat and threatened to call the police. Mrs. O disappeared in panic, delighted nevertheless that for once justice had been done.

Nothing in these idiosyncratic internal rule-books may ever be called into question, for if doubted the system runs the risk of falling apart, leaving emptiness in its wake and terror at the threatened loss of identity feeling. The character trait that leads the person to blot out other people's psychic reality also makes it difficult for him to grasp his own, and can give rise to veritable thinking difficulties; it is as though he lacks the elements necessary to further reflect on his many predicaments in the way that Bion (1963, 1970) conceptualizes the thinking process in terms of *alpha* functioning. Thus such a patient has difficulty in grasping and thinking through a problem such as the question of otherness and all it implies. Although this gives rise to considerable irritation with others, especially those who manifestly threaten the person's inner system of weights and balances, he is on the whole *unaware of his own suffering,* unaware of his psychic fragility and his loneliness. In consequence, he can neither think nor talk about these problems. As the years go by, there is no relief from the accumulated pressure. In order to render more clearly the incipient danger of remaining out of touch with one's personal psychic pain I shall choose an analogous image from another field.

There exists a rare physical illness in which the person afflicted suffers from his *inability to suffer* in that he is incapable, for physiological reasons, of registering and thus feeling sensations of pain. This is potentially a very grave illness in that it endangers physical survival—unless of course the sufferer is able to learn *certain basic rules* that he must follow to the letter since they replace the normal biological alarm signals. If he should perceive that blood is flowing from a wound in his body, he must learn to bind it rapidly. Should he accidentally place his hand in the fire or on a burning surface, or run a sharp instrument through his hand, he must remember to withdraw his hand or to pull out the damaging instrument immediately and then deal with the resulting wounds. In addition he must constantly be on the look-out for such physical hazards since he has no in-built warning systems, and must therefore follow a careful set of rules which would seem incomprehensible to other people. Otherwise he runs the risk of burning, or bleeding to death, without warning. To stay alive he must learn to act like an *automaton*. Because of his disability he will tend to seem unsympathetic to other people's physical suffering, and perhaps even deny that it exists. Our robot analysands have developed a psychic insulation of this order. The analytic process has little chance of acting upon this impermeable protective layer, since the person concerned senses that his psychic life may be endangered should he change any one of the rules by which his affective and objectal life, and indeed his philosophy of life in general, is governed. Like the subjects of the above-mentioned physical illness, these patients give the impression of being in excellent health. Their seeming normality may be a danger signal, a problem I shall deal with extensively in the final chapter of this book. Afflicted with inner wounds whose pain they do not feel, they run the risk that their psychic hemorrhages may continue unrecognized and unabated.

The construction of such an infallible psychic system gives to the ego the strength of a computerized robot which in turn becomes the invincible guardian of the subject's psychic life—but at the price of a certain inner deadness. Vital contact with others must be avoided, and they will tend to be held at distance through the system of denial and repudiation we have been examining, as though death emanated from the Other. The dilemma of the analyst is twofold with the anti-analysand: not only must he realize that his very presence, his otherness, the very reason for which the patient came to see him in the first instance, is itself felt as a dangerous situation; he must also accept that he is struggling with anti-life forces in his patient, forces that will strive to reduce to zero every movement susceptible of awakening instinctual desires, of reanimating hope—all of which may draw the individual into libidinal relationship. Freud's concept of the *death instinct* finds its place here. Might we conceive of certain people whose only means of survival is to employ the forces that eventually lead to death?

At this juncture I should like to explore the question of psychosomatic potentiality with patients of this kind. Clinically they display many similarities to the gravely ill patients studied by Marty, de M'Uzan, and David (1963). In their book, *L'investigation psychosomatique,* the authors stress the following characteristics: a detached form of object relating; marked poverty of verbal expression, and concern with things and events rather than people;

absence of neurotic symptoms; gestures in place of emotional expression of a verbal kind; a notable lack of aggression, even when circumstances seem to call for it; a general climate of inertia that requires vigorous handling on the part of the investigator if a stalemate is to be avoided. Further research by Fain and David (1963) points to the meager fantasy and dream life of psychosomatic patients.

Our anti-analysand demonstrates a similar form of relating to others, the same poverty of verbal expression and absence of emotional response, and a similar lack of conscious fantasy and of dream life. From my reading of the above texts I would add that everything points to a notable lack of unconscious (repressed) fantasy which would tend to deprive an individual of a potential psychic capital to buffer himself (through the formation of sublimations, or indeed of neurotic and psychotic symptoms) against life's inevitable frustrations and occasional catastrophes, while at the same time enabling him to maintain viable contact with others.

The robot analysands differ from the psychosomatic patients in three important respects: they do not suffer from manifest psychosomatic maladies;[1] they do not demonstrate the typical inertia in the interview situation observed in psychosomatic investigation; they show no conspicuous lack of agggression and, on the contrary, express aggression in what might often be considered an inappropriate fashion. I shall explore these points of divergence more fully.

The question of the "somatization" of psychic conflict is fraught with complexity. In discussing my anti-analysands with an analytic colleague who played for many years an important part in psychosomatic research in France, I gave a detailed description of their character traits and system of relationships. "These are typical and indubitable psychosomatic patients," my colleague insisted. I protested that the patients in question showed no marked propensity toward psychosomatic afflictions. "Just wait. They'll get them!" he retorted. Although I am prepared to believe that these analysands may well be in danger of falling ill in this way, this does not afford me an explanatory hypothesis, nor define their present status and form of psychic functioning. To make a somewhat rudimentary analogy, let us say I am seeking to define what kind of animal a dog is. If I were told that a dog is an animal that has fleas, I might protest that my dog has none. Even though I

1. Since this chapter was written, I have observed that many of these patients suffered in intermittent fashion from various *allergic conditions,* possibly facilitated by similar factors in the psychic structure.

am assured that with time he will get them, this still does not tell me what a dog is. What is a "psychosomatic patient"? If this architect, at present in his forties, were to have a myocardial infarction or suffer from essential hypertension at the age of sixty-five, is he a psychosomatic sufferer? And at what point could this be said of him? Perhaps in the long run we all die for psychosomatic reasons. And in the short run it is possible that the apparently "normal" individual, the man-in-the-street, who would not dream of seeking an analysis, is more exposed to psychosomatic hazards than the neurotic.

Coming now to the inertia displayed by the psychosomatically ill in preliminary interviews, it may be said that this in no way characterizes the anti-analysands in their *initial* contact with the analyst. On the contrary they are particularly active in pleading their cause as future analytic patients. However, the inertia appears later in the course of the analysis, and is particularly discernible in the lack of response to interpretative attempts, or when the patient is invited to imagine situations which might be linked to or underlie his daily conflicts. Faced with a conspicuous void in fantasy production with my patients, I have frequently resorted to offering personal fantasies based on the details of family relations and childhood events furnished by the analysand in the course of his associations. Such initiatives, if they are not rejected out of hand as absurd, may bring forth a brief flowering of images and daydreams, but these die rapidly away. This is rather like getting a broken alarm clock to work by shaking it. It will produce momentary ticking sounds only to stop again. To think you have repaired it is mere illusion. In this situation, although the analysand does not display inertia and shows no wish to leave analysis, the *analyst* tends to get discouraged and finally to become inert. His repeated efforts to interpret, to identify, to question, to innovate, in order to set the analytic process in motion are liable in the last resort—and not without reason—to make the patient feel persecuted. Although these feelings of being criticized or otherwise attacked by the analyst are apt to bring forth new material for a short while, the insights thus gained tend to be wiped out and later denied. The analyst who has succeeded in being perceived for a brief period as Other, as possessed of a different psychic space and psychic reality, will eventually be denuded of his otherness and reabsorbed into the patient's psychic world.

One of Mrs. O's sessions provides a limpid example of such a phase. She had fulminated throughout the session, much as she had done for three years, against the injustices inflicted against women, but had finally broken down in tears (which was unusual for her). I suggested that the fact of being a woman was felt as an inarticulate threat and perhaps based on painful and depressing fantasies that were still to come to light. "What rubbish! I won't buy that. This is not a personal problem of mine—it applies to all women," replied Mrs. O. That night, however, she had a nightmare in which she was watching a play. On the stage, two "colossal females" were holding down a young girl in order to force into her throat a large egg without its shell. The egg was disgusting, dripping, and stained with blood. This object of disgust was at the same time a blood-stained sanitary napkin. In her dream Mrs. O remarked to an unidentified and invisible person that the young girl would shortly be having her periods. Among the many possible interpretations of such a dream, certain themes are immediately suggested by the manifest content alone: the overwhelming female figures would appear to effect a castrative attack upon the young girl in order to make her bleed correctly and become a woman. This is a maternal castration of an oral-sadistic and archaic kind, a situation of "forcefeeding." At the same time, the accession to adult female sexuality is depicted as a brutal and disgusting anal incorporation. There is in the awesome threesome a hint of a telescoped primal scene. Finally, it might be presumed that at one level the unknown listener to whom Mrs. O explains the horror that is occurring on stage is the analyst, whom she has tried hard to convince with regard to the miserable situation of womanhood. All this and much more is potentially inscribed in the condensed dream scene. Mrs. O had no associations to this strange dream, so with extreme caution I suggested that perhaps it depicted the painful fashion in which she might have experienced getting her periods and becoming a woman. "Well I certainly remember nothing of the sort. So you won't get me to *swallow* that!" replied Mrs. O firmly. I then proffered the only interpretation I felt she could accept, namely that the overbearing women of the dream represented myself with my analytic interpretations, trying to get her to "swallow" (to reintroject) many thoughts and feelings she did not consider to be true. In my mind there was no doubt that Mrs. O had in fact suffered great emotional pain, perhaps from early childhood, over being a girl, and perhaps over having to "swallow" many other unpalatable ideas as well, but that she did not wish to re-experience this pain nor even think about it. Her rule-book said that in talking of the difficulties of being a woman she was simply commenting on universally acknowledged facts. What right did I have to thrust my analytic "insights" down her throat? Mrs. O considered with interest the idea that she might feel I was thrusting interpretations down her throat like the forceful dream women, but then dismissed it as preposterous.

The defensive psychic structure of these analysands aims at keeping the destroyed affects out of reach, at maintaining the paralyzed sectors of their inner lives, and the hampered wishes, where they are. A definitive solution to mental pain has been found, so why suffer needlessly. The palpitating center of all that may happen in the exchange with others, whether for good or bad, has been extracted leaving only an outer shell, impervious to pain. Thereafter the external world will tend to be peopled with those who fulfill well-defined functions, and if necessary each object will be replaceable.

What occurs within the analyst who finds himself the helpless witness of this paralyzing process? He suffers of course by being reduced to impotence with regard to his analytic function, but the fact that a patient by reason of his psychic structure prevents our doing constructive and creative work with him does not seem sufficient explanation for the specifically painful feeling these patients arouse in the majority of analysts. After all, many analysands are not able to make extensive use of their analytical adventure. In addition, we are accustomed to protecting our patients from our own therapeutic ambitions, which we know from experience may be harmful rather than helpful to the analysis. Our distress with the anti-analysands goes beyond the question of professional failure and narcissistic injury. It is true that our interpretative work, far from promoting the analytic process, falls into a bottomless pit, leaving us bereft of an echo and therefore threatened in our analytic identity. But again this is a familiar problem; many patients put up forceful resistance to the analytic work and the analyst's endeavors for long periods of time. With the patients I am discussing here I suspect that something more specific is involved. Although our attempts to identify with the different dimensions of their obscure enigma and their throttled psychic pain are vigorously rejected or rendered insignificant, this still does not prevent us from identifying introjectively with both the ego and the inner objects of our analysands. Since the analyst's work always has as its goal the observation and understanding of psychic reality—his own as well as that of his patients —he is obliged to capture certain objects of analytic observation, namely the love, hate, rage, anguish, and other kindred emotions that lie behind the words, largely through his countertransference reactions, if these important affects have been detached from their original objects and representations. I have referred to this type of transmission of experience in analysis as "primitive communication" to indicate that the analyst's function is similar in this respect to that of the mother's with her as yet nonverbal child (McDougall, 1975). Faced with the robot analysand, out of touch with his own suffering, the analyst will point out sooner or later his observation that the patient is cutting himself off from his affective and instinctual roots. But with these particular patients such interventions go unheeded. The analyst must stand helplessly by watching his analysand psychically hemorrhaging, allowing himself to be crushed to death for an unknown cause. This unequal struggle with a deathlike force brings to the countertransference a measure of intense anxiety, and a wish to protect oneself from it. Thus one is tempted in such a situation to shrug one's shoulders and say of the patient that it is his problem, we have done our best and that's that. But whether we want it or not, it is also our problem. Not only does the enigma require understanding, but this death-bearing force must exist somewhere within us all.

Thus we are left with that which is legitimately ours to work with—our countertransference affect of pain and anxiety—as the sole means for furthering our understanding of these patients' psychic reality, other than our theoretical sources of information from other fields.

In reflecting on the impression of intolerable pain and bereavement that these analysands, in spite of themselves, communicate (and it might be noted that several, though by no means all, had known early loss of parental figures) I found myself thinking of the children studied by Spitz and also by Bowlby, who at a very early age lost contact with a parental object, whether through death, abandonment, or hospitalization. Bowlby and his research team have recorded their observations of a repeating pattern of behavior demonstrated by such traumatized children. Following a period of protest and anger, they become depressed and withdraw into themselves for a variable length of time. Once this period of detachment is over, they appear to have completely *forgotten* the loved or essential object which has failed them. In the most serious cases, the child from then on will invest solely inanimate objects, and henceforth only people who give him concrete *things* may be allowed to count. Unfortunately for our purposes, Bowlby, who describes so sensitively the conduct of these children, does not investigate the intrapsychic processes implied in the maturation of object relations. His ''attachment'' model, fruit of meticulous observation, gives little insight into the libidinal economy involved. It is evident that the small child, because of his psychic immaturity, can with difficulty, if at all, accomplish the work of mourning. His urgent *need of the object* does not permit of his introjecting it in its absence and thus securing inwardly an object that otherwise is constantly disappearing or definitively lost. Instead massive denial and displacement will occur, and this must inevitably distort the identification processes. In addition to the elimination from the inner world of well-elaborated whole objects of a living kind, there is the subsequent danger that all aggressive impulses will be turned against the self and set in motion a potentially destructive process. At the same time the cutting of the outer object ties and their affective links further impoverishes the inner object world with consequent diminution of imagination and fantasy life. The anti-analysands resemble these bereaved children. Like them, they appear to have mummified their internal objects (whether good or bad), and attach themselves predominantly to factual and concrete aspects of interchange with others. Experiences coming from the "outside," including the experience of analysis, find no symbolic resting place in the inner world and as a result rapidly lose their affective charge.

At this point I come to the third area of divergence with the typically psychosomatic patients—the absence of aggressivity. In this respect, the anti-analysands are more like the grieving children in the first phase of their detachment cycle. The robot analysands possess a considerable fund of hostility that can, and in general is, projected onto others, thus creating a solid, if ill-tempered, link. The extensive irritation so often expressed toward the important others in the patients' lives reveals that, to this extent at least, the Other may be envisaged as a valuable *container,* even though somewhat of a garbage pail. This recalls the analytic function that Meltzer (1967) has named the "toiletbreast," with the exception that these patients seem unable to establish a "nourishing" exchange; their deep and, in a certain sense, positive attachment to their hate objects is unconscious. The consciously vented anger maintains an affective link with its object, and this may be one of the reasons why these patients appear to strive toward a chronically angry relation with their entourage. It is important to emphasize that this constant feeling of being ill-used and the reiterated hostility may be regarded mistakenly as an indication of *psychic suffering.* It may be more accurate to consider this way of relating to the world as a bulwark against self-destruction and a safeguard against terrifying emptiness and the shadow of psychic death. It might even be that this aggressive screen serves as a protection against psychosomatic explosion.

Be that as it may, the constant activity of these analysands in the service of their negative feelings does give many signs of being a manic defense, though poorly structured, against an unelaborated depression stemming from early psychic trauma and of which the subject is unaware. The early break between the self and its important objects would seem to have destroyed not only the continuing capacity for libidinal investment but also the desire to explore, to question, to know more. *This is the death of curiosity*. The ravaged child will no longer seek to know what is happening within himself, nor what takes place inside the others. The "dark continent" of woman is no longer peopled with fabled monsters or fairylike creatures, and the *passion for knowledge* which finds its earliest source in the small child's wish to burrow inside, to take possession of the mother's body and all its contents, suffers a paralyzing blow. The magic book of fantasies about all that links one human being to another has been firmly closed—and in its place come the rules of conduct and an operational relation to the external world.

Two theoretical approaches seem to me germane to this type of psychic functioning. The violent splitting off from the inner object world and the instinctual roots of feeling, whose damaging effects we have been following in these patients, recalls what Bion (1963) describes as "minus-K phenomena," and what he also refers to as "ego-castration" or the "castration of meaning." The representations are there, undistorted, but denuded of their significance, and thus cannot be used as elements of conceptual thought. Another approach to similar phenomena is that of Lacan (1966) in his concept of "foreclosure," following on the Freudian concept of "repudiation" from consciousness, which unlike repression, treats the psychic events in question as though they had never existed. Such events or representations are thus excluded from their place in the symbolic chain. Freud considered that this defense mechanism was predominant in psychotic structures, and the work of Bion and of Lacan would support this point of view.

However our anti-analysands are not psychotic. The denial of psychic separateness is not compensated through delusional formations; instead these patients remain, if anything, excessively attached to external reality but on the condition that affective links with others remain severed and the interpenetration of ideas severely controlled. By these means the patient may hope to protect himself from intolerable hurt, but at the price of cutting any tie that might draw him within the circuits of desire and the orbit of other people's wishes, fears, and refusals. It is not surprising that in the analytic situation the transference is destined to be still-born.

But the anger and irritation and the reiterative search for fictive enemies who may be held to blame for the treachery and abandonment of the earliest objects remain. The analyst becomes in his turn a fictive enemy to be warded off. Are we within our rights in attempting to decipher and pull apart this precious rage? The question is difficult to answer since in the majority of cases the analysand does not give us the opportunity to do so. The cancellation of libidinal investment, and even of the vital anger, in the relation to the analyst, and the recurring elimination of the attempts to find meaning to his deep unsatisfaction, tend to create a cold and sterile space between the two partners to the analytic relationship, which eventually extinguishes the analyst's ardent desire to know more. It is indeed sad to note that the analyst risks becoming, like the patients themselves, indifferent, even to their psychic pain.

Perhaps this tragic result has dynamic significance for the patient nevertheless, in that he may implicitly ask to be allowed to protect his angry tie with the external world. The persecutory objects contain a part of himself and are thus a living receptacle for a vital dimension of his personal identity. As for his unrecognized suffering, does he not ask us to contain this without reacting and, to the extent that we identify with it, to keep it to ourselves? Is this finally the successful realization of his analytic project?

Yet this facile explanation is not a satisfactory one, for it is obvious that these analysands cling tenaciously to *their* analytical adventure, more than many a normal-neurotic patient does—and this in spite of obvious stagnation. It has sometimes seemed to me that they cling to the analysis like a drowning man to a lifebelt, even though he no longer believes he will ever reach the shore. I would suggest as a hypothesis that such patients hold to the hope that somewhere inside them there *is* a hidden universe, an unconscious mind, another way of thinking and feeling about themselves and about others. Even if the patient does not himself believe this, he knows that his analyst believes it, and he thus clings to this faint source of hope.

REFERENCES

Bion, W. R. 1963. *Elements of Psycho-Analysis*. London: Heinemann.
———. 1970. *Attention and Interpretation*. London: Heinemann.
Bouvet, M. 1967. *La relation d'objet*. Paris: Payot.
Fain, M., and David C. 1963. Aspects fonctionels de la vie onirique. *Rev. Franc. Psychanal.* 27: 241–343.
Lacan, J. 1966. *Ecrits*. Paris: Seuil.
McDougall, J. 1975. Countertransference and primitive communication. In *Plea for a Measure of Abnormality*. New York: International Universities Press, 1980, 247–98. Reprinted from *Topique* 16, Paris.
Marty, P., and M'Uzan, M. de. 1963. La pensée operatoire. *Rev. Franc. Psychanal.* 27: 345–56.

Marty, P., M'Uzan, M. de, and David, C. 1963. *L'investigation psychosomatique*. Paris: Presses Universitaires de France.

Meltzer, D. 1967. *The Psycho-Analytical Process*. London: Heinemann.

Strachey, J. 1934. The nature of the therapeutic action of psychoanalysis. *Internat. J. Psycho-Anal*. 15: 127–59.

20. A Special Variation of Technique

Annie Reich

In recent years the pathology of the ego and superego has increasingly become the centre of psycho-analytic interest. There exists as yet no systematic classification of the forms of ego pathology and character disturbances; hence there cannot be any systematic description of variations in technique or parameters, to use Eissler's term, necessitated by this pathology.

Methods of giving initial support to a weak ego, so as to strengthen it for the task of facing instinctual conflicts, have been most frequently discussed. E.g., it has been described how the violence of anxiety in these cases often necessitates all sorts of supportive measures, such as to 'nurture' some positive transference by giving the patient the feeling that the analyst is always there for him and can be called in a situation of panic, etc. Sometimes his relation to the analyst may become the first really reliable object relationship in the patient's life, a contingency which of course entails the danger that it may seriously interfere with the possibility of the transference ever being analysed.

I shall concentrate on a special variation of technique dealing predominantly with a particular form of superego pathology in a certain group of patients who can be defined as impulse-ridden characters or acting-out hysterias. The ego disturbance in these cases appears to be a secondary effect of the defective superego. Such patients are a helpless prey to uncontrollable outbursts of libidinal and/or aggressive impulses, which cause violent anxiety and guilt reactions. Between these powerful drives and a relentless superego the ego seems weak, almost non-existent, so to speak; but it may manifest itself very forcefully in negative ways, i.e., as inhibitor of normally ego-syntonic, important gratifications and activities. Such an ego is of little help to the analysis. Repetitive acting out occurs outside and within the analysis, cannot be stopped, and threatens to make the treatment impossible.

In cases of this kind, the analyst frequently finds himself in the same role

Reprinted from Annie Reich, *Psychoanalytic Contributions* (New York: International Universities Press, 1973), 236–49 by permission of International Universities Press, Inc. Originally published in 1958.

as the child analyst who has to observe the conflict going on outside the analysis, between child and parents or siblings. It appears that this undesirable situation also has a positive aspect, because the violence of the conflict is so intense as to make analytic work impossible. The analyst remains outside for a time—and is not completely the butt of unsatisfiable libidinal demands and aggressive impulses, until slowly, with the progress of the analysis, a shift of cathexis and the establishment of a genuine transference can be achieved.

Within the analysis these patients try, *via* their acting out and the ensuing guilt-ridden anxiety, to force the analyst into the role of a primitive superego against which an endless and tumultuous war of ambivalence is being waged. The superego is insufficiently internalized and is constantly reprojected. It is as though no real love objects existed and no integrated ego, but only externalized superego figures; as though the pathological superego, like a parasite, had usurped the place of all other psychic structures.

The roots of this pathology are found in a premature, overstrict enforcement of superego demands while simultaneously the normal development of object relationship was severely interfered with by a too extensive and too early repression of libidinal as well as aggressive strivings under the impact of too-forbidding early objects. The disintegration of the pathological superego, which is necessary in order to achieve restructuring of the personality and establishment of normal object relationship, should be brought about by a careful analysis of the dependent and highly ambivalent relationship to these early objects. But the violence of the acting out makes this impossible. To break this impasse it proves useful to take sides with the patient, in a rather unanalytic way, against the object: demasking and dethroning it, so to speak. It is this active intervention, this stepping out of his natural role by the analyst, which I should like to describe. It is, I believe, a variation of classical technique that is often necessary in cases of this kind.

I shall give some fragments of the material from a long analysis of such a case, to illustrate the structure of the pathological superego as well as the ways and means by which its virulence finally was abated.

The patient, Abigail, a strikingly elegant and attractive although not beautiful woman, was in her forties when she came to analysis. She presented a curious mixture of very upper-class social graciousness, impeccable manners, and uncontrolled aggressive outbursts. She suffered from alcoholism and addiction to barbiturates which were taken during the day, so that the patient spent most of her day in bed. In the evening, before her husband returned home, she would get up, longing now for his affection and companionship. At this point, in order to dispel tension and to be able to be gay, she would begin to drink. Invariably she felt the husband's response to be insufficient. She felt 'misunderstood and left alone'; and sooner or later she would have a temper tantrum, attacking him physically and provoking him to such a degree that he also would resort to violence.

By and by it became clear that the barbiturates were taken to permit withdrawal into sleep, which was needed to allay the unbearable anxiety Abigail experienced when left to her own devices. When she was alone it was as though she were no real person. There was nothing she wanted to do; it was as though she were paralysed in all her ego functions. She was like a little girl needing to ask every few minutes, 'Mother, what shall I do?'. Indeed, it turned out that as long as there had been somebody telling her what to do, Abigail had been much better. There had been no temper tantrums, hardly any drinking, no sleep addiction. All these symptoms started to appear following her marriage, a few years before she came for analysis, to a man of wealth and social standing who was twenty-five years her senior.

Abigail stemmed from a socially prominent family; there was more prestige than money. She had lost her father at the age of fifteen. In order not to be financially dependent on her mother, the complicated relationship with whom will be described later, she did the most revolutionary thing in her life: instead of having a 'coming-out party', she insisted upon getting a college education and training as a social worker. Being a person of high intelligence and sensitivity, Abigail was able to function very well under the pressure of school and job. She worked until the age of forty, when her mother died. Only then was she able to marry. The husband clearly was a parent figure. Before they were married, he had been her boss with whom she had had a thrilling flirtation. After marriage she was completely frigid and reacted to his sexual advances only with anxiety and disgust.

Now Abigail lived under conditions of which she had always dreamed. She finally had a husband and a lovely house, although owing to a hysterectomy she could have no children. She was wealthy and did not have to work any more, but could do whatever she pleased. Yet there was nothing that she felt she wanted to do. It transpired that empty boredom had already been predominant in her early childhood. As far as she remembered, she had been unable to do anything on her own. She had started very late to walk and talk. She could not play by herself; neither could she play with other children. When brought together with them Abigail would stand in a corner, in despair,

388   TYPES OF CHARACTER PATHOLOGY AND TREATMENT TECHNIQUES

not knowing what to do or how to talk with them. Clad in a lovely white lace dress, she spent many hours just sitting motionless and stiffly in the parlour, in a chair much too big for her, while her mother entertained her lady friends. Much later it emerged that this was exactly how her mother had wanted her to behave. Her near-paralysed state was thus the expression of obedience to the mother, whose demands she had taken over so completely that it was as though she had no impulses of her own. She therefore needed constantly to be told what to do. When in later childhood she found herself in a situation where she had to make a decision, she was able to do so only by 'consulting' her stomach. If between two alternatives she thought of the one that was really not pleasing to her, she would feel somatic discomfort within her body: in this way she knew what she wanted.

The same pattern was repeated in the analysis. She wanted me to tell her what to say; free association for a long time remained impossible. More and more, she saw me in the role of an imaginary companion who would constantly accompany her and advise her what to do. It was as though the analyst represented a personified superego.

In the presence of her husband, on the other hand, Abigail was overcome with vehement emotion, longing, and rage. She was then completely unreasonable in her demands; the docility and good manners would fall away from her, and in rebellious defiance she would give rein to her violent outbursts.

The superego problems led back to the mother. To describe the latter, as she emerged in the analysis, one could best characterize her as being 'a lady' in the truest Victorian sense. Most important for her were good behaviour and the opinion of other people. Life was narrowed down to a pleasantness of voice and manner. Any expression of emotion, of deeper feelings, any activity beyond the scope of church, charity and good society, was considered not to be 'ladylike'. Any unrestricted play that might be accompanied by noise, by dirtying of clothes and hands, was unacceptable; any abandon, any spontaneous expression of affection. Whatever was connected with sex in any way could not be mentioned and should not be seen. Pregnant women were shameless if they went out in public. One of the patient's terrifying, originally repressed memories was how as a very little girl she had once put her hand into a box in the dark cellar and, to her horror, touched a litter of newborn kittens that had been hidden away from her; of course, no explanation had been offered her.

Another example was an incident which Abigail remembered late in the analysis, under extreme anxiety. When she was about five years old, she was riding with her mother in a horse-drawn carriage when her mother suddenly seized the child's head and pushed her face into her lap. The horse, without any consideration for the ladies, had lifted his tail and followed his natural urge. Little girls just could not look at such disgusting things as a horse's anal productions. The mother's attitude with regard to anal training followed this pattern. The patient was trained at an incredibly early age and had to be constantly spick and span. It was most important that the child produce every morning at a regular hour, lest she becomes ill with appendicitis. On the other hand, any interest in anything not perfectly clean—by looking, touching, smelling—was completely out of the question.

The mother's inability to accept bodily contact extended to Abigail even when she was still a baby. She could not tolerate the child snuggling up to her or, as a toddler, clinging to her hand in the street. Even endearing words were considered vulgar.

Most important for the patient's pathological development was the relationship between her parents. They slept in separate bedrooms, the mother having banished the father from her bed. Abigail, an only child, owed her existence to a night spent in a hotel, on the way to a vacation spot, when the father had been too stingy to take two rooms. The latter, a judge in the juvenile court and a kindly man who could tear himself apart for a juvenile delinquent, met his wife only at the dinner table and then took revenge upon her by behaving in the rudest manner he could devise. He would eat in a disgusting fashion, spit in a wide curve into the floral centerpiece, and break into violent outbursts of temper against the mother, who through all this would remain silent, gentle, well-behaved, and saintly. The parents would not talk to each other. For the little girl, the father was almost a complete stranger; as he was so unacceptable to her mother, she dared not love him. During endless dinner hours the child would just sit there, silent and motionless, unable to eat or to talk.

The mother, never raising her voice, always gentle, had achieved an almost total repression of instinctual forces in the child, including all wishes for affection. This was combined with a complete lack of interest in or with direct disapproval of any timid attempts at sublimation, most of which were condemned as 'not ladylike'. The result was a grave interference not only with the child's libidinal vicissitudes and object relations, but also with her ego development. Abigail's inability to function independently gave the impression of there being a serious intellectual defect.

Later in adolescence, by a great effort of will, the patient consciously forced herself to behave 'as if' she were outgoing, cheerful, charming. This artificial, gracious behaviour proved very helpful: she became 'popular'. But it was based on continuous effort. She had to sense what people wanted and to behave, not as she really felt (which she did not know), but as she thought others wanted her to be. She had many friends now, but could tolerate these only for a short time. To be with them demanded a terrific effort of her. Thus after a short while she could not bear her friends any more and wished only to get rid of them again.

After moving to college and away from her mother's presence, she became able to do all kinds of things that were anathema in the mother's eyes. She flirted around, acquired many admirers, and permitted them to neck and pet with her, only to disappoint them when it became in any way serious.

The patient thus behaved, indeed, like the classical 'as if' case described by Helene Deutsch. She had no real object relations. Her friends represented to her mere temporary superego figures. Trying to divine their commands, she found it impossible to live up to this relentless task. The superego demands were not only excessive, but were not really integrated into the personality; they were experienced as coming from outside objects, and her tremendous ambivalence against these superego objects prevented any real relationship with them.

After her marriage, the tenuous balance of this 'as if' existence proved insufficient. The husband clearly represented the mother—and the maternal superego. He became too much of a temptation for Abigail. Everything she had warded off all her life now broke through; she became childishly de-manding. The husband was expected to shower her continually with love and affection (which had been so severely denied by her mother). He was sup-posed to share all kinds of things with her (which, as we understood much later, were derivatives of infantile activities, genital as well as pregenital). She succeeded in experiencing his behaviour as an endless repetition of maternal condemnations of her unconscious strivings, to which she reacted with uncontrollable temper tantrums facilitated by the effects of alcohol. These outbursts alternated with desperate anxiety and clinging to a superego figure.

While thus acting out in her marriage, she was unable to carry these emotional storms into the analytic hour and to face what she felt or associate to it. She could not lie on the couch because she had to watch my facial expression, 'to find out what I wanted her to say'. Whatever childhood material emerged was offered because she knew this was expected of her. In the absence of an integrated ego with whom to form an alliance, the patient's deadlock between impulse and guilt could not be broken until I finally resorted to the aforementioned very active form of intervention, which is my reason for presenting this lengthy case history. This method can be described as a frontal attack on the original superego model; i.e., as a systematic devaluation of the idealized mother.

From the bits of material about the mother that were reported here, it might appear as though an analysis and solution of the patient's mother relationship would have come about by itself and led naturally to a disintegration of the pathological superego. But this was not so; if such an impression was created it may be due to the difficulty of presenting the material of a long analysis. The mother had actually imposed herself as an absolute ideal on the child. This ideal, like a malignancy, usurped the place of an independent ego as well as of any genuine love object and had to be undermined before either could be restored. The patient felt so overwhelmed by guilt as to be incapable of critical judgement. The mother was seen as a saint, and her opinions as moral law. Hence it was only with my active help in demasking the mother that this patient could develop something completely new: tolerance and understanding of her libidinal and, eventually, also of her aggressive impulses. Only then could a mass of repressed material be recalled and finally experienced as belonging to the past; only then did the patient become an integrated person. Only then could she become aware of what she felt and wanted. In this way a diminution of her emotional violence could be achieved, and the acting out was then controllable.

What I did, concretely, was to put together for the patient the fragments of information I had about her mother and, so to speak, to analyse the mother for her. I went even further and expressed value judgements in regard to the mother.

I could show her that mother indeed was no saint. Mother was not kind. Mother had not been able to give love to anyone. Mother had driven her husband as well as her only child close to breakdown and had brought endless misery into their lives. Mother wanted the girl to behave like a grown-up when it so suited her, but treated her as a baby when this was what happened to suit her. Mother herself, in fact, was a very neurotic person, which caused her not only to frustrate the father so completely, but also to frustrate Abigail as a young infant in her most natural demand for closeness. Mother's neurosis made her utterly narrow, self-centered, and selfish.

Slowly the patient became able to see the mother clearly, and many confirmatory memories emerged. The most impressive of these was the following. As a small child, she had run into a glass door; her face was badly cut and had to be bandaged for weeks. Her mother's main concern was: 'What will people think of you!' Thus the mother became divested of her halo, and as a result the patient succeeded in breaking through her defences.

Of the wealth of repressed material that became available after the mother's demotion, not more than a hint can be given here. In the beginning, this material centred exclusively around the mother and consisted in an intense, pregenital-type longing for love and for sexual activities 'shared' by the mother. Gradually it emerged that because of the utter frustration of her need to touch, to see, and to understand, curiosity had played a tremendous role in the child's fantasy life. While sitting motionless, and apparently doing nothing, she was filled with wishes to put her fingers into all holes, all body openings; to tear everything apart, the mother's clothing, the mother's body. Thus she finally progressed to the father and her inability to understand the difference of the sexes.

The complete blocking of any outlet into active play and the unusual amount of pregenital frustration had led to an inability to bind and modify any aggression. It was not surprising, therefore, to find a particularly sadistic coloration of fantasies. She finally remembered how, again while sitting still and doing nothing, she had been simply boiling with rage and hatred, wanting to tear her mother into small shreds. The dinner hours would be filled with a repetitive fantasy: she imagined the big oak chest behind the mother's chair, in the dining room, falling on the mother and smashing her. All these fantasies were extremely frightening to the child, because thus her only love object would be destroyed and she would be left all alone.

The thorough analysis of these conflicts enabled us finally to unearth the repressed love for her father, and brought to light a wealth of material referring to childhood masturbation and feminine sexual wishes. The way in which this patient was eventually able to analyse and the very gratifying therapeutic results convinced me that despite her apparent borderline pathology she was, after all, a hysteric who had already in childhood reached a genital, heterosexual level from which she had then so impressively regressed.

Impulse-ridden characters not infrequently belong to this group of acting-out hysterics. It seems to me that in cases of this type, which are characterised by an intolerant but insufficiently internalized superego and by oscillation between breakthrough and guilt, such active attack upon the superego pathology is often very helpful.

On the other hand, a closer scrutiny of this method shows that its use involves something more, which is not a part of classical technique either. When the disintegration of a pathological superego is undertaken in this way, value judgements of the analyst come to the fore, expressions of his understanding, tolerance, and different moral attitude, which usually have no place in the analytic process. To a certain extent, the analyst offers himself as and becomes a new object of identification to the patient. Evidently this is permissible only if it is combined with a careful analysis of the conflict. Were the 'technical advice' to predominate, we should be educators and not analysts.

PART V

THE ROLE AND SIGNIFICANCE OF THE ANALYST'S CHARACTER IN THE ANALYTIC PROCESS AND THE ANALYTICAL SITUATION

21. A Silent Partner to Our Practice: The Analyst's Character and Attitudes

Francis D. Baudry

My hope in writing this paper is to sensitize therapists to look at a neglected area in our technique: the relevance of the analyst's character. I will arbitrarily divide the structuring effect of the analyst's character into three areas which overlap somewhat: (1) general attitudes; (2) analytic style proper; and (3) the analyst's reaction to specific situations. I will then focus on two narrow issues—the issue of parameters, and that of the transference neurosis.

Occasionally, we take the liberty of making simplifying assumptions in order to conduct experiments or research. Only later (at times, at the cost of bitter experience) do we become aware of the liability of such a strategy. In the Dora case, Freud made such assumptions. He unwittingly took the position that attitudes and the character of the patient (and himself) could be safely ignored and that he could count on her cooperation in his search for the meaning of her symptoms and dreams. It is a tribute to Freud that he could learn from his errors and make major discoveries as a result of the difficulties his nonverbalized assumption created for him; in this case, the loss of the patient allowed him to discover the concept of transference.

A large bulk of our technical writings adopts the simplifying assumption of the average expectable analyst who will "apply" appropriate technique of principles, such as the rules of abstinence. This approach bypasses the character and subjectivity of the practitioner in order to focus on the content of the method. I do not believe I am overstating the case in seeing the purpose of technique and its structure as an effort to tame the personality of the analyst so as to allow psychoanalytic work to be done. The issues in this paper can be seen both as the impingement of character on technique and as the impingement of technique on the analyst's personal attributes.

Reprinted from the *Bulletin of the Association of Psychoanalytic Medicine* 21 (1982): 100–109 by permission.

THE ANALYST'S CHARACTER AND ITS EFFECT ON TECHNIQUE

By character, I refer to the broadest attributes of a person, ones that are generally self-syntonic. This list includes values (ethical and otherwise), therapeutic stance, and general traits (such as impulsivity and optimism) which are specific and stable. Some of these traits may be more conflictual than others; others may merge on the symptomatic.

In what follows, I will closely examine issues of technique with the analyst's character as an organizing factor. One advantage of the concept of character is that it subsumes both the normal and the abnormal and includes both what is stylistic (the form of the analyst's manner in contrast to its content) and what is generally subsumed under the label of countertransference. Bearing in mind the neutral aspects of character, we are not forced to make premature judgments about the pathological aspects of a particular response.

In the title of this paper, I have purposely used the terms *character* and *attitudes* because character (in the sense of character traits) is primarily something observed from the outside by another person. Attitudes, on the other hand, refers to a mind set—primarily, internal attributes. Thus, an attitude will determine behavior which will then be perceived by an outside observer. The latter will then infer (correctly or not) some character trait.

Character traits are combined to form the character organization—a stable, coherent structure. It is possible to describe the latter along a variety of axes, depending on one's preferences—object relations, drives, defenses, developmental, adaptational and the like. Because of the ambiguity of the term character, I will sometimes consider the analyst's character as referring to an external attribute—something the patient observes, and sometimes consider it from the inside realm—a structure which lends form to the analyst's perceptions and shapes his view of the world.

How does the analyst's character permeate his technique? This broad topic may, for the sake of convenience, be broken down into three sections: (1) his self-syntonic general ways of being, which express the analyst's values and attitudes: pessimism or optimism, permissiveness, tendency to gratify or frustrate wishes; rigidity or flexibility, degree of activity, degree of warmth vs. distance, passivity, and so forth; (2) analytic style proper—formal attributes apart from the content of interpretations; such things as tone, manner, verbosity, use of humor, authority, and readiness to make interpretations or reconstructions; (3) the analyst's specific reactions to affects of the patient such as anger, criticism, love, or problems in treatment (for example, stalemate).

THE ANALYST'S GENERAL ATTITUDES

It is very difficult to disentangle an analyst's professional behavior from his character. Although technically speaking, his behavior as an analyst reflects his professional and therapeutic stances, its very stability is by definition part of his character. These attitudes color the ways he conducts the analysis as a whole. Permissiveness and gratification of wishes are good examples. An analyst who, in a given instance, does not answer a patient's questions and clearly frustrates him, may do so for a variety of motives which only analysis (or self-analysis) may reveal. He will hopefully do so because he believes it is in the patient's best interest even though the patient experiences rage or anxiety as the result. In accordance with the principle of multiple function, such behavior will also have its unconscious significance, often not, by the way, dealt with by the training analysis.

The analyst may unconsciously express his sadism or possibly take revenge against what he perceives as an ungiving patient. The opposite might also be true; an analyst who is too ready to answer questions may do so out of a fear of provoking aggression. We would expect that a reasonably well-analyzed therapist would be somewhat cognizant of the influence of his unconscious motives. To the degree he is not, these motives could then cause difficulty. In the case cited, they might interfere with a proper therapeutic stance: the therapist might remain silent when it is more appropriate to interpret, rationalizing his stance on the basis of the rule of abstinence. Even knowledge of one's own unconscious motives and character attitudes does not necessarily put the analyst in a position to do something about them. Character responses seen from the inside are, for the most part, forced choices of an automatic nature not open to question. They are like a pair of colored glasses one is not free to remove. It is possible to describe these general attitudes both as mind sets—predilections for certain reactions—or as sensitivities to certain constellations and the readiness of their being evoked in the analyst. This includes both cognitive and affective reactions.

Values characteristic of the person's *Weltanschauung* may have been especially influenced by early experiences. For example, childhood illness or trauma which was surmounted may promote a belief, not clearly masochistic, that certain sufferings are valuable and growth promoting or that given a choice, the hard way is preferable.

There must be a complicated relationship between the way an analyst was treated as a child (for example, strictly or permissively) and his adult attitudes, varying with the outcome of his analysis and the resolution of infantile identifications. There is still another step concerning his adult attitudes to his analytic demeanor. A "strict" personal predilection may, because of many different motives, lead to a permissive stance. Reaction formations may color the end result.

A number of separate attitudes will converge to determine a particular stance; for example, how silent the analyst ends up being is determined by a combination of attitudes of permissiveness, rigidity, gratification of wishes, and activity, to name but a few. I am leaving out for the purpose of this presentation the learning the analyst has acquired during his training and the identification he may have made with his supervisors and the thoughtful integration of the above into what will eventually turn out to be his personal style. I am also leaving out the major impact of the identification with the training analyst—his values and attitudes and the degree to which the analysand accepts or rejects them and works through this aspect of his professional identification. These last purposive acquisitions may themselves be involved in conflicts. It is common knowledge that as an analyst gains more experience, his professional attitudes change. He often can become less rigid, less concerned about rules and their infractions, and more willing to reveal certain personal attitudes.

THE PROBLEM OF ANALYTIC STYLE

I have not ceased to be amazed by both stories and vignettes of what well-known teachers and respected analysts could do within the limits of their style without apparent major difficulties. One now-deceased senior analyst was well known to touch certain depressed patients during the course of therapy. As an expression of love, warmth, and caring, this parameter may have been very useful and when applied, it was very likely experienced as nonintrusive. I could imagine a student trying to learn technique copying this analyst's approach and getting disastrous results. Another analyst who used to share a suite with a fellow therapist confided how often he would hear his colleague yell at his patients through the soundproof door. To him, this did not sound like anger, but rather in this instance a demonstration of loving and concern. The problem with such issues of style is that they are hardly, if ever, analyzed, and the patient's responses to them are often misunderstood or glossed over.

What are the components of analytic style, the subtle formal aspects in contrast to the content of interpretations? Many variables exist, such as intonation (degree of uniformity), manner, humor, drama, verbosity vs. pithiness, conviction vs. tentativeness, use of authority, and many more. Such elements are the counterpart of the patient's style and it is important for the analyst to be aware of their presence and potential impact. The degree of tonal uniformity, to take but one limited example, may be described in very different ways: even, bland, lackluster, stable, restrained, neutral. The choice of these adjectives carries with it a value judgment: "neutral" the least and "bland" or "lackluster" the most. This is true in general of all descriptive terms applying to character. We tend automatically to see a trait as good or bad. Yet even the term neutral can be thought of as signifying both a negative (absence of criticism, judgement and the like) and as positive (making understanding possible implies certain therapeutic values). There are clearly instances where a departure from a neutral tone is called for, especially with patients whose style superficially mirrors this stance. An example is the stubborn obsessional isolator who uses the analyst's tone to further his own distance from the interpretations. "You remain neutral so why shouldn't I?"

STYLE AND RESISTANCE

There are important differences in the degree of activity of the analyst not explained by rules. I have heard the humorous epithets of hunters vs. trappers in describing two extremes of stylistic approach! On a personal note, my second analyst's rather loquacious manner allowed me to take distance from and realize the impact of my first analyst's scant verbal pronouncements — clearly a stylistic difference which had a major effect on the course of the treatment. For some patients, the analyst's style seems to matter very little; it is hardly ever mentioned in the treatment. This may or may not represent an avoidance on the patient's part. I have in mind two patients. The first patient felt very needy of help and quickly developed an intense transference neurosis characterized by the emergence of a new symptom, impotence; he was able to associate well and dreamed profusely. He was in many ways an "ideal" analytic patient. He did not make chronic repetitive battles out of the formal aspects of what I said although, amusingly enough, he picked up almost in passing a small grammatical error I had made in the recording of my voice on my answering machine! In contrast, a second patient, generally mistrustful and cautious, focused very early in the treatment on one aspect of my personal style. As English is not my first language, my speech is often a bit precise, stilted, and clearly enounced. She latched on to this quality which she began to attack mercilessly, and would giggle and laugh at occasional pronunciation errors I might make or grammatical oversights (a very provoking attitude on her part I might add). In fact, the content of what I said was hardly ever the focus of her concern. No matter how I tackled this attitude— its functions in the here and now, such as turning the tables on me, focusing on my imperfection, dreading a closeness to or fearing to be influenced by me—the treatment made little progress. A certain similarity between my speech and that of her mother served as a hook for a very sticky transference which could only be very partially resolved. It would be too easy to dismiss this case by saying that the speech problem was coincidental or that the patient would in all likelihood have focused on some other issue to maintain her character defenses. I suspect that the accidental similarity between my speech and her mother's made it more difficult for the patient to see her attitude as essentially transferential, a point I will return to later. I believe patients are often intimidated by aspects of our style which they sense are invested with considerable narcissistic libido and are therefore not open to question. A patient once told me he was afraid of freely expressing his thoughts because of what he understood to be the "No Trespass" sign of his previous therapist's attitude towards all his patients: he would never get up and greet the patients in the waiting room but would simply leave his door ajar as a signal, making it the patient's responsibility to keep watch on the door's position.

Gill has written on the value of paying close attention to resisted aspects of the transference; however, our own taking for granted certain self-syntonic aspects of our style requires a constant vigilance on our part not to miss the way patients react to it.

THE ANALYST'S REACTION TO SPECIFIC SITUATIONS

This category—the analyst's reaction to specific situations—is the more familiar countertransference examined from the characterological point-of-view. How does the analyst typically react when he feels attacked, criticized, loved, idealized, or stuck? Such issues are more often taken up in the personal analysis than the other categories because they lead to obvious conflict in the analyst. I shall have less to say about them as there is a vast literature on the topic. Glover in his textbook on psychoanalysis refers to the silent resistances and counterresistances—the most dangerous—for obvious reasons. He gives a clue as to their appearance—when the analyst is tempted to or does actually depart from his usual way of doing things. Examples include the way patients are ushered in or out of the office, the ways bills are handled and so on. I will deal, however, with one specific aspect, that of parameters.

In what situations does an analyst feel the need to introduce a parameter in an ongoing analysis? The answer is fairly obvious. It is in those situations in which the treatment appears stuck and where, in the opinion of the therapist, interpretation is useless or harmful. Often there is some state of crisis or stalemate. Let me cite a well-known example, looking at it from the point-of-view of the analyst's character structure.

A deceased well-known colleague once told a group a most fascinating vignette about a very wealthy patient he had been treating in Paris before the war—some time in the early thirties. Money meant nothing to her. After some time, the treatment seemed stuck. All the interpretations of the patient's resistance, aggression, and contempt failed to resolve the impasse. The analyst then announced one day to the patient that until further notice, he had decided not to charge her a fee! Surely, a very dramatic gesture, which, as he tells the story, had a dramatic impact. The patient was very much shaken and the treatment moved forward again after months of stalemate. It would seem to me to rob our understanding of this intervention if one failed to take into account certain "characteristic" attitudes of the analyst in question which became apparent as I came to know him over many years—his willingness to sacrifice himself, his capacity for *le beau geste,* and many other traits. We can only imagine what he may have experienced prior to the introduction of the parameter—chagrin, anger, frustration, helplessness, or some variation of these affects according to his particular sensitivity and character structure, along with curiosity, puzzlement, and so on. His casual comments about the incident left no doubt that even in an informal setting he did not think it of much relevance to refer to his own personal attitudes in discussing either the crisis or its resolution, leaving his audience in an affective state combining awe, admiration, and envy! My point is not simply to identify character traits for their own sake, but to demonstrate what we lose in our explanatory and descriptive potential when we leave them out of our formulation. Consideration of character leads, of course, to thorny, perhaps unanswerable questions which need to be asked. Was the above situation stuck because of the analyst's blind spot and could one say that the dramatic gesture represented his (preconscious?) solution to his characterological problem in the treatment?

It is very instructive to read the early cases in the analytic literature, as they often illustrate very well the point I made early in the paper: the absence of a well-developed technique has as its counterpart the greater flourishing of more personal (that is, characterological) reactions on the part of the analyst. The principle of neutrality is in a sense a safeguard for the analyst against too personal an intrusion.

CHARACTER AND TRANSFERENCE NEUROSIS

The topic of character and transference neurosis deserves close attention. The concept of transference neurosis as developed by Freud between 1910 and 1920 did not consider character issues but concerned itself more with neurosis; that is, an encapsulated illness in an otherwise normal personality organization. Symptoms were its hallmark. For the purposes of this presentation, I will dwell on the analyst's contribution to the development of the transference neurosis as seen from the point-of-view of his *character* and *attitudes*. I refer to both terms, as the problem of transference neurosis can be studied both clinically (how is it experienced by both participants) and theoretically (how do we conceptualize its structure). The transference neurosis is not limited to symptoms, yet it is not clear which attitudes of the patient will become manifest and which aspects of the analyst's attitudes will become the target of the patient's attacks. I would like to think that the more conflictual aspects of the patient's character traits will occupy center stage. Freud (1916) wrote: "What opposes the doctor's efforts is not always those traits of character which the patient recognizes in himself and which are attributed to him by people around him. Peculiarities in him which he had seemed to possess only to a modest degree are often brought to light in surprisingly increased intensity or attitudes reveal themselves in him which had not been betrayed on other relations of life."

Brian Bird (1972) makes, amongst others, the following points: Only when the analytic situation becomes, in a sense, an adversary situation, should we expect the kind of transference neurosis to develop that can admit to it a representation of destructive impulses strong enough and faithful enough to permit this aspect of the patient's neurosis to be effectively analyzed. The analyst, through the analytic process, must somehow enable the patient to extend his intrapsychic conflicts to include the analyst (p. 295). In order for this to happen, Bird believes the analyst's own transference involvement is necessary. For one thing, his own transference may be the factor that enables him to accept an adversary role in the patient's neurosis (p. 296). When the transference neurosis finally develops, neither patient nor analyst may realize for a while that it has. What they will very likely realize is only that the analysis has been caught up in a stalemate, a negative therapeutic reaction, a strong unmovable resistance, or some other seemingly impossible negative struggle between patient and analyst.

I am in full agreement with Bird's findings, but would like to restate them in characterological terms. At the point just mentioned by Bird, there is a particular engagement between the character attitudes of the patient and the character attitudes of the analyst. At those times, I transitionally often experience a certain helplessness, as though I were caught up in the patient's way of subtly distorting the situation between us. When I examine myself further, I often find the kernel of truth in the patient's accusations which leads me to be caught up in his subjectivity ever so briefly.

SOME CLINICAL EXAMPLES

An example will clarify. A psychotherapy patient with homosexuality and a severe masochistic perversion came to sessions at times somewhat inconvenient for him. I could have changed his hours, but had not on the basis that I did not think the inconvenience that great for him and wanted to keep open the more desirable hour for a case in more intensive therapy. One day, the patient, somewhat to my surprise, exploded in a paranoid-like rage, saying I was taking advantage of him in not attempting to change the hour and that I must have known I could push him around and that he would do nothing about it. Some self-reflection immediately confirmed the kernel of truth in his accusation; namely, if he had categorically stated the hours were impossible and interfering with his work, my attitude might have been different. One could say that his sudden outburst—a repetition of life-long fights he had had with his psychotic mother, triggered off some transitory guilt reaction in me, temporarily blinding me to the other components behind the patient's attack (for example, the self-loathing). This was possible because of my transiently accepting an identification with a bad object, in this case, the mother who mistreated him.

When Bird is referring to the transference neurosis, I believe, as I have written elsewhere, that one has to include in the term a character portion for it to have any meaning. It is at this point that analyst and patient really "lock horns." There is a strong mutual affective involvement in contrast to that occurring during aspects of the analysis of the transference which does *not* involve the analyst in the same intense way.

By the term "locking horns" I believe Bird means that the analyst has to feel that in some way the patient is "getting to him" for the work to really come alive for the patient in the experience of the transference neurosis. I suspect that the analyst's real character traits serve as hooks on which patients can "hang" their transference reactions. In fact, patients hungrily seek out the analyst's character—in part, as an effort to reach out, to make contact as compensation for the analyst's abstinence. If the patient engages the character of the analyst at a point in which the latter is vulnerable or sensitive, the treatment may not make progress at that point.

I recall also an incident from the analysis of my first treatment center patient. For considerable parts of the analysis, she came late, missing anywhere from ten to forty minutes. Although I attempted to "analyze" her lateness, the treatment made little headway on that issue. My supervisor and I puzzled on this until one day in my personal analysis, I confronted the fact that first, I enjoyed the lateness of this patient as it allowed me to catch up on other work and that further, I felt it almost my due; that is, it served as a compensation for the negligible fee (one dollar) she was paying me and the considerable skill with which she was demonstrating my greenness as a student analyst. I am not sure I could pinpoint exactly what changed in my analytic listening or interpretations, but shortly afterwards, the lateness ceased. As best as I can reconstruct it, the consequences of my awareness of my resentment were that I was able to effectively combat a slight withdrawal from the patient. I could be more sensitive to important nuances of her communication by focusing less on her aggression towards me—real enough, but which I had overly interpreted as a screen for my own resentment towards her. My withdrawal had mirrored in some small way her narcissistic mother's treating her like an object. A conflict was, therefore, played out rather than analyzed.

THE PRINCIPLE OF COMPLEMENTARITY

It is in the nature of characterological behavior that it stimulates in the audience a specific reaction. This reaction is a combination of the demand that the behavior makes and the recipient's sensitivity and characteristic mode of functioning.

This is the principle of complementarity first written about by Helene Deutsch in 1926 and elaborated by Waelder. Briefly stated, a character attitude in one person has as its effect to stimulate either a mirror or an opposite reaction in the other person who is the target of it, this depending on the latter's character style. Sadistic or aggressive behavior may stimulate counter-aggression or compliance. Procrastination or stubbornness may stimulate a form of nagging; whining or helplessness may stimulate aggression or caring. This is in part the appeal function, generally unconscious.

In writing further on the range of identifications an analyst makes with his patients, Helene Deutsch differentiates two types: one is the so-called concordant identifications, which enable the analyst to put himself in the place of some aspect of the patient in the service of the wish to understand; in contrast, there are the complementary identifications—those are made with the patient's internal objects according to the prevailing transference fantasies. This occurs largely out of the analyst's control.

The former identifications pose no danger to the analyst's objective attitude of observation, whereas in the second type, the analyst is emotionally involved in the situation. The experience is felt by him with great intensity as a "true" reality. The analyst may respond to this situation by perceiving his reactions and using them in his interpretive work or by acting out alloplastically or autoplastically (such as by feeling guilty or by acting angrily or defensively in the case of an attack by the patient). Such activation of the analyst's character traits and complementary identifications, far from being a hindrance to analysis is, in my view, a central part of the transference neurosis experience. This is particularly true in patients with sadomasochistic features, in which the analytic situation will at some point involve an adversary relationship.

To a minimal degree, the activation of a character response in the analyst puts him at a crossroad in the paths of acting out versus understanding. The analyst's ability to do the latter is a function of his inclination to anxiety, guilt, pathological defenses and the like. There is, unfortunately, a possibility that the function of certain of the analyst's character traits either block or distort his perception of the patient's communication or affects or that the analyst perceives correctly but that he can only react neurotically. The question may be asked, "What motivates a particular character response in any person?" The answer has to be some aspect of the situation for which the character reaction is a solution. This is as true for the analyst as it is for the patient. One of my supervisees had developed certain passive compliant attitudes as a solution to an aggressive conflict with a dominant parent. Whenever a patient behaved in an aggressive demanding fashion, the form of the supervisee's response would be clearly compliant regardless of its content.

SUMMARY

At present we are lacking a proper framework to describe the impact of the analyst's character on the analytic process. I believe that our character shapes our work more than we are willing to admit beyond the usually considered countertransference reactions. I have attempted a brief overview of this topic including issues of style, general attitudes, and introduction of parameters. I have also begun to explore the role of the analyst's character in the development of the transference neurosis and have appended a few clinical illustrations.

REFERENCES

Bird, B. 1972. Notes on transference: Universal phenomenon and hardest part of analysis. *J. Amer. Psychoanal. Assn.* 20:267–301.

Freud, S. 1916. Some character-types met with in psycho-analytic work. *Standard Edition,* 14:309–33.

22. Therapeutic Problems in the Analysis of the 'Normal' Candidate

Maxwell Gitelson

I

In order to consider the problems of the psychoanalytic situation in which the 'normal' candidate becomes involved, it is necessary to have in mind a conception of mental health. Only when we know what our goal is can we consider the technical problems confronting the training analyst. We assume that it is not simply a question of freedom from symptoms or of 'social' adjustment. It is understood that we are concerned with normality from the standpoint of psycho-analysis.

Ernest Jones approached the question in an essay which was originally intended for general readers.[1] He referred to two main groups of definitions of normality: (a) those depending on the criterion of *happiness* and (b) those depending upon *adaptation* to (psychological) reality. The latter 'does not necessarily imply the acceptance of environmental standards, but it does imply a sensitive perception of them and a recognition of their social significance'. This depends on a 'feeling relationship' with other human beings, which 'is to be estimated by the internal freedom of such feeling' as distinguished from surface attitudes of conciliation or self-assertion.

Midway between the concept of happiness and the concept of reality adaptation Jones introduced the concept of *'efficiency'*. This concept depends on a number of factors: normality cannot tolerate a state of excessive influence by others; nor can it dispense with sensitiveness to others; it is dependent on what Jones calls *'gusto';* it is not concerned solely with external success, but it does require the fullest use of a given individual's powers and talents. The one is born of confidence, the other of fear.

Against this background Jones came to the conclusion that the state of

Reprinted from Maxwell Gitelson, *Psychoanalysis: Science and Profession* (New York: International Universities Press, 1973), 211–38 by permission of International Universities Press, Inc. Copyright 1973 by International Universities Press. Originally published in 1954.

balance in relatively stable persons can be 'unsuspectedly precarious' and that this applies to 'apparently normal candidates' in whom 'one is often astonished to observe how a comparatively good functioning of the personality can exist with an extensive neurosis or even psychosis, that is not manifest'.

Up to this point we have been considering truisms. However, Dr. Jones went further toward what is particularly relevant to the topic of this paper: He stated that while a thorough analysis leads to changes of character and intellect in the direction of increased tolerance and open-mindedness, 'there is no motive as a rule to make use of the work done by applying it in detail to the conscious and pre-conscious layers of the mind'. Thus the only thing which distinguishes analysed people, 'including psychoanalysts', from others is 'their greater tolerance in sexual and religious spheres', and the modification of attitudes on subjects directly connected with analytic problems (e.g., mental responsibility for crime). 'In other spheres they seem to form their judgments, or rather to maintain their previous convictions and attitudes, on very much the same line of rationalized prejudices as unanalysed people do'. In short, in his consideration of 'normality' Jones has given us the most difficult of psychological problems, but one which in the training of an analyst we must face, whether we solve it or not, and that is: 'the assessing in the "normal" of the relation between the interests of the individual and those of society'.

Heinz Hartmann, in his more recent discussion of the question of mental health,[2] was, like Jones, convinced that the more we begin to understand the ego and its manœuvres and achievements in dealing with the external world, the more do we tend to make these functions of adaptation the touchstone of the concept of mental health. 'Psycho-Analysis', says Hartmann, 'has witnessed the development of a number of theoretical concepts of health which often lay down very severe standards'.[3] These have taken two directions— on the one hand emphasizing rational behaviour; on the other hand, instinctual life. This two-fold orientation reflects the two-fold origin of psychoanalysis in the history of thought: rationalism and romanticism. Freud recognized both, but the fact is that theory has often assigned undue prominence to one standpoint at the expense of the other. Hartmann is sceptical of the supremacy of biological values. When this criterion of mental health is dominant we approach dangerously near to that 'malady of the times whose nature it is to worship instinct and pour scorn on reason'. On the other hand, the concept of the 'perfectly rational' man presents us with this complication: 'recognition of reality is not the equivalent of adaptation to reality. The most rational attitude does not necessarily constitute an optimum for the purposes of adaptation'.

Hartmann turned to the co-ordinating or integrative function of the ego as a solution for this dilemma. 'The rational must incorporate the irrational as an element in its design'. Progression in one direction entails regressions in other directions. Applying Waelder's criterion of freedom from anxiety,[4] he stated that 'the mobility or plasticity of the ego is certainly one of the prerequisites of mental health . . . (but) . . . a healthy ego must be in a position to allow some of its most essential functions, including its "freedom" (from anxiety) to be put out of action occasionally, so that it may abandon itself to "compulsion" '. In other words, it is neither defence nor instinct which are in themselves normal or pathological but rather their contextual balance or imbalance which is the criterion. Thus mechanisms have a positive value for health; withdrawal from reality may lead to an increased mastery over reality; there are progressive and regressive modes of adaptation. The work of conducting an analysis, as well as undergoing it, are examples of the latter.[5] Thus, 'a system of regulation operating at the highest level of development is not sufficient to maintain a stable equilibrium; a more primitive system is needed to supplement it'.[6] In the balanced operation of the personality we expect to find an emotionally 'open' system of communication between the various institutions of the mind, operating through a fluid process of checks and balances among the instinctual and defensive tendencies, so that none is fully isolated, self-operating and self-sustaining.[7]

It is because we have looked upon health in contrast to neurosis that we have failed to appreciate how much these mechanisms and modes of reaction are active in healthy individuals. This is why it is precisely the analysis of conduct adapted to reality which is of such importance.[8]

In the end Hartmann came to the conclusion that 'a more attentive examination of the phenomena of adaptation may help us to escape from the opposition between "biological" and "sociological" conceptions of mental development'. There is 'an organization of the organism' which in the mental sphere eventuates in the synthetic and differentiating functions of the ego and is a prerequisite of successful adaptation. Adaptation must be considered against the background of the environment in which it develops. It can be 'appropriate only to a limited range of environmental conditions; successful efforts at adaptation towards specific external situations may, in indirect ways, lead at the same time to inhibitions in adaptation affecting the organism'; and the reverse may be true.[9]

II

It is generally agreed that the neuroses which come to the psycho-analyst today are different from those of fifty years ago. The manner in which the ego admits, repels, or modifies instinctual claims depends on how it has been taught to regard them by the outside world. The changes which have occurred in moral and ethical outlook reflect themselves in the inconsistency of early educational influences on the child with the consequence that the boundaries between license and deprivation have become blurred and the personality itself has become the carrier of the symptom.[10]

The change in the form of the neuroses has been from those of the transference type, based on ego-id conflicts, to the narcissistic type, based on ego-superego conflicts. It has been stated that the transference neurosis with its intrapsychic symptoms represents an autoplastic regression which is harder to treat than the character neurosis, which is looked upon as directed towards an alloplastic (i.e., 'living out') solution of conflict.[11] However, this apparent alloplastic conflict with reality is made up of pathological projections and displacements which are connected with the wishfulfilling orientation of the narcissistically regressed ego; the conflict is not only *truly* intra-psychic, but, in addition, is deprived of that impulsion of the instincts toward objects in the outer world which occurs in the transference neuroses and assists in their cure. The very fact that in the narcissistic neurosis the ego maintains its capacity to perceive and to deal 'adaptively' with external reality makes it possible for the intra-psychic conflict to be laid out on the framework presented by the environment, and to follow there a course which has the aspect of 'normality'.

In 1924 Freud asked the question as to what circumstances were conducive and by what means the ego succeeds in surviving conflicts without falling ill. His own answers are well known: 'The outcome of such situations will assuredly depend upon economic conditions, and upon the relative strength of the forces striving with one another. And further, it is always possible for the ego to avoid a rupture in any of its relations by deforming itself, submitting to forfeit something of its unity, or in the long run even to being gashed and rent. Thus the illogicalities, eccentricities and follies of mankind would fall into a category similar to their sexual perversions, for by accepting them they spare themselves repressions.'[12] I think it follows that one of the important factors in the support of the ego's conflict with the superego, i.e., the maintenance of the narcissistic character defence in the guise of normality, is to be found in the acquiescence of our culture in the phenomena of this defence.

All this by itself would not merit special consideration in a Symposium on Training, since we take it for granted that in the analysis of 'normal' candidates we are confronted by the problem of character analysis. However, because the increase in our knowledge of the economics of the psychic structure has greatly complicated the differential diagnosis between the normal and the pathological, some analysts have begun to despair of the suitability of 'normal' candidates for a career in psycho-analysis. Then, the recent history of the psycho-analytic movement has literally dropped the problem at our doorstep. And finally, as an aspect of that history, the particular ecology of recent candidates has added special problems.[13]

Sachs unequivocally ruled out a group with 'too few neurotic symptoms', who were well adapted to reality and outwardly well integrated, but whose narcissistic organization produced too firm a repression of conflict. While they might indeed have a good intellectual grasp of mechanisms and be therapeutically eager, he felt that psycho-analysis could not possibly satisfy their ambition or 'assuage their compassion' while it was very likely to injure their self-esteem and drive them towards one of the schools of 'improved techniques'.[14]

Kubie stated: 'Some analysts feel that the persistence of frank symptoms is less important than is the persistence of masked neurotic personality traits. Yet precisely here is where the therapeutic goal becomes most difficult of attainment. . . . It is easy to say that the goal is to spread the domain of conscious control in the student's life, and to shrink to a minimum the domain of unconscious control. But a bright and intelligent student will sometimes unconsciously disguise his subtle neurotic trends, and even make them appear as assets. For some the training analysis is like a successful courtship, during which the student feels happy, relieved, and free from tensions; he is on his way towards his professional goal; he is full of warmth and gratitude to his training analyst. Under such circumstances subtle neurotic mechanisms can be temporarily inactivated (*sic!* I should say: *remain concealed*) only to reappear in later years after the analyst has faced the stresses of his professional life. This is where the therapeutic leverage of the training analysis (of the "normal" candidate) is so often far less than is the leverage of the analysis which has no training implications, even when the instructor is on the lookout for just this difficulty'.

In contemplating this problem 'some instructors and some Institutes feel that the preparatory analysis should be a purely therapeutic venture, undertaken individually by the would-be student . . . and that no application for admission should even be considered until after the candidate has completed a therapeutic analysis. Other analysts feel that we should admit quite frankly that in most instances the preparatory analysis achieves little therapy except perhaps where there have been frank and painful symptoms'.[15]

On the basis of an experience with a patient 'who gave the impression of being relatively symptom-free and well adjusted' and who wanted treatment 'only for professional reasons' Eissler decided for a time that he 'would never again try the analysis of a "normal" person'.[16]

Knight, in his Presidential Address[17] before the American Psychoanalytic Association, last December [of 1952], said among other things: 'Another factor which has been operating in the past decade to alter the character of analytic training and practice also derives from the great increase in numbers of trainees, especially in the postwar period, and from the more structured training of institutes in comparison to the earlier preceptorship type of training. In the 1920's and early 1930's those who undertook psycho-analytic training were of a somewhat different breed from the current crop of candidates. There was in those days less emphasis on selection procedures and many analysts were trained who might today be rejected. Many training analyses were relatively short, and many gifted individuals with definite neuroses or character disorders were trained. They were primarily introspective individuals, inclined to be studious and thoughtful, and tended to be highly individualistic and to limit their social life to clinical and theoretical discussions with colleagues. They read prodigiously and knew the psychoanalytic literature thoroughly.

'In contrast, perhaps the majority of students of the past decade or so have been "normal" characters, or perhaps one should say had "normal character disorders". They are not introspective, are inclined to read only the literature that is assigned in institute courses, and wish to get through with the training requirements as rapidly as possible. Their interests are primarily clinical rather than research and theoretical. Their motivation for being analysed is more to get through this (sic) requirement of training rather than to overcome neurotic suffering in themselves or to explore introspectively and with curiosity their own inner selves. Many have had their training largely paid for by the Federal Government, and this factor has added to training problems. The partial capitulation of some institutes arising from numbers of students, from their ambitious haste, and from their tendency to be satisfied with a more superficial grasp of theory, has created some of the training problems we now face'.

III

Now, let us glance at the social-cultural situation. I have referred to the fact that while character, ultimately, is rooted in the instincts, its formal qualities belong to a large extent to the external reality of the culture in which it develops and operates. We take for granted that the character and personality of the putative analyst are the product of the interaction of his instincts with the general cultural characteristics of his developmental time and place. However, in the context of the problems of training, we must remember also that the characters of our present-day candidates are also determined, at least in their secondary aspects, by the particular circumstance that they have grown up in an atmosphere of psycho-analysis. Their pre-analytical training goes on in the midst of psycho-analysts and their 'psycho-analytically oriented' colleagues, and under the influence of the various derivations and applications of psycho-analysis, as well as psycho-analysis per se. In short, psycho-analysis has become respectable and 'normal'; it has become a part of the milieu.

The consequence is that a number of artifacts enter into the defensive organization of the ego of candidates which, to say the least, create an additional layer of ego-syntonic resistances. Under the influence of reading, lectures, and sometimes 'wild analysis' by psychiatric colleagues and instructors, candidates now tend to develop a façade of pseudo-normality, due in part to 'inexact interpretations'[18] resulting in gratifications and repressions, in part to the development of counter-phobic and denial mechanisms, and in part to the intellectualization of symptoms.[19] As regards the last, for example, it is not an unusual experience to encounter applicants for training who will make the most of mild situational tensions and depressive reactions, since it has become current that 'it is all right' to have some neurotic symptoms while 'character problems' are suspect. What may be overlooked is that such an apparent acceptance of the facts of life may actually be the presenting sign of far-reaching character resistances based on submissiveness and acquiescence to authority. It would seem, indeed, that one of the unconscious imagos of authority is now the field of psycho-analysis itself. This appears to be the case even with candidates who sincerely affirm their intellectual acceptance of analysis.

Another artifact which complicates the analysis of all candidates, but I think especially the so-called normal, is the disappearance of the incognito of the analyst. Not only are candidates intellectually immersed in psycho-analysis but also they are surrounded by analysts during their pre-analytic training and often enough in their social activities. Even more pervasive is the fact that in the small world of the training centre the analyst lives in a glass house of gossip, of rumour, and of some known facts. Out of this stem still other consequences:

First of all we encounter phenomena connected with the choice of analyst. To the extent that freedom of choice exists, we see decisions tending to be based on the impression the candidate has had of the analyst in terms of his own neurotic needs. For example, these may be based on the unconscious recognition of a prospect of gratifying unconscious wishes; or the person of the analyst does not threaten the character defences, or even promises to sustain them.[20] However, 'choice of analyst' is largely an academic consideration. In most instances this is not feasible and the consequences of the pre-analytic situation are reflected in the phenomena of the analysis itself.

Another situation is this: It is well known that regardless of the rationalizations presented, the choice of psychiatry and psycho-analysis as a career is in the end determined by the person's search for his own integration. In the early days of analysis this was more obvious. To-day, because of the factors I have already discussed and because analysis has been accepted as a valid medical discipline, we see more candidates who cannot be so frank and for whom such frankness is unnecessary. They unconsciously attain and can consciously maintain the attitude that they wish to become analysts because they are interested in psychosomatic medicine, or because they are interested in human beings and in what makes them tick. As an added fillip, of course, they may add (with unconscious truth) that they are not quite satisfied with themselves and would like to find out why. What it amounts to, however, is that an unconsciously erected façade of professional or scientific interest is now found to be a usual first line of intellectual defence against unconscious conflict.

Then we must consider that the 'paranoid' defence and the 'manic' defence are more extensively elaborated in the so-called normal character. I have previously alluded to its pseudo-alloplastic nature. Under the circumstances of the opportunity given by such realities as I have described, these defences can attain actual or apparent validation for their still deeper entrenchment. For example, in the cases of candidates with whom I have had professional contacts of the most routine sort prior to their coming into analysis with me, I have seen the largest incidence of first dreams in which I appeared in undisguised form. Such dreams, as I have shown in a previous paper, are prognostic of a difficult, if not impossible analytic situation, due to the fact that the analyst is quite literally reacted to as if he were in fact an ancient and dangerous imago.[21] This has been the case when a pre-analytic teaching situation has resulted in anxiety of expected criticism or suspected disapproval. On the other hand, I have tried to analyse former students whose idealization of me became a difficult initial defence which covered a still more serious resistance in the form of identification and omnipotent denial. The apparently 'normal' activities of such patients often characterized by considerable 'practical' effectiveness, are displacements *or* denials of the unconscious object to which libidinal regression has occurred. This is perhaps most clearly seen among those 'phallic characters' for whom the phallus is really an instrument of orality and whose ambition is a substitute for the regression to the oral triad.

The general situation which obtains in the structure of the 'normal character' defence is the basis for these consequences. The libidinal and the hostile tendencies, as well as the defences against them, are assimilated into and fused in the ego-system so that the person's way of life aims at once to satisfy the instinctual tendencies, to preserve the ego from anxiety, and to fit in with the pattern of the environment. For example, among 'scientifically minded' medical students the attitude of 'critical scrutiny' is highly developed and valued as an important integrative ego function. This certainly belongs to the realities of a career in medicine. However, we know also how effective an instrument it is, often quite subtly used, for ventilating hostility in the service of defence. We are also familiar with those therapeutically oriented and practically ambitious students who live out their reparation and their denial. This makes them more useful citizens perhaps, but their treatment becomes harder. Candidates of this type have great difficulty in surrendering themselves to the uncertain gratification and postponed solutions which effective analysis requires of them. On the other hand, as Sachs has shown,[22] they become deeply involved in the prospect of the magical solutions for their guilts and anxieties which certain modifications of analysis seem to offer them.

The distortions and disguises through which the various libidinal and hostile impulses express themselves in the character defence are supported by the very common existence of these tendencies in the present day. These defences favour compromise and ersatz. Their mutual interpersonal utility creates a situation in which the character defence can remain unrecognized as such and can even flourish as alleged normality. Thus in a social setting in which aggressiveness, ambition, and hard work have a high premium attached, a gifted analysand can live through his analysis as he has lived through his life, cleverly disguising his neurosis.

To sum up thus far, we see that the analysis of the 'normal' candidate confronts the analyst with a situation in which the basic conditions of his work are spoiled:

(1) Normality, a symptom, actually is not suffered from as such. On the contrary, it is capable of earning social rewards of which the first is acceptance as a candidate. To no other symptom does such a large quota of secondary gain attach.
(2) The defensive system is supported by the general culture and, besides this, is reinforced by the pre-analytic professional experiences of the candidate.
(3) The analytic situation is contaminated and distorted by adventitious external factors which interfere with the normal development of the transference.

IV

We come now to a consideration of some clinical problems presented by these candidates. First of all, despite overt manifestations of anxiety, they come into their analyses with the psychic mobilization which they have maintained in their general life situations. Their emotional position from the beginning appears in the analysis as a special case of the general character defence and, as I have previously indicated, complicated by special current factors.[23]

Despite the best intentions, which in some cases are felt as a desire for a better personal integration, the student-patient attempts to accomplish in his relationship to the analyst the same things that he has accomplished in the world at large. In this attempt he follows the pattern which has been more or less successful hitherto in mastering the vicissitudes of his emotional development.[24]

The various libidinal and hostile impulses do not reappear as themselves, but in their established distortions. As Anna Freud has said, 'in extreme cases the instinctual impulse itself never enters into the transference at all but only the specific defence adopted by the ego against some positive or negative attitude of the libido'. Insistence on the fundamental rule of free association is quite ineffectual with these patients.[25]

Fenichel[26] has stated that the formation of the character traits and their maintenance corresponds to a single massive act of repression which makes possible the later avoidance of single definite acts of repression. Thus separate anxiety situations are avoided because such chronic anchorages of instinctual defence are worked into the ego and not experienced as ego-dystonic. This is what produces the relative constancy of the defensive attitude, and which establishes the 'sign' of the personality, no matter how different are the demands from the unconscious and from reality.

Fenichel also has cautioned us against taking at their face value that behaviour of the allegedly normal which appears to give the impression of satisfying instincts rather than repressing them. Thus we know how inhibitions may lead to counterphobic attitudes and these, in turn, to other inhibitions or reaction formations; while the maintenance of the defence of one instinct may involve the expression of another. As an example, we have observed how the ego can assimilate genital sexuality with apparent normality while actually employing it in the service of pregenital instincts which are themselves repressed.

It was Fenichel's opinion that the distinction between the rigid character defence, which I have been discussing, and a mobile transference resistance is dependent, in the first instance, on a fixation on part objects (and indifference to the whole object) which themselves are used only to relieve an endopsychic conflict and, in the second instance, on relationships to whole objects.[27] In other words, the analysands with whom we are concerned suffer from narcissistic problems which render them at first incapable of developing a true transference neurosis. They are regressed from the genital position and, to begin with, they not only continue their defences against pre-genital impulses, but also, against the transference, in which these would, of course, have to appear.

A technical digression may be worthwhile here: The resistance to the transference which I have just referred to arises (as Anna Freud stated in her contribution to the Eitingon Memorial Volume) from the threat that analysis brings to the ego that it may be deposed from its hard-earned seat on the

throne of reality. It is necessary to remember, however, that in such situations the resistance is quite often an id resistance, that is, it is a defence
against giving up the clandestine gratifications of the oral triad[28] which the
'normal' in particular succeed in repressing. This is achieved behind the
façade of normality.

Another technical consideration at this point is concerned with the superego's role in the analysis of such candidates. If they are looked upon as
students rather than patients, and 'active' measures are taken (even if this be
only a tensional attitude of 'concern' or impatience on the part of the analyst)
in the hope of accelerating the analysis, there will be a serious interference
with the normal development of the transference neurosis. In effect, the
analysand is under a constant superego injunction to be 'up and at 'em'. The
therapeutic split, which permits the patient to regress libidinally in the transference while ego regression remains minimal, is made difficult if not impossible. We find here the chief indication for passivity in technique. All of this
faces us with the need for analysing the 'living out' of the neurosis in the
atmosphere of the training situation and the 'training analysis'.

Now, we must consider the problem which Freud first discussed in 'Analysis, Terminable and Interminable',[29] in its bearing on the clinical problem
presented by the 'normal' candidate. As you will remember, Freud raised
these questions regarding the obstacles to cure. He asked: (1) Is it really
possible to resolve an instinctual conflict; (2) Can we inoculate patients
against any other instinctual conflicts in the future; and finally he asked: (3)
Can a pathogenic conflict be stirred up for prophylactic purposes? His answer
to all these questions was in the negative.

But Fenichel saw it differently. He felt that instincts are invulnerable only
when barred from discharge. It is a question of the relative strength of the
instinct and this can be diminished through the partial satisfactions which
occur in analysis. While admittedly it is not possible to resolve all the
unsettled instinctual claims of the past, the more insistent remaining claims
can be settled. When these are solidified in the structure of the character,
then it is necessary to tackle them at the beginning.[30] Fenichel is here
referring to the whole technique of ego-analysis *which, in the case of candidates, includes as a first step the meticulous effort to resolve that part of
their defences which has gained strength from the ecology of their pre-
analytic experience. This includes the analysis of the very choice of psychoanalysis as a career.*[31]

This brings us to the most serious of the questions raised by Freud: Are we ethically warranted and is it technically possible to turn an unconscious conflict into a conscious conflict? Unless there is already evidence which forces us to decide to terminate the analysis, and to advise the patient to give up the idea of training, we must consider the possibility suggested by Fenichel that it is not a matter of creating new conflicts but of mobilizing latent ones.[32] Of these there are always *small signs* even though the ego ignores them. By treating these signs as resistances it may be possible to demonstrate ultimately the fact of conflict and to bring it into analysis.[33]

In recent years there have been various technical proposals made to accomplish this end. Most prominent are those that have had as their objective the *active* mobilization of latent conflicts. These have been characterized by manoeuvres intended to manipulate the transference, or as has been recently stated, 'to change the therapeutic environment as required in order to activate trends in the patient which may lead to the necessary therapeutic experience'. It has been proposed that 'only thus can we bring the doctor-patient into the situation where he will accept himself as just another patient in analysis'.[34] This type of endeavour leads only to the deeper entrenchment of the narcissistic defences since it, in effect, reduplicates parental manipulations which in the first place play a large role in the creation of the neurosis of the 'normal' adult.

The type of candidate whom I have been discussing comes to his analysis prepared to deal with its problems in the same way he has dealt with his developmental vicissitudes and with their repetitions in his later adult life. If the analyst is to obtain therapeutic leverage he must try to correct for the analytic situation the 'spoiling' which I have suggested occurs in the pre-analytic milieu. He cannot do this by carrying into the analytic situation the attitudes and techniques of that milieu. The hope of the analytic situation lies in the possibility of effecting a differentiation between it and the atmosphere of the candidate's past life. This idea must not be confused with the idea of the planned creation of a 'corrective emotional experience'. The latter is narrowly conceived as being directed against the presumptive pathogenic effect of a significant figure of the patient's childhood. The correction to which I refer has to be applied against the distortion of reality produced by the culture in which the details of the character defence have been acquired. It is, therefore, concerned with the institution of a learning process which goes on during a prolonged initial period of 'testing', during which the validity of the analytic situation establishes itself. The patient must prove its *'difference'*.

I have seen such testing go on for several years before the patient dared to allow himself to experience the transference situation as we see it in the transference neurosis. One such patient at last exclaimed, 'It's a tremendous realization to see finally that you really mean this!' He was referring to the fact that he had in the end not succeeded in exploiting the relationship with me as he had in his previous relationships. He had carried concealed in him the deep conviction that analysis was really not what it 'pretended' to be, that it was 'just another racket', though a fascinating one.

It is during this initial phase of the analysis, but only after the patient's testing of the analytic reality and of the analyst's integrity has gone some distance, that one begins the cautious analysis of the various ego derivatives of the instincts. Only as the patient begins to believe that the analyst 'means it' does the analyst begin to stand in the position of an auxiliary ego which *enables the patient to take that distance from himself,* which makes possible the analysis of the 'small signs'.[35] The 'normal' candidate is, to begin with, characterized by the shortness of this distance. He believes that he wants to be an analyst; he believes that he wants to do research; he believes that he wants to help people. He does not feel ill. Nevertheless, one such candidate who came for a second analysis said to me: 'This time I want it to be for me'!

Another candidate, in a second analysis, who still adhered to the attitude with which he had gone through the first one, namely, that he wanted it only to qualify for his examination, at last presented the following dream:

> *The patient enters the office for his hour. The chair and couch are interchanged and the foot of the couch is towards the chair. The analyst is already seated, and to his right, in the other half of the room, is a class of students. The issue for the patient seems to be whether to lie down with his head or feet towards the analyst. The analyst tells the patient that the latter has been tried by others before but that it does not work.*

The fact is that my office is arranged so that there is an 'analytic half' at one end of an elongated room and a 'consultation half' with several chairs at the other end, my desk being in the centre. The analysand knew that students whom I saw in supervision sat in the chairs of the 'consultation half'. In the dream the reversal of the analytic chair and the couch has resulted in putting me 'in the middle' between the couch and the class of students.

Associations

A female patient, who was presented at a diagnostic seminar, had reported that after unsatisfactory intercourse she scratched various parts of her body until orgasm occurred. During the seminar, when the instructor had momentarily left the room, my analysand had acted as if it was immaterial whether he was there or not and had taken up the interrogation of the patient. Looking back upon the episode it struck the analysand that it would have been a compliment to the instructor for him to have waited for his return.

When the patient was very young he used to lie in bed with his mother when she was resting, and often she would hold his hand and drum on it with her finger tips. During his early teens, when his mother was resting in bed, he followed the example of an older brother and would lie on top of the bed clothes, with his head at the foot of the bed, and carry on conversations with her.

In a recent conversation with another young analyst, who was also in his second analysis, the latter had said it was practically inevitable that the first analysis should be contaminated by the fact that it was looked upon as a learning process rather than a treatment. Another young colleague had responded to this with a statement to the effect that it was up to the analyst to be aware of this attitude and to force the student-patient to deal with it as a defence.

The night of the dream the analysand's wife had playfully put her feet on his abdomen. This was the precipitating event for the dream.

Somewhere he had heard an older analyst make an exceedingly keen remark—that it was harder to love one person than to love everybody. To love everybody means nothing at all; to be able to love one person fully means everything.

Lying with his feet toward me brings to mind the idea of stamping on me and, as he says this, he jerks his feet, which reminds him of the characteristic kicking together of his feet when he has felt annoyed with interpretations connected with passive attitudes towards me. Then he speaks jokingly of wanting to play footsie with me and at this point his left ear, the one towards me, begins to itch and he has the impulse to scratch it—which again reminds him of the patient who produced orgasm by scratching. The class of students now reminds him of the times when he had attended conferences conducted by me.

It seems unnecessary to point out that this patient has mobilized his old 'student' defence against the classical transference situation which was beginning to develop in the context of a consistent management of the character resistances. In this context too the hostile denial of the libidinal transference also appeared.

This case example brings up another problem of particular importance with the 'normal' candidate. That is, there are disadvantages in the effort to deal with the type of ego-defences they present, when their analyses are conducted by 'teacher-analysts'. I have sometimes tried to deal with this problem by saying at the beginning of the analysis that, first of all, I was interested in the patient's health. But I have found that the candidate has taken this with a grain of salt and incorporated it into his defensive doubt of my sincerity. In the end he has had to discover for himself that I 'meant' it.

V

The problems in the analysis of the 'normal' candidate may now be summed up as follows:

(1) There is an actual disturbance in his 'feeling relationship' (Jones). He lives in terms of a façade whose structure is patterned by his environment. This provides opportunistic gratification of his instincts by virtue of their imbrication with the demands of his environment.
(2) This is the final consequence of the development of an 'adapted' personality— 'an organization of the organism', as Hartmann put it, whose adaptation is appropriate to its culture and thus passes as normal. But it is not adapted to psycho-analysis which needs to be free from the gravitational pull of a particular culture and which is incompatible with opportunism and compromise.
(3) It becomes the task of analysis to provide first of all an opportunity to test out a new reality—the analytic situation, to establish its integrity, and to prove its relevance to the basic nature of the person. In this context, and looking upon the culturally determined 'normal' behaviour as itself a resistance, we may attempt to mobilize conflict made latent by the culture and thus, in the end, analyse the vicissitudes of the libido itself.

This is a large order. We may not be able to fill it. But our candidates, as we find them, are the future of psycho-analysis. We cannot sidestep our responsibility for trying to insure that future.

NOTES

1. Jones, Ernest: 'The Concept of a Normal Mind', *Int. J. Psycho-Anal.*, 23, (1942). First published in Schmalhausen's *'The Neurotic Age'* (1931).
2. Hartmann, Heinz: 'Psycho-Analysis and the Concept of Health', *Int. J. Psycho-Anal.*, 20, (1939).
3. He would approach the problem from the empirical side and examine, from the standpoint of their structure and development, the personalities of those who are actually considered healthy 'since theoretical standards of health are usually too narrow in so far as they underestimate the great diversity of types which in practice pass as healthy'.
4. Waelder, Robert: 'The Problem of Freedom in Psycho-Analysis and the Problem of Reality Testing', *Int. J. Psycho-Anal.*, 17, (1936).
5. In advance of the fuller development of my topic, I may suggest that capacity or incapacity to tolerate regression is one of the criteria of mental health which is involved in the problem of the type of candidate whom we are discussing.
6. Hartmann: *Op. cit.*
7. Gitelson, Maxwell: 'The Emotional Position of the Analyst in the Psycho-Analytic Situation', *Int. J. Psycho-Anal.*, 33, (1952).
8. Hartmann: *Op. cit.*
9. Hartmann: *Op. cit.*
10. For example, in a previous paper (Maxwell Gitelson, 'Intellectuality in the Defense Transference', *Psychiatry*, 7, 1944) I have described a character neurosis in a patient in whom intellectuality was a leading defence. His mother had brought up her children with much serious and earnest discussion and appeals to reason. Anything that could be rationalized could be condoned. For years the patient escaped punishment for a variety of hostile acts against his sister because of clever explanations which were acceptable to the mother. Despite a prudish surface attitude toward sexuality, the mother's self-deluding character had made it possible for the patient to indulge himself erotically with her by engaging her in deviously solemn discussions of the facts of life. His erotized and barren intellectuality was the end result.
11. Alexander, Franz: 'The Neurotic Character', *Int. J. Psycho-Anal.*, 11, (1930).
12. Freud, Sigmund: 'Neurosis and Psychosis', *Collected Papers*, Vol. II.
13. In an extension of a report made to the International Educational Commission in Paris in 1938, Anna Freud reviewed in some detail the psychodynamics of the training analysis in comparison with the therapeutic analysis of the neurotic patient and examined the dynamics as they are influenced by the total training situation. This article ('Probleme der Lehranalyse') appeared in a volume commemorating Max Eitingon and was published in 1949 in Jerusalem by the Israeli Psycho-Analytic Society. It was unknown to me until I read it in a translation prepared and loaned to me by Dr. Paul Kramer of Chicago some months after the present essay had been written, and presented at the 18th International Congress.

    There is a degree of overlapping in the theme and in the elaboration of the theme in Anna Freud's paper and mine, particularly as regards what I have called the 'ecology' of present-day candidates. However, in this paper I have given particular attention to the problem introduced into training by the type of candidate who presents a pseudo-normal façade. Thus, Anna Freud (as translated by Dr. Kramer) says that 'the most difficult part of the work (in training analysis) is the process of making the unconscious conscious against the power of the ego resistances'. On the other hand: 'In the analysis of the seriously impaired neurotic the difficulty is mainly that of overcoming of the Id resistances through the activity of working through'.

It is the fact that 'seriously neurotic' persons become candidates and that their analyses are further complicated by *ecological factors* which they exploit and of which the training analyst does not take adequate cognizance, that I am attempting to demonstrate.

14. Sachs, Hans: 'Observations of a Training Analyst', *Psa. Q.*, 16, (1947).
15. Kubie, Lawrence: *Special Problems of the Preparatory Analysis.* (Presented mimeographically to the participants in a Panel on Psychoanalytic Training, Chairman: Karl Menninger, Annual Meeting of the American Psychoanalytic Association, May 1948. Not published.)
16. Eissler, Kurt: 'The Effect of the Structure of the Ego on Psychoanalytic Technique', *J. American Psychoanal. Assn.*, 1, (1953).
17. Knight, Robert: 'The Present Status of Organized Psychoanalysis in the United States', *J. American Psychoanal. Assn.*, 2, (1953).
18. Glover, Edward: 'The Therapeutic Effect of Inexact Interpretation', *Int. J. Psycho-Anal.*, 12 (1931).
19. Reider, Norman: 'The Concept of Normality', *Psa. Q.*, 19 (1950).
20. Thompson, Clara: 'Notes on the Psychoanalytic Significance of the Choice of the Analyst', *Psychiatry,* 1 (1938).
21. Gitelson, Maxwell: 'The Emotional Position of the Analyst in the Psycho-Analytic Situation', *Int. J. Psycho-Anal.*, 33 (1952).
22. Sachs: *Op. cit.*
23. As an example, I may cite an analysand who had known about me for some time and whom I had encountered socially on two occasions prior to his beginning analysis with me. For years the patient addressed me by the short form of my given name. This familiarity happened to be an index to a general character defence which, at the nearest level, served against his castration anxiety, and more deeply, as a 'handle' by means of which he negated his separation fear. Characterologically it had entered into his false self-esteem and his cynical depreciation of others.
24. Thus an analysand whose previously successful career had been characterized by an attitude of eagerness to be useful and co-operative presented the following first dream: *The patient enters the analyst's office and sees him, as himself. He is suffering from a toothache. The patient comforts him.*
25. Freud, Anna: *The Ego and the Mechanisms of Defence.* (Hogarth Press, 1937.)
26. Fenichel, Otto: 'Ego Disturbances and Their Treatment', *Int. J. Psycho-Anal.*, 19 (1938).
27. *Ibid.*
28. Lewin, Bertram, D.: *Psychoanalysis of the Elations.* (New York, W. W. Norton and Co., 1950.)
29. Freud, Sigmund: 'Analysis Terminable and Interminable', *Collected Papers,* Vol. V.
30. Fenichel, Otto: 'Problems of Psychoanalytic Technique', *Psa. Q.*, 8 (1939).
31. For example, a candidate whose training was finally interrupted, had come to his analysis with the common enough claim that he had no symptoms; his family life was satisfactory; he had been very successful in another field of medicine; he had become interested in psycho-analysis while in the army, through seeing analytically trained psychiatrists at work; he had been an avid psychiatric resident. He wished nothing else than to become an analyst and within three months was requesting that he be permitted to start didactic work. This request was chronic throughout the two and a half years of his analysis, despite the fact that there was no dynamic progress and the patient's external gains were based exclusively on identification with me. The focus on analysis as a career constituted a resistance which was

not solved. I could not continue the attempt at its solution because of threatening developments which made a compromise advisable.

32. *Ibid.*
33. An example is the case of a phallic character who had successfully lived out his denial of castration fear and was looked upon as 'normal' by himself and others. His first analysis seemed successful until difficulties in his work, which he valued highly, forced him into a second analysis. Only then was it possible to enlist him in the analysis of a smile which had been the occasional preface to the first verbalizations of his hours. This symptom, previously not admitted as such, now became a source of conscious discomfort. Its analysis led to his previously unconscious hatred and fear of women and the oral-sadistic fixation to his mother.
34. Grotjahn, Martin: *Recent Trends in Psychoanalytic Training;* presented at the Panel on Training, 1953 Annual Meeting, American Psychoanalytic Association.
35. Sterba, Richard: 'The Fate of the Ego in Analytic Therapy', *Int. J. Psycho-Anal.*, 15 (1934).

23. Psychoanalytic Technique and the Analyst's Unconscious Masochism

Heinrich Racker

Psychoanalytic cure consists in establishing a unity within the psychic structure of the patient. Most of what is ego alien must be relinquished or
reintegrated in the ego. For this unity to be achieved the analyst must, in the
countertransference, achieve a kind of unity especially with what the patient
rejects or splits off from himself. The analyst is able to do this to the degree
to which he has mastered his own ego defenses, and in so far as he is able to
recognize what there is or was of himself in the patient.

   Every object-imago is psychologically a projected part of the subject. The
psychoanalytic process in one sense consists, for both patient and analyst, in
restoring the unity broken by this division of one into two or more. To be
cured is to have the integrity and mastery of one's personality restored; and
to cure is to integrate the patient's psyche by integrating one's own, re-
establishing the equation nonego (you) = ego. To understand is to overcome
the division into two, and to identify oneself is, in this aspect, to restore an
already pre-existing identity. To understand, to unite with another, and hence
also to love prove, at root, to be one and the same. Therefore, understanding
is equivalent to positive countertransference, taking this term in its widest
sense to mean love and union. The disturbances of positive countertransference, its 'negative' aspects, are thus disturbances of the union and equivalent
to disturbances of understanding. Hence the continual analytic utilization and
solution of every manifestation of negative countertransference and the re-
establishment of positive countertransference are decisive factors for the
favorable development of the psychoanalytic process. To the degree to which
negative countertransference is a response to a negative transference, the
negative countertransference must be resolved if the negative transference is
to be resolved. Only by resolving the negative countertransference can we
rediscover and re-establish positive transference, which is in one sense the
patient's union with himself, and his cure.

Reprinted from the *Psychoanalytic Quarterly* 27 (1958): 555–62 by permission.

During the last few years psychoanalysts have become increasingly aware of the importance and meanings of countertransference, both as a hindrance and help for the analytic work. I may mention the publications of Lorand, Rosen, Winnicott, Heimann, Annie Reich, Little, Gitelson, Weigert, Fliess, Spitz, Zetzel, Money-Kyrle, and others. In my own paper, The Meanings and Uses of Countertransference,[1] I started from the thesis—transference, upon the analysis of which the cure so essentially depends, always exists. Normally the analyst responds to it in two ways: he identifies with the patient's ego and id; and he identifies himself with the patient's internal objects which the patient places within the analyst. These internal objects, projected by the patient into the analyst, range from the most primitive persecutors and idealized objects to the parents of the genital œdipus complex and their heir, the superego. The patient treats the analyst as he would the objects he places within the analyst, who feels treated accordingly. Thus the analyst normally identifies himself, in part, with the objects with which the patient identifies him. The identifications with the patient's ego and id I have suggested calling 'concordant identifications'; those with the patient's internal objects, following an analogous term introduced by Helene Deutsch, as 'complementary identifications'. In the ideal case the analyst carries out all these identifications, perceives them, and utilizes them for understanding and interpretation of the processes of the patient's inner and outer world. This ideal is accepted by all analysts in so far as it refers to the concordant identifications, but not, I believe, in what concerns the complementary ones. In other words, it is taken for granted that the analyst must coexperience, to a corresponding degree, all the impulses, anxieties, and defenses of the patient, but it seems to be less readily assumed that he also coexperiences or should coexperience, to a corresponding degree, the impulses, anxieties, and defenses of the patient's internal objects. Nevertheless, if this occurs, the analyst acquires a further key of prime importance for the understanding of the transference, In my paper I also pointed out which transference processes usually provoke in the analyst depressive or paranoid anxieties (in Melanie Klein's terminology), which ones provoke guilt feelings, aggressiveness, submissiveness, somnolence, and other states, and how the analyst can deduce from his own specific countertransference feelings what is going on.

We can, however, use countertransference and, in particular, the complementary identifications in this way as a technical aid only if the identifications in question are true ones (and not projections of the analyst's own problems onto the analysand), and if the analyst keeps a certain distance from all these processes within himself, neither rejecting them pathologically nor 'drowning' in them by falling into violent anxieties, guilt feelings, or anger. Both repression of these internal processes and 'drowning' in these feelings hinder or prevent the analyst from opening a breach in the patient's neurotic vicious circle by means of adequate transference interpretations, either because the analyst does not himself enter far enough into this vicious circle or else because he enters too far into it. In such cases it may also happen that the analyst's attitude toward the patient is influenced by his neurotic countertransference; then the patient is faced once again (and now within the analysis itself) with a reality that coincides in part with his neurotic inner reality. But adequate countertransference experience of these situations and understanding of them afford the analyst increased possibilities of interpreting the transference at the opportune moment and of thus opening the necessary breach. Adequate countertransference experience depends on several factors, two of which are particularly decisive: the degree of the analyst's own integration and the degree to which he is able, in his turn, to perform for himself what he so often performs for the patient, namely, to divide his ego into an irrational part that experiences and another rational part that observes the former.

In the present paper I will confine myself to one specific problem, one of the most important disturbances of countertransference, of the analyst's understanding, and of the successful evolution of psychoanalytic treatment: I refer to the analyst's own unconscious masochism. By this I mean masochism as a universal tendency which exists in every analyst. Nevertheless, the description that follows will refer more to analysts with predominant traits of a masochistic character than to those of other characterological types. Just as we differentiate, among patients, between neuroses and characteropathies and their various corresponding transferences, so also must we differentiate, among analysts, between 'countertransference neurosis' and 'countertransference characteropathy'. The latter also includes the analyst's characterological counterresistances, analogous to the patient's characterological resistances. A characterology or characteropathology of the analyst and his corresponding countertransference would be of great practical value.

In terms of object relations the analyst's masochism represents one of the forms of unconscious 'negative' countertransference, the analyst putting his sadistic internal object into the patient. The unity between analyst and patient is thus disturbed from the very outset and gives place to a duality with a certain degree of predominance of thanatos (sado-masochism) and a certain degree of rejection of eros.

It should be stressed, first of all, that the analyst's masochism aims at making him fail in his task. We should, therefore, never be too sure that we are really seeking success and must be prepared to recognize the existence of an 'inner saboteur' (as Fairbairn says) of our professional work. We must likewise reckon with an unseen collaboration between the masochism of the analyst and that of the patient. In so far as the analyst's activity signifies to him, for instance, an attempt to destroy the father, the œdipal guilt feeling may express itself in a moral masochism conspiring against his work. We are dealing here with a pathological (for example, a manic) signification of the act of curing, or more precisely, with a 'pathological desire to cure' in the analyst. Psychological constellations of this kind may constitute, to a variable degree, a 'negative therapeutic reaction' of the analyst. In such a case the analyst is partially impeded in achieving progress with his patients or else he feels unconsciously compelled to annul whatever progress he has already achieved. I have, for instance, repeatedly observed how a candidate or an analyst, after having given a series of good interpretations and having thus provoked a very positive transference, thereupon becomes anxious and has to disturb things through an error at his next intervention.

The analyst's masochistic disposition is also an unconscious tendency to repeat or invert a certain infantile relationship with his parents in which he sacrifices either himself or them. The analyst may, for example, seek to suffer now, through his analytic 'children', what he had made his own parents suffer, either in fantasy or in reality. The transference is, in this aspect, an unconscious creation of the analyst. This tendency may manifest itself, for instance, in the unconscious provocation of a preponderance or prolongation of certain transference situations. That one's fate is, in some respects, the expression of one's unconscious tendencies and defenses holds good for the analyst and his work. Just as countertransference is a 'creation' of the patient[2] and an integral part of his inner and outer world, so also, in some measure, is transference the analyst's creation and an integral part of his inner and outer world.

As is well known, masochism goes hand in hand with the paranoid disposition, and hence our masochism not only makes us seek failure but also particularly fear it. Masochism creates, therefore, a special disposition to countertransference anxiety over the patient's masochism which conspires against the task of therapy. Furthermore, it predisposes the analyst to feel persecuted by the patient and to see mainly the patient's negative transference and his aggression. Masochism and paranoid anxiety act like smoked glasses, hindering our perception of the patient's love and what is good in him, which in turn increases the negative transference. Our understanding becomes a partial one; while we clearly perceive the present negative transference, we easily become blind to the latent and potential positive transference.

The masochistic analyst also has, analogously, an unconscious preference for perceiving the patient's resistances, which he experiences as aggressions, and thus the patient turns into a persecutor. The analyst tends to overlook the valuable communications, the 'contents', the 'good things' that the patient transmits to him together with his resistances. The classical rule according to which the analyst should direct his attention in the first place to the resistances can, in this sense, be unconsciously abused by the analyst's masochism. Moreover, the masochistic analyst is inclined toward submission to the patient, and particularly to his resistances. He tends, for instance, to 'let him run' too much with his associations, sometimes with the rationalization of showing him 'tolerance' and giving him freedom. The truth is that the neurotic is a prisoner of his resistances and needs constant and intense help from the analyst if he is to liberate himself from his chains.

In this sense, the masochistic analyst is also inclined to misapply another good psychoanalytic rule: the one recommending passivity to the analyst. This is a very elastic concept and our masochism may make ill use of it and lead us into being exaggeratedly passive and not fighting for the patient. The masochistic analyst tends to renounce parenthood, leaving the direction of the analysis overmuch to the patient. Excessive passivity implies scant interpretative activity and, this, in turn, scant working through on the patient's part with a consequent reduction of therapeutic success.

Masochism can also give rise to a certain affective detachment in the analyst with respect to the patient and his communications, since approach, union, and even reparation may be too gratifying because to the analyst's unconscious they signify gratification of a concurrent aggressive tendency such as the desire for triumph over a rival. Masochism may also cause stiffness, overobedience to rules, and other similar traits in the analyst's methods.

The patient's resistances and negative transference manifest themselves also in the patient's attitude to the interpretations. The importance of this attitude is very great; upon it depends to a high degree the success or failure of the treatment. The masochistic analyst is predisposed to bear passively the patient's negative relation to the interpretations, or he may become anxious or annoyed by them when the proper thing is to analyze the patient's œdipal or preœdipal conflicts with the interpretations and his paranoid, depressive, manic, or masochistic attitudes toward them. Masochism here induces the analyst to allow the patient to manage the analytic situation, and even to collaborate with his defenses, preferring, for instance, to let himself be tortured and victimized rather than frustrate the patient.

A change in the analyst's masochistic attitude to the act of analyzing, to the patient, and to the patient's communications can considerably increase the success of the therapeutic work. Such a change can bring an awakening, a greater readiness for battle and victory, a fuller acceptance of our new parenthood, a closer approach to the patient, a struggle for his love along with greater confidence in it. It can bring willingness to see the positive transference behind the negative, to see the good things together with the bad ones, and the content offered us by the patient together with the resistances. It likewise implies a constant striving for rediscovery and recovery of the positive countertransference through continual solution of the negative countertransference. This point is fundamental, for it implies one's experiencing the patient as one's own self, the basis of understanding. On this ground the analyst is always *with* the patient, he accompanies him in each of his mental movements, he participates in every detail of his inner and outer life without fear of him and without submitting to his resistances, he understands him better, and for everything he receives he tries to give by communicating to the patient as far as possible all that he has understood. There is then a greater activity in the empathic and interpretative work, the analyst gives more (albeit with certain exceptions), and thus really becomes a 'good object', remaining all the while attentive to how the patient is taking what he gives him and how he is digesting it. With this greater activity and freedom the analyst includes himself more in the psychoanalytic process, and likes to do so; thus the transference and countertransference experiences become more intensely mobilized and enriched. His passivity gives place to a greater interchange of roles with the patient, analyst and patient oscillating to a higher degree between listening and speaking, between passivity and activity, between femininity and masculinity; and thus the infantile psychosexual conflicts are analyzed as they are manifested in these aspects of the analyst-patient relationship as well as in the other ways with which we are familiar.

The previous therapeutic pessimism changes toward a more enthusiastic and optimistic attitude which gains strength through the improvement in the therapeutic results and the satisfactions afforded by the reparatory work.

The struggle with the resistances for the sake of the patient's health thus acquires a certain similitude to the famous wrestling of the Biblical patriarch Jacob with the Angel. This continued undecided the whole night through, but Jacob would not yield and said to the Angel: 'I won't let you go unless you bless me'. And finally the Angel had no choice but to do so. Perhaps we shall also finish the struggle, as Jacob did, somewhat lame-legged, but if we fight as manfully as he, we no less shall enjoy from our own inner being a blessing of a sort—and the patient will as well.

NOTES

1. Racker, H. 1957. The meanings and uses of countertransference. *Psychoanal. Q.* 26: 303–57.
2. Heimann, P. 1950. On countertransference. *Int. J. Psa.* 31:83.

24. Some Limitations on Therapeutic Effectiveness: The "Burnout Syndrome" in Psychoanalysts

Arnold M. Cooper

Problems of maintaining psychoanalytic therapeutic effectiveness during a professional lifetime are discussed. Psychoanalysts are subject to paradoxical emotional and characterologic demands, uncompensated by the usual gratifications available in the healing professions. Problems arising from the analyst's character and the paucity of data in the field are discussed. "Burnout" syndromes are liable to occur in those working in a setting of great emotional intensity demanding high degrees of affective awareness and control, empathy and tolerance of uncertainty. Masochistic and narcissistic forms of "burnout" syndrome are described as they occur in psychoanalysts. The profession, as well as the individual, can help to prevent these syndromes.

In this paper I will discuss some sources of the psychotherapeutic limits which are inherent in the experience of being a psychoanalyst. I shall suggest that carrying on psychotherapy or psychoanalysis is an endless exercise in paradox. The psychoanalyst is required simultaneously to maintain opposing attitudes and ways of thinking, and he loses therapeutic effectiveness if the paradox or balancing act cannot be maintained.

I will discuss several topics: the contradictory attitudes required in our analytic stance; aspects of the analyst's character and their relationship to therapeutic limitations; the negative effects on the analyst of the lack of data and research in our field; the difficulties in knowing what our goals ought to be; and the perils of therapeutic burnout.

THE THERAPEUTIC STANCE

Long experience with psychoanalysis seems to teach that most analyses, although not all, go best over the long run if the analyst maintains an attitude

Reprinted from the *Psychoanalytic Quarterly* 55 (1986): 576–98 by permission.

which, paradoxically, includes both therapeutic fervor and therapeutic distance. In gloomy moments it has sometimes seemed to me that the life course of too many analysts begins with an excess of curative zeal and proceeds in the latter part of their careers toward excessive therapeutic nihilism. Both are serious handicaps to therapeutic effectiveness. The task is to extend the period of more or less ideal balance.

The peril of an excess of *furor therapeuticus* is that it places the analyst in the parental position. The patient's failures become personal failures for the analyst who demands that his patient get well. This, in turn, creates an irresistible unconscious temptation for the patient to manipulate this powerful control over the analyst. The patient's knowledge that he can torture his analyst for all the old real or imagined crimes of parents creates a therapeutic impasse. It is a necessary piece of the analyst-patient relationship that both parties, at some level, are aware that although the analyst's dedication to his patient may be total, his emotional involvement is limited. That is, he will make his utmost effort to do everything to help the patient but should he fail, the analyst may be sad, will examine his responsibility for the failure, may mourn, but he will never feel as if it were his child whom he had lost. The patient is one of many; the analyst will go on doing his work, temporarily sadder and perhaps permanently wiser. Analysts cannot carry out good treatment if they have the same sleepless nights over their patients that parents may have over their children. Simultaneously, the analyst cannot do his job well if he is not basically optimistic and dedicated to the work he is conducting with his patient. One aspect of therapeutic efficacy arises from the patient's perception that an analyst will not easily be discouraged, is extraordinarily persistent, will stick by the patient almost no matter what, and really believes the seemingly bizarre or stupid interpretations he keeps insisting upon. Since analysis is not always rewarding, either immediately or in the long run, the dangers of therapeutic discouragement or disillusionment are great and occur with considerable frequency. The analyst who no longer believes in the efficacy of his methods, who is bored with his patient, who no longer listens carefully or puzzles over his patient's communications, cannot provide the basic elements of the therapeutic situation which are required for optimal treatment.

The suggestion that optimal therapeutic efficacy depends on maintaining a stance which includes both zeal and distance, both devotion to the patient and exclusion of the patient from one's personal life, leads to the self-evident conclusion that this optimal stance will be difficult to maintain. It is this difficulty of maintaining the balance of therapeutic determination and remoteness, of deep empathy and emotional detàchment, of shared responsibility between patient and analyst, of therapeutic persistence and willingness to let go—it is these difficult balances that give rise to appropriate therapeutic modesty. It is wise to be aware of how easily we can become de-skilled and of how difficult it is for us to maintain an optimal balance as analysts.

THE ANALYST'S CHARACTER

Another set of therapeutic limitations involves the relationship of the analyst's character to the treatment situation, as I have discussed earlier (Cooper, 1982). A purpose of the analyst's analysis is to enable the analyst to be aware of his range of responsiveness, even if he cannot change it. I will not enter into an extended discussion of character, but in a psychotherapeutic era in which we all acknowledge the emotionally interactive nature of the therapeutic process, it is clear that the analyst has an obligation to know a good deal about what frightens him, what makes him angry, what seduces him, what brings out his sadism, and what lulls his interest. We all know analysts who seem reluctant ever to let a patient go, and we all know analysts who seem unable to retain certain kinds of patients in treatment. Winnicott (1965) wrote about analyses which were false because the analyst never engaged the true self of the patient, and a potentially endless charade was carried out between the two. We also know analysts who cannot abide severe obsessionals or who hate to treat manipulating histrionic patients. It is not always clear, however, whether these kinds of situations should be labeled technical, that is, better training would enable the analyst to overcome them, or whether they are, at least for certain analysts, characterologic and are not alterable by education. Rather, they require a characterologic change in the analyst.

Waelder (1960, p. 245) once wrote of the impossibility of analysis for certain kinds of revolutionaries because the analyst's ego ideal and the ego ideal of the patient were too far apart. He implied that the analyst's empathic capacity would inevitably fail under such circumstances. I would suggest that Waelder was describing a special case, true for him, of the more general proposition that psychoanalysis will fail if the analyst cannot find points of empathic contact with his patient. I think I am more likely to have difficulty with a child abuser than with a revolutionary. In discussing the complex issue of the limitations of the analyst's character, I would like to separate several dimensions: character, values, theory, rules of technique, and analytic style. These characteristics of the analyst are not clearly separable but it may be useful to discuss them separately.

Character

We usually mean two different things when we talk about character. We say admiringly of someone that that man or woman has character and pejoratively that he or she lacks character. When we say someone has character, we imply that there are qualities of perserverance, a capacity to endure, a core of belief which does not readily change, perhaps an ability to sacrifice for beliefs, and a consistent identity. It is important to recognize that a person can, in this description, be a person of character and yet be someone we detest, if in our opinion his or her beliefs are detestable. No one ever suggested that Charles de Gaulle lacked character, but not everyone found him an admirable person.

We also speak of persons having good or bad character, depending upon whether they have attributes such as honesty, loyalty, industry, respect for culture, and so on. We expect of analysts both that they should be persons of character and that their character should be good. Our demands are rather heavy. We expect the analyst to be empathic, benevolent, reliable, dedicated, steadfast in his analytic endeavor, flexible, and so on. It is unlikely that many of us have either as much or as good character as we would like.

I am convinced that any long-time analysis reveals the analyst's character to the patient. However, character is, fortunately for our patients and ourselves, not a simple fixed quality. Rather, it is state-dependent. Many of us are much better persons with more reliable and more desirable character traits in the analytic situation than outside of it. The analytic situation is so constructed that the analyst's safety is assured—we need not answer embarrassing questions, we need not speak when spoken to, and our quirkiness is hidden behind our technique. In this atmosphere of safety and limited responsibility—we ultimately give the patients responsibility for their lives—we have every reason to be good characters. Many of us know that we can be more empathic, forgiving, benevolent, and consistent toward our patients than we can be toward our families.

However, basic characterologic flaws will show through in the analytic situation and will seriously handicap analytic work. Psychoanalysts with sociopathic or severe narcissistic tendencies are likely unconsciously to communicate these characterologic deficits and will deprive the patient of opportunities for idealization, core identifications, and the firming up of consistent superego qualities. I believe, however, that this situation is rare. A larger danger comes from the analyst's inability adequately to be alert to his own core characterologic make-up. The analyst's analytic ego must allow him to see the interactions of his own characterologic qualities and his patient's behavior and to use these as the engine of the treatment. Transference emerges most usefully in the gap between the patient's correct observation of our character and his distortion of that observation. We must be able to acknowledge, at least to ourselves, the correctness of the patient's observation if we are to be able most effectively to point out the distortions.

Those of us with more than our due share of narcissistic needs or anal, controlling, sadistic qualities or characterologic reaction formations—the list is endless—will find ourselves with certain patients with whom we are periodically enjoying the treatment too much or not enough. We look forward to the hour, or dread it or forget it. I believe the issue is not one of characterologic match or mismatch—should sadists treat masochists or vice versa—but rather the specific modes with which any patient of any character manages to carry out resistances by consciously or unconsciously fitting or thwarting the analyst's characterologic needs. Our job is to know how and when this is occurring, and when we are out of our depth. Clearly, we cannot treat patients we dislike. Equally clearly, we cannot treat patients whom we love too much.

Values

An analyst's value systems, usually interwoven with his character, are a more likely overt source of therapeutic difficulty. Which of us has not had to bite his tongue when hearing a patient proclaim political views that make us see red. While the situation has changed dramatically in the last decade, it is still not uncommon to discover analysts, both male and female, with value systems concerning the feminine role which they unhesitatingly urge upon their patients in the name of therapeutic help.

We analysts may be blind to our value systems or may be unable to maintain therapeutic neutrality in the face of a challenge to our value system. It was, after all, only a few decades ago that analysis was held to be a value-free enterprise (Hartmann, 1960, pp. 20–21), and not all of us have rid ourselves of that illusion. The blend of values and characterologic needs is deep and may be subtle. Helping a passive masochistic male to understand his pathology may easily blend into expressions of macho contempt from the analyst, who is defending against recognition of his own passivity. The harsh unfriendliness of a competitive female patient toward her young male analyst may expose him to narcissistic castration anxieties which lead to his angry exposition of his patient's phallic competition and create a silent, angry, therapeutic stalemate. The analyst, however, thinks he is helping his patient become more "feminine." I know of several instances in which analysts inadvertently, or casually, revealed their contrary views about a political issue or an issue of social values to masochistic patients who were secretly hurt and enraged but too intimidated to work through what, for them, was a traumatic event. Rather than being a minor difference of opinion it was, for these patients, an actualization of a narcissistic, mocking parent contemptuously dismissing the opinions of a child. These kinds of situations, often transparently clear to a consultant or supervisor, can be completely masked by the pseudotherapeutic zeal with which the analyst protects his values, which serve important defensive functions.

Theory

The analyst's character inevitably relates to his version of psychoanalytic theory. In the United States today, significantly different theories are being advocated and advertised, and analysts have a choice. We must choose whether we wish to be so-called "classical," cognitive, object relational, self psychological, Kleinian, interpersonal, and on and on. It is obvious that after discounting the effects of specific training and indoctrination, and without clinical data which clearly support one theory over another, analysts will choose the theory that best fits their character and value systems. While all self-respecting theorists claim, perhaps correctly, that their theory allows for a full range of flexible therapeutic attitudes and behaviors, it does seem to be the case that, in practice, different theories coincide with particular therapeutic attitudes and behaviors. It is also the case that therapeutic flexibility is a quality with which not all analysts are equally endowed. Let me give an example: Kohut (1977, pp. 249–261) claimed that there is a group of patients with narcissistic character disorders and damaged selves who require the analyst's vivid presence and activity to help counteract the early lack of mirroring and the withdrawn qualities of their internalized objects. He derived this therapeutic recommendation from his theory and explicitly stated that the classical technique of muted responsiveness, derived from the classical theory, was the wrong treatment for these patients. It is my impression that, regardless of any intrinsic merit, Kohut's theoretical position appealed to analysts who were eager to interact with their patients and who welcomed a theoretical justification. I believe it is also the case that numbers of analysts, while overtly rejecting Kohut's theory, accepted his permission for a more interactive stance. Conversely, I suspect that one bit of the more violent response to Kohut came from those who could not tolerate the prospect of a requirement for personal liveliness in the conduct of treatment.

Even where theories do not clearly dictate a set of treatment attitudes, they surely indicate the content of interpretations. Unless one believes that interpretations are merely metamessages through which patient and analyst establish a mode of discourse, and the actual content of the interpretation is not important, then theories will powerfully influence what we do. If we subscribe to Kernberg's (1975, p. 241) view of pathological narcissism, we are likely to interpret the patient's rage early. If we believe Kohut's (1977, p. 92) view, we will bypass the rage and examine the enfeebled self. Some analysts are more comfortable dealing with rage, and some are more comfortable dealing with victimization, and this must influence one's choice of a theory.

In a field in which every communication from the patient is so filled with meanings, in an era in which alternate theoretical claims are actively competing, and without experimental data to demonstrate the correctness of a theory, there can be a great comfort in adhering tightly to a single theory which provides a consistent explanation of phenomena and which justifies our personal needs. We may even continue to cling to our theory although the patient seems to fit it poorly or not to be benefiting. No one can operate without theory. It is desirable that we know what our theory is, how it suits our character, and how each theory limits us in some direction. I am quite certain that the universal theory which will supply correct meanings and attitudes for all treatment events is not yet at hand.

Rules of Technique

Technical rules come in two forms: there are rules which are clad in theoretical language and rules which speak directly to clinical behavior. An example of the former is the rule of technical neutrality—the analyst maintains a stance equidistant from ego, id, and superego. An example of the latter is that the analytic situation requires the use of the couch. Both types of rules present problems. The rules cast in theoretical language are subject to multiple clinical interpretations. Fairbairn (1958), for example, as he developed his object relations theory, became convinced that the use of the couch represented a reproduction of the infantile trauma of maternal separation and deprivation and, therefore, was not technically neutral. In the name of technical neutrality, he decided toward the end of his career that his analytic patients would sit up and be able to face him. The peril of rules that dictate clinical behaviors is that they may not permit the full range of therapeutic behaviors that suit a particular patient.

Rules of both kinds are necessary, and, like all rules, they can be broken. The experienced analyst breaks them, but, one hopes, not unknowingly, unwittingly, or without having made the decision to break the rule. Certain gifted analysts have always been able to fly by the seat of their pants and define the rules later. For most of us, it is better to know what we are doing. Less able analysts are likely to cling to rules blindly or to flout them without knowing that they are doing so. Anyone who has ever taken tennis lessons knows the difference between trying to *think* of how to make the stroke— keep your eye on the ball, bring your racket back, turn perpendicular to the net, shift your weight, etc., etc., etc.—and having mastered the stroke. With mastery, one does more or less what the rules indicate, but one adapts to the needs of each situation and the rules are broken whenever necessary. Rules get people started, impose outer limits on behavior, but fade in importance as each analyst develops his own integrated technique. It is to me an astonishing failure of our education of young analysts that silence, or support, or any other activity, is so often believed to be a core behavior rather than a technical device in the service of one's deeper goals. We all know the plight of the analytic candidate with his first analytic case, sitting silently behind the couch, unable to help his patient explore the new, strange situation in which the patient finds him or herself, because the budding analyst is afraid that breaking his personal vow of silence will mean that he is not doing analysis (Cooper, 1985).

In discussing theories and rules, we are, of course, aware that not only will analysts choose the theories and rules which already suit their characterologic needs but that a major purpose of theories and rules is to provide analysts with assistance in curbing their nontherapeutic characterologic tendencies.

Analytic Style

It is all too rare that we have the chance to actually observe analysts at work. When we do, we often discover that they have an analytic style which we might not have predicted from knowing them outside of the analytic situation. Many people, when they are being analysts, speak in a different tone of voice, abruptly change their level of vivacity, change their facial expressions, and so on. Under optimal circumstances, this therapeutic style represents the integration of character, theory, values, rules, and experience. It is the way in which the analyst is comfortable performing the task he has set for himself. Style, in my view, is generally the least important aspect of the analyst's behavior, although for the patient it is likely to be the aspect of the analyst of which he is most conscious. I have been impressed that successful analyses are carried out in circumstances in which the patient feels his analyst was not all that bright, or had terrible taste in furniture, literature, or clothes, or spoke bad English, or lacked a sense of humor, or was too bourgeois, and so on. All of these opinions provide grist for the analytic mill and are not in themselves significant difficulties.

Two situations involving the analyst's style do, however, present serious problems. One is when the analyst cannot tolerate the harsh critique of his style by certain astute patients, especially if they are also able mimics. The second is when the analyst's personal style is congruent with a traumatic aspect of the patient's difficulties and the actualization of a past trauma becomes so vivid that opportunities for analyzing it are seriously handicapped. When the patient says he does not like something or other about an analyst, it may be extremely difficult to know whether the patient's complaints about the analyst really represent a misfit or are analyzable and unavoidable aspects of the transference. In general, I would suggest that patients who respond initially to their analyst with powerful negative feelings that cannot be understood and moderated within a few sessions are probably well advised to find another analyst with whom they feel more comfortable.

PROBLEMS OF THE DATA-FREE FIELD

The paucity of reliable research data is a significant source of the anxieties of and of the limitations upon the analyst, which tend to erode our confidence and enthusiasm. Three kinds of data are needed: data supporting theoretical propositions, psychoanalytic outcome data, and psychoanalytic process data.*

THERAPEUTIC BURNOUT

I would like, finally, to address a peril of the profession—the "burnout" syndrome as it appears in psychoanalysts. Freud unhesitatingly identified psychoanalysis as one of the impossible professions, along with teaching and government. I have discussed a number of hazards of our field. Let me describe them in a slightly different light.

1. Analysts operate in a climate of extraordinary isolation. a) The full-time analyst suffers the loneliness of social isolation. He is likely to spend a full day seeing no one but his patients and sometimes, literally, not even seeing them. While this social withdrawal is a comfort for some analysts, it is, for most, a terrible strain. b) As I have indicated, we operate isolated from data. We require strong belief systems in order to maintain the vigor that our work requires and this, historically, has led to certain intellectual perils. The isolation from scientific data has cost us dearly. c) With rare exceptions, we are isolated from outcome knowledge of our own patients. Few of us are likely to have significant contact with many of our patients after the completion of treatment. Having been intensely involved for many months or years, convinced or hoping that the result has been a good one, we may never again hear from the patient and cannot accumulate either the confidence that our work was well done or the knowledge that would come from a careful review of our errors. Our separation from our patients' futures is another significant isolation.

2. Analysts carry on their work with very little opportunity for the usual rewards present in the healing arts. Most psychoanalysts see very few patients in their lifetime. Our emotional investment in each of our patients is large, our propensity for disappointment is great, and our opportunities for reward are deliberately limited. Not only do we not continue to see our grateful patients, as does the internist, for example, but the treatment situation is designed to inhibit the patient's tendencies to reward us except through fees. In general, we do not receive gifts, we do not become social friends with our patients, and we do not enjoy the atmosphere of continuing idealization from our patients, either in analysis or after it, as most other healers

*[Pages 587–91 from this article have been deleted. The reference for the complete article is *Psychoanalytic Quarterly* 50 (1986): 576–98.]

do. The psychology and sociology of our defenses against this isolation and lack of reward is a well-known topic which I will not elaborate.

Confronted with the many difficulties and strains of doing psychoanalysis that I have described, it is not surprising that burnout syndromes are liable to appear in analysts and constitute serious limitations on our doing our best work. I shall describe two manifestations of the burnout syndrome: masochistic defenses and narcissistic defenses.

The masochistic defenses to which analysts are prone appear as discouragement, boredom, and loss of interest in the psychoanalytic process. Self-reproaches are translated into projected aggression against the analytic work. The various tensions, uncertainties, and sources of self-doubt that plague every analyst are, for these masochistically inclined individuals, an unanswerable source of inner guilt and self-recriminations, as well as an unconscious opportunity for adopting the role of victim toward their patients and their profession. Faced with these inner accusations and masochistic temptations, these analysts are unable to maintain their self-esteem and cannot sustain their claim that they are doing all that any analyst can do—i.e., to try his best to help his patient with the theories and skills available to him. For combinations of reasons related to character and to training, they cannot produce inner conviction that what they are doing in the conduct of analysis is sufficient for a clear conscience. It is an evidence of both the attraction of masochistic victimization and of the harshness of the superego of the analysts involved that they are willing to doom themselves to a relatively pleasureless professional existence, for the sake of the deflection of the inner reproach against their talent or skill. Feeling helpless against their inner conscience which charges them with not helping their patients, they say, "Don't blame me, blame psychoanalysis." The extent of the cynicism that may be part of this defense can be startling in its depth. I know analysts who have refused to permit members of their own family to enter analysis because they did not regard the treatment as helpful. Obviously, anyone going through the motions of a treatment in which he lacks faith has lost the power to maintain his own self-esteem. Conscious self-pity over the difficulty of the work or the shortcomings of psychoanalysis is matched by unconscious acceptance or even welcome of the opportunity to enact an endless infantile drama of being unloved or unappreciated or overwhelmed. Depression is always on the horizon for these analysts, apparent in their lack of pleasure in their patients or in the profession of psychoanalysis, both of which have let them down by not adequately protecting them from their unconscious conscience.

A corollary of this discouragement is boredom. Boredom is an affect of which we are all capable and which is probably a part of every treatment. In itself, it is a valuable clue to transference and countertransference events. What I am speaking of here, however, is chronic boredom. I have heard analysts say that all patients seem the same to them, the patient's story lacks interest, struggling to unravel meanings seems either too difficult or unchallenging, and the analyst struggles through his patient's sessions unstimulated and uninterested. Clearly, treatment cannot be optimal under such circumstances. The odd thing, however, which raises questions about the therapeutic factors in the treatment situation, is that certain patients seem to get better even under these conditions. Some patients are self-healing and seem not to require very much from the analyst. This knowledge is a useful check on therapeutic hubris.

A consequence of discouragement and boredom is, of course, loss of inventiveness. The analyst, frightened of not succeeding, discouraged in advance by the harshness of his superego reproach that it is grandiose for him to think that he can help someone else understand his unconscious desires and conflicts, especially when he is aware of his own neurotic shortcomings in the conduct of the treatment, gives up his active inquiring role. The analyst no longer puzzles, plays with the data, tries out interpretations, finds excitement in deciphering new meanings of old data and new connections which previously had escaped him and his patient. Playful inventiveness is a necessary part of the analytic dialogue, and its loss deadens treatment. These secretly frightened, consciously bored analysts may resort to stock answers, bullying patients with what they were taught were correct interpretations, often unconsciously parodying their teachers in secret vengeance. They find it difficult and threatening to maintain close contact with the patient whom they perceive primarily as a source of inner reproaches for their professional incapacity.

Finally, these masochistic defenses of the discouraged analyst lead to chronic anger at his patients, his profession, his colleagues, and himself. The patients of these analysts, when later they see someone else, sometimes report an analytic atmosphere of sarcasm, denigration of the patient, devaluation, and lack of appreciation. This pairing of masochistically angry, discouraged analyst and masochistic patient may last for many years.

It has long been my view that narcissistic and masochistic pathology are closely intertwined, representing two different defensive faces of the same constellation. The narcissistic defenses of the burned out analyst take a different form. The image of the great analysts of the past, or even of the imagined present, is often a significant factor in the ego ideal of these analysts. However, lacking adequate capacity for sustained positive identification, or unable to sustain genuine efforts at emulation that do not provide rapid affirmation or gratification, they seek other means of narcissistic comfort to avoid the humiliation they experience if they have not met their unrealistic perfectionist goals. Convinced they cannot be as creative as Freud, they can only carry on a secretly ironic imitation of the analyst ensconced in their ego ideal.

Unable any longer to restrain his narcissistic needs in the isolated, unrewarding setting he experiences analysis to be, the narcissistic analyst abandons efforts toward neutrality and increasingly uses charismatic behaviors to elicit the patient's overt admiration. These analysts intrude into the patient's life, give guidance and advice, are grossly directive and paternalistic, and attempt to maintain the patient in childlike devotion. Should the patient be famous or rich or live an interesting life, these analysts are liable to attempt to enliven their own inner deadness by living through their patients' success or fame. They are prone to lure the patient into amusing and interesting them and to abandon discretion and confidentiality in social situations. The tales of the success or glamour of their patients give the analyst a sense of a richer life than in fact he has. These analysts are also prone to use the profession as a badge of social distinction, allying themselves with groups or theories for the sense of narcissistic power such alliances may provide. Because their beliefs and identifications are often shallow, based on narcissistic need rather than on intellectual and emotional conviction, any challenge to their professional role produces severe defensive responses. In narcissistically threatening situations they are prone to respond with attitudes of superiority and superciliousness, toward both their patients and their colleagues.

I assume that all of us are subject to one or both of these tendencies during the course of a given treatment or during a given period in our careers. The tendencies are self-observable markers for attending to our psychoanalytic well-being. When they become chronic, however, it is obviously time for a return to analysis. It is to the credit of the profession that many analysts do exactly that. Sadly, however, some do not.

CONCLUSION

Good psychoanalysis involves many paradoxes. We must maintain therapeutic fervor and therapeutic distance. We must maintain belief in our theories and an experimental attitude. We must be firm in our character and flexible in our therapeutic approach. We must believe in our therapeutic effectiveness and be prepared to admit therapeutic defeat and to suggest that someone else might do the job better. We must obtain satisfaction from the work while labeling as exploitation the usual modes by which healers obtain satisfaction from their patients. Indeed, this is an impossible profession. But I have been discussing only the difficulties; I could write at even greater length about the gratifications of the profession. Many of us are unable to imagine anything else as interesting, exciting, important, challenging, or gratifying. No other profession provides us the opportunity to know human beings so well, to touch their suffering so closely, to have the opportunity to help. To realize that we have at least been a factor in bettering lives and perhaps releasing creativity and joy where none existed before are great satisfactions and privileges. There is even the opportunity to add to the sum of human knowledge. I also believe that doing psychoanalysis is good for the mental health of the not-too-neurotic psychoanalyst.

We surely need research to strengthen our enterprise. We cannot be self-satisfied about our own assessment of our own activity. Studies are needed for our well-being and for our patients' well-being. But I think we are fortunate in being analysts at this time. Not since the earlier days of psychoanalysis has our field been so exciting. Theories compete, theorists are boldly breaking out of old molds and making suggestions which are productive and interesting and would not have been seriously considered two decades ago. Psychoanalytic research is achieving new levels of productivity and sophistication. The data from infant observation have begun to penetrate our clinical theories, and productive ferment surrounds us. We have every reason to believe that our knowledge and effectiveness will vastly increase in the future. It has been my hope that by considering some of the difficulties and perils of our professional lives, we will be better prepared to overcome them. I am optimistic that we will shortly be in a position to prove Freud wrong. We will discover that our profession is *not* impossible; merely difficult.

REFERENCES

Cooper, A. (1982). Discussant: A special issue: problems of technique in character analysis. (Delivered at scientific meeting of The Association for Psychoanalytic Medicine.) *Bull. Assn. Psychoanal. Med.*, 21:110–118.

———. (1985). Difficulties in beginning the candidate's first analytic case. *Contemp. Psychoanal.*, 21:143–150.

Fairbairn, W. R. D. (1958). On the nature and aims of psychoanalytic treatment. *Int. J. Psychoanal.*, 39:374–385.

Freud, S. (1937). Analysis terminable and interminable. *S.E.*, 23.

Hartmann, H. (1960). *Psychoanalysis and Moral Values*. New York: Int. Univ. Press.

Kernberg, O. F. (1975). *Borderline Conditions and Pathological Narcissism*. New York: Aronson.

Kohut, H. (1977). *The Restoration of the Self*. New York: Int. Univ. Press.

Smith, M. L., Glass, G. V. & Miller, T. I. (1980). *The Benefits of Psychotherapy*. Baltimore: Johns Hopkins Univ. Press.

Waelder, R. (1960). *Basic Theory of Psychoanalysis*. New York: Int. Univ. Press.

Winnicott, D. W. (1965). Ego distortion in terms of true and false self. In *The Maturational Processes and the Facilitating Environment*. Studies in the Theory of Emotional Development. New York: Int. Univ. Press, 1965, pp. 140–142.

Name Index

Subject Index

P   C

21 (P.D.)   8

7 (FAD) 60 items 7

2 (IMS, IPA) 2

   25   25   17 variables

30 variables

indiv score

fam score

role score

$$30 \times 2P = 60 \text{ var. per couple}$$

34 var. per kid

94 var. per fam.

$\times 100$ fam

9400

$\times \underset{3 \times 5}{\quad}$

2823

$\cancel{30}$

$\times \cancel{3}$

90

7. let self re-experience the longing, need + love

expressed to therapist

let self experience the rage of anticipated

narcissistic injury

express murderous rage to therapist